The Best I Can Do

A True Story of Navigating the Complexities of Mental Illness and Homelessness

Cheryl Landes

Tabby Cat Communications

The Best I Can Do is a work of nonfiction. The names and identifying details of certain individuals have been changed to protect their privacy.

© 2024 Cheryl Landes

All rights reserved. No part of this book may be reproduced, stored in a retrieval system, or transmitted in any form or by any means without the advanced written approval of the publisher, except by a reviewer who may quote brief passages in a review to be published in a newspaper, magazine, journal, or online.

Published in the United States by Tabby Cat Communications in Camas, WA

Cover design by Ryan Forsythe
Tabby Cat Communications logo design by Charlie Okada
Inside pages design and layout by Cheryl Landes

Paperback ISBN: 979-8-9895450-2-5
Ebook ISBN: 979-8-9895450-3-2
Library of Congress Control Number: 2024903192

Advance Praise for *The Best I Can Do*

"Cheryl Landes accomplishes something very difficult: describing the journey into ambiguous loss—the pain, confusion, and emotional chaos of loving someone with an untreated mental illness—while retaining her sense of self and her empathy. This is the story of a woman trying to hold the pieces of her life together as her world is becoming dismantled one day at a time. This is also a story of courage, healing, and finding peace in impossible circumstances—a story of doing the best we can and knowing that it is enough."
~ Valentina Stoycheva, PhD, co-author of *The Unconscious: Theory Research, and Clinical Implications*

"In candid, evocative prose, Cheryl Landes reminds us of how mental illness can gradually destroy even the most seemingly-secure life. *The Best I Can Do* is storytelling at its best—poignant, sometimes humorous, and always full of surprising compassion."
~ Melissa Hart, author of *Better with Books: 500 Diverse Books to Ignite Empathy and Encourage Self-Acceptance in Tweens and Teens*

"Mental illness can shatter a perfect marriage into hardship and homelessness, but Cheryl Landes alchemized her gut-wrenching reality into a fierce advocacy for her husband, and finally for herself. She is living proof that we can find grace in chaos. When she says, it's *The Best I Can Do*, I believe her. I am better for having read this book."
~ Laura Munson, *New York Times* bestselling author of *This Is Not The Story You Think It Is* and *Willa's Grove*, and founder of the acclaimed Haven Writing Retreats

"I've had the privilege to know and work with Cheryl for many years as colleagues in our professional association, the Society for Technical Communication. She is a consummate professional and is one of the strongest, most courageous, resilient people I have ever met. If these events could happen to her, they can happen to anyone, at any time. The tragedy of a loved one's severe mental illness, exacerbated by our society's lack of support for mental health care, compounded by the dot com bust and the recession in the early 2000s, created a perfect storm. While this story is a tribute to the resilience of the human spirit in the face of terrifying and overwhelming challenge, it is also an indictment of the way mental health is viewed and managed in our society, and the difficulty in getting (or even knowing how to access) resources when you need them most. A must-read."

~ Kit Brown-Hoekstra, Principal, Comgenesis, LLC

This book is dedicated to all the caregivers of loved ones struggling with mental health conditions. You're doing your best regardless of the circumstances you're facing. Never forget this.

Table of Contents

Home in the Snow	1
Our Fifth Anniversary	3
Darkness in Magnolia	8
Night Shift at the Ski Area	18
The Black Box	21
Tom's Layoff	26
The Cat in the Birdbath	32
The Hotel Suite	35
The CFP Exam	41
My Scouting Trip	47
The Holidays	57
The Move to New York	64
My Dot-Com Retreat	77
Escapes	89
Another Layoff	99
Interviews	103
Job Offers	111
The September 11 Attacks	125
The Hit and Run	135
My Revelation	142
The Swans	146
A Reunion with Friends	156
Counseling	165
Tiger's Grief	176
Deaths in the Family	178
The Breaking Point	192
Stepping Forward, Sliding Backward	200
An Encounter with the Police	219
Tom Returns to Seattle	225
Reconnecting with Nature	244
More Financial Struggles	254
Hitting Bottom	264

Tom Becomes Homeless	274
The Proposal	280
The Hearing	290
Home Again	296
Homeless Again	308
Don's Death	317
Final Journeys	323
Appendix	333
Acknowledgments	339
About the Author	342

Home in the Snow

Massachusetts, January 2005

My ringing travel alarm jolts me from a deep sleep. I peek at the windows. They are covered in snow. I'm grateful for the thick comforter I salvaged from the storage unit before the auction. The skin on my face stiffens and stings from the frigid air.

How long have I been here? The limit is eight hours.

I throw back the covers, slip into my jacket and boots, and get out of my Honda CR-V. Big dry flakes glide through the air.

I walk through a foot of snow to the back of my car, open the hatch door, and retrieve a snow broom underneath two folded blankets. A tow truck driver stops a few feet away and watches me brush the snow off my car.

Please don't tow me! I can't afford another bill. Just go away!

Maybe the tow truck driver heard my thoughts, because he moves on. I sigh with relief.

The snow smells fresh. Aside from muffling the sound, the newly fallen flakes make everything look and smell clean—even in this dreary rest area thirty-five miles northwest of Boston. I long for a place to call home, but this is the best I can do for now. I moved into my car four weeks ago, when I couldn't afford the rent anymore. I'm ashamed that I have to be homeless and frustrated that I can't keep up with the bills, but I feel fortunate that at least I can use my car for shelter. So many people who don't have places to live must sleep on the streets, under bridges, or anywhere else they can find.

The bathrooms are locked at the rest area for another hour, so I drive to the nearest Mobil station in Westford. I pull a change of clothes from a garbage bag in the back of my car, stuff them into a tote bag with my toothbrush, toothpaste, and comb, and carry them into the bathroom inside the convenience store. This is where I change and freshen up for the office. I don't want anyone at work to know what's happening to me.

When I'm done, I buy a croissant sandwich with bacon, egg, and cheese and a cup of coffee with cream at the Dunkin' Donuts counter. I don't have to buy lunch today because I left a half-eaten Chinese dinner in the refrigerator at the office. That's the perk about eating Asian—stretching leftovers.

During the drive to the office in Acton, I think about my long day ahead and feel overwhelmed. I need to finish writing a manual for the latest product. It's due today, and some of the features won't be ready. I need to talk to the engineers again to get whatever information I can to make the manual as complete as possible. It will have to do until the next release.

I can't forget to turn off my cell phone before entering the office. If I do, the creditors will bug me all day. They're never happy, even when I can make my payments on time.

Why don't they understand I'm doing the best I can? They treat me like I'm some deadbeat who's hiding a pot of gold somewhere that I don't want to give to them.

After a full day at the office, I will change again for my second job at the restaurant at the ski area. Hopefully the snow will attract more skiers tonight so I can earn enough tips to spend the night at the Motel 6 in Leominster. Maybe I can even pay a small bill or two. If not, I'll return to the office and take a shower before heading to the rest area for another night. No one uses the fitness center that late, so it's safe to shower without anyone knowing I'm there.

How did I wind up living in my car? I wish there were an easy answer. There's so much going on, and it's overwhelming. I've lost almost everything except for my car and I'm living in it. I'm struggling financially, and Tom, my husband, disappeared. He isn't the same loving man I knew. He's now in his own world, trying to escape people he believes are constantly following him. I wonder whether he will ever return to his old self and we can resume the happy life we lost.

Our Fifth Anniversary

London, September 1994

Tonight, Tom and I are as excited as two four-year-olds whose parents just said we're going out for an ice-cream cone. We're sitting in the back seat of a taxi, riding to London's West End. We've seen live theater at home in Seattle, but this is the first time we'll go to a big production in one of the most famous performing arts centers in the world.

If we were sitting any closer to each other, one of us would be in the other's lap. I'm staring out the back passenger window with my hand on Tom's knee. His hand is on my knee, and he's leaning over my shoulder to see the sights. I can feel his breath tickling my ear.

The black Fairway we're in reminds me of a car from the 1950s. The classic look fits in with the stone and brick buildings, many centuries old, we pass as the driver navigates the narrow, curvy, wet streets. Lights shine through windows of pubs and cafés, where people talk and laugh while eating a meal or enjoying a pint or two. A couple strolls along the sidewalk, sharing an open umbrella, deep in conversation.

I'm trying to remember everything I see, but I'm approaching sensory overload just like Tiger, our Maine Coon cat, when he spends too much time studying the view through the two picture windows in our living room.

How appropriate, I think. *We're on our way to see* Cats. *What would Tiger think of that?*

I look at Tom and smile. He smiles back. I love those beautiful, sparkling hazel eyes. That's the first thing I found attractive about him when he was a regular customer at the 7-Eleven where I worked as a clerk when we were students at the University of Oregon. And his smile. His smile and sparkling eyes complement each other, always caring and comforting. He's a handsome man with a stocky muscular frame, two inches taller than I am, with short, straight light-brown hair parted on the right side. He's clean shaven, because he says when he tries to grow a mustache or beard, the hair grows unevenly. I've never seen him with a mustache or beard, but I tell him he doesn't need facial hair to enhance his appearance. He's four years older than I am, but he looks much younger.

In smiling, I can feel my eyes sparkle as well. "I still can't believe we're doing this," I say.

"Me, too," Tom says. "This show has been sold out for years."

"Maybe someone heard it's our anniversary."

"Time flies, doesn't it? It seems like we got married yesterday." Tom smiles again, his face beaming with love. I squeeze his hand and lay my head on his shoulder. He wraps his arm around me.

The taxi driver stops in front of the New London Theatre on Drury Lane. Tom pays the fare and tip, and we thank the driver for his excellent service. On the marquee, the bright-yellow *Cats* logo and eyes flank the words "Now and Forever" in bold white block letters on a black background. The entrance is under a big banner reading, "Welcome to the Jellicle Ball," which matches the marquee's lettering and background.

Tom holds a door open for me as I walk into the lobby. He helps me remove my jacket and drapes it over the back of my seat.

Always the gentleman, I think. Four years of dating and five years of marriage haven't changed that. I'm the luckiest woman in the world for having Tom in my life. Before he showed up, I'd given up looking for a man to share the rest of my life with. I'd had too many bad experiences. Tom showed me there are males who still exist who aren't complete jerks. They can be caring, supportive beings who are more than spouses; they're best friends. With the right people, a couple can be a true team. That's what we are.

The theater is laid out like a target, with the stage being the bull's-eye and the sections of seats in rings surrounding it. Every seat has an unobstructed view of a junkyard. When we bought the tickets at the central box office today, the agent said the stage and orchestra pit rotate. We've never seen a rotating stage at a theater.

I wonder how the actors and musicians can focus on their parts while on a rotating stage, but after the show starts, I discover the movement is barely noticeable. I think about our anniversary dinner last year at the top of the Space Needle in Seattle, where the restaurant makes one full rotation in an hour. We dined on fresh grilled salmon, roasted red potatoes, and steamed asparagus while the sun slid behind the Olympic Mountains, painting the sky with abstract swathes of red, orange, and purple. Ferries resembling double-decker wedding cakes glided across the water to downtown Seattle from Bainbridge Island and back again. We were so focused on our conversation, the delicious food, and the scenery that we didn't pay attention to the floor moving below us.

We live like this. Life turns and we turn with it. I never have to worry that we don't.

We return to the bed-and-breakfast near Victoria Station at eleven at night. When Tom unlocks the door to our room, he pokes his head inside and looks around. I stand behind him.

"What's wrong?" I whisper.

"Just checking," he says.

"Checking for what?"

He doesn't reply.

I peek over his shoulder and scan the room. A streetlight shines through the window and outlines the two oversized twin beds with cast-iron headboards, a small nightstand with a pot-bellied lamp between the beds, and a chest of drawers. Everything I see looks the same as before we left to see *Cats*, except now it's mostly dark.

What's stopping him from going inside? I wonder.

Then I remember what happened earlier today. After a full morning of touring, we returned to our room to take a nap. We usually don't take naps in the middle of the day, but the eight-hour time difference between Seattle and London caught up with us. We've been in London for only two days, and it's taking longer than we expected to recover from the jet lag.

We cuddled in one of the beds and fell asleep. Twenty minutes later, we awoke to the sound of a key turning in the lock and the door opening. We shot up, speechless, as the gray-haired innkeeper poked his head inside, glancing at the sink next to the door and a small adjoining room that contains only a water closet. Then he saw us sitting up in the bed with the covers wrapped around us, staring at him with startled looks on our faces.

"Sorry," he said quietly in a beautiful British accent while lowering his head. He backed into the hallway and gently closed the door.

Tom looked at me with clenched jaws and lowered eyebrows. "Why would he come in here in the middle of the afternoon?"

"He was probably checking on whether we need fresh towels, soap, and toilet paper."

"He should have knocked."

"He assumed we weren't here. Most people are out during the day, seeing the sights."

"Well, I don't like it!"

"I'm sure he didn't mean any harm."

Tom frowned at me. I couldn't understand why he was overreacting but decided I shouldn't talk about it anymore. This was the first time I'd seen Tom act this way. If I tried to continue our conversation, would he become more agitated? I didn't know, so I decided it was best to let it go.

Now I wonder whether our experience this afternoon makes Tom believe that someone might be in our room tonight. But why would anyone be here this late at night? Why would anyone be here at all?

Another minute passes, which seems like hours. Tom reaches in, flips on the light switch above the sink, pushes the door open, and waits for me to go inside. We're silent while dressing for bed. I'm still bewildered by his behavior when he climbs into his bed and rolls onto his side, his back facing me. I turn out the light, climb into my bed, and say, "Good night. I love you." He doesn't respond because he's already asleep, softly snoring.

When we awake the next morning, Tom is back to his usual calm, pleasant demeanor. This puzzles me, but I rationalize that maybe he was tired from our full day yesterday and the persistent jet lag. After a good night's sleep, he probably realizes he overreacted.

Our nine-day adventure continues. We tour Leeds Castle, the ancient city of Bath, and Kensington Palace. We ride bright-red double-decker tour buses while listening to guides talk about London's history and landmarks and hop off at a stop to snap pictures of Big Ben. We take turns posing for pictures next to an old-fashioned cast-iron phone booth matching the color of the double-decker buses. We take the Tube to Little Venice for a lunch cruise of

Regent's Canal on a rainy day. We buy tickets to see two more plays, *Five Guys Named Moe* and an Agatha Christie mystery. We admire the beautiful stained glass and architecture of St. Paul's Cathedral and explore the Tower of London with a guide whose storytelling talents bring its history to life. We take long walks along the River Thames, hand in hand.

I never dreamed we could be this happy, but we are.

Darkness in Magnolia

Seattle, January 1996

Lord, please let these publishers hire me to index their books! I pray while pushing batches of stamped nine-by-twelve-inch manila envelopes through the mail slot at the post office, a tiny corner room at the State Farm Insurance office in our West Seattle neighborhood. The envelopes, addressed to publishers I found in *Writer's Market*, contain cover letters, résumés, and two samples of indexes I created.

I haven't worked for almost three months and it's wearing me down. I'm wondering whether I'll ever work again. An agency in downtown Seattle had hired me to revise a report for an environmental consulting firm the Monday after I returned home from the Society for Technical Communication (STC) conference in Portland back in October. On the day before the conference, shortly after I arrived in Portland, I got the call from the vice president of the department where I worked as a technical writer, when he said the maritime company cut fifty percent of its workforce. I was among them. What's worse, he called on my birthday, the same day before I spoke in front of my peers for the first time in my career. Somehow I pulled off the presentation, but I'm still astonished I could through my shock, frustration, and anger.

The last batch of envelopes slide down the chute while I look at the post office counter, an arch-shaped window with a wooden lip at the base, and debate whether I should buy some stamps in case I find more good publishing leads. I haven't seen or heard anyone inside the post office since I arrived. Maybe the clerk took a long break.

I decide to buy stamps later. It's more important to go home in case the phone rings. Oh, how I'm hoping someone calls me today about a job!

My thoughts continue wandering after I leave the post office. I walk past familiar sights during my six-block walk—from a restored movie theater built in the mid-1930s, mixed-use buildings, gas stations, a Safeway store, and fast-food restaurants, to streets of well-kept homes dating from the 1920s to 1940s.

All I can think about is getting a job. That project for the environmental consulting firm lasted only two weeks. The recruiter said she would have more work for me, but then didn't. I check in with her every week, and still nothing. Why would she say she has more work when she doesn't?

I worry about Tom. I feel like I'm a burden, although we've managed with his income and my weekly unemployment checks since my layoff. I'm not used to depending on someone. Before we married, I took care of myself. Our marriage is a partnership, where we contribute equally. We treat each other as equals and support our personal dreams and professional goals, but it feels like my job loss has tilted the scales.

He has been so supportive since this happened. When I called him from Portland, he didn't get upset. He was sad and sympathetic. He called me back after he finished his sales rounds that day to check on me. He made me feel like everything would be okay, although I wasn't so sure. And the next day after work, he drove all the way to Portland. He fought a twenty-five-mile backup from the Southcenter Mall to the Tacoma Dome on a Friday afternoon and other stops and starts along the way just to be with me. I didn't ask him to come, and he didn't tell me he was coming, but I was glad he did.

The traffic light at the intersection turns red. I push the chrome button to trigger the walk light and wait until it illuminates to cross the street.

Throughout our relationship, Tom has surprised me when I've hit hard spots. He seems to enjoy cheering me up. I remember the first time, a month after we started dating. When he heard that I got a C on a marketing midterm that I had studied hard for, he asked me to meet him on campus between classes and handed me a bouquet of white carnations. His thoughtfulness touched me so deeply that I cried. Then he worried that I was sad. I had to explain that I was crying happy tears, which made him feel better.

I turn onto the street to our house. The sun peeks through the clouds long enough to warm my face, then hides again.

Although Tom never complains about my struggles, I sense something is wrong. He has been quieter lately. Sometimes when he returns home from work, he's edgy. He mentions a few times that George, his manager of four years at his *Fortune 500* employer, is more demanding, so he's feeling pressure to sell more.

I think about those conversations, which don't vary much. Tom starts them with, "I saw someone following me today."

"Was it George?" I ask.

"No."

"What did the car look like? Could you see them?"

"I didn't recognize them." He doesn't describe the car, which puzzles me. If he believes someone is following him, why wouldn't he talk about the car? Could he see who's in the car? He knew it wasn't George, so he must have had a good view of them.

"Why would someone follow you?" I ask.

Tom doesn't reply.

The sales managers routinely audit the grocery stores in each sales rep's territory to check the company's market shares of products on the shelves, but they've never followed the reps anywhere. I wonder whether Tom's job stress is becoming overwhelming and hope I can find steady work soon to relieve his pressure.

By the time our house, a 1920s-era cottage with cream-colored siding and brown trim, is within view, I'm feeling sadder than ever. I'm trying not to give up, but today, I really want to. It would be easier to crawl into bed and sleep all day than continue this frustrating job search, but I never take the easy way out.

My mother and grandparents taught me that if I work hard and am reliable, my efforts will pay off. I learned those lessons early from helping them on a forty-acre farm in the Missouri Ozarks. We raised purebred Angus cattle, chickens, and pigs, and had three gardens that produced most of the food we needed. The only items we consistently bought from the grocery store in the largest town in the county, nine miles from the farm, were sugar, flour, salt, pepper, and spices.

When I was growing up, I loved school and studied hard to get straight As. Grandma encouraged me and was proud that I kept up my grades. She also encouraged me to go to college because she believed getting a degree would lead me to a prosperous career. She was sensitive to this because Grandpa, who was almost twenty years older than her, couldn't finish school. He had to quit in the fourth grade to help his widowed mother take care of the rest of the family. He couldn't read, so Grandma took care of anything that required reading discretely. No one knew outside our family about Grandpa's inability to read. Despite this, Grandpa worked steadily in a variety of blue-collar jobs throughout his life until his health forced him to retire. That's when Grandma and Grandpa decided to move from my birthplace of San Jose, California, to the farm in the Ozarks, about sixty miles from where they grew up and married. My mother, a single parent, decided to join them with me and Julie, my younger sister.

I settle into our office, turn on the computer, and surf the Internet, hoping to find some openings I haven't applied to. Nothing new today.

Tom returns from his sales rounds a few hours later, carrying a sheet of paper. He hands it to me. "I saw this in one of the grocery manager's offices and asked him if I could make a copy."

I look at the black-and-white drawing on the paper while Tom watches me. A stork stands on the bank of a pond with a frog's rear sticking out of its mouth. While the stork tries to swallow the frog, the frog grips the stork's neck with its four feet. The words, "Never Give Up," are centered across the top of the page.

I look up at Tom with watery eyes. "You don't know how much I needed to see this," I say. "It's been a tough day."

Tom smiles at me. "I thought about you when I saw it. I knew you needed some encouragement."

He hugs me and kisses my forehead.

"I'm taping this to the side of the file cabinet in our office," I say. "We'll always see it when we're working on the computer. It will inspire both of us."

Tom smiles again.

A week later, I'm at home mopping the floor in our compact, functional kitchen that hasn't been updated since the seventies. The color scheme gives it away: an avocado refrigerator and electric stove in a bank of maple-stained cabinets forming an L-shape along the walls. The cream countertops match the linoleum. The dishwasher leaks because the landlord doesn't want to spend money to fix it, so we wash our dishes by hand in the stainless-steel sink next to the dishwasher. We've stopped contacting the landlord for repairs because he raises the rent after he's finished. If anything we need breaks, we fix it ourselves if we're able or hire someone else to do it if we can afford it. Tom's experience working for his dad in cabinetmaking and construction while he was growing up and during holiday and summer breaks in college transformed him into a great handyman.

I'm feeling down again today. Like that leaky dishwasher, I can feel the energy draining from my body. It's now exactly three months since I've been laid off. No one replies to my job applications and inquiries. It feels like I'm sending my résumés to a black hole. Heck, I feel like I'm being sucked into a black hole. Why won't anyone contact me?

At least the mopping makes me feel like I'm in control of something, and I can see the results—a clean kitchen floor.

I hear chattering in the living room. Through the doorway, I see Tiger crouching on top of the bookshelf under the windowsill, staring at a squirrel grabbing a peanut from the wooden box Tom nailed to the trunk. The squirrel jumps on a branch and nibbles the peanut. Tiger's puffy tail swings like a pendulum on a clock, brushing the top of the bookshelf.

I can always rely on Tiger to distract me. Does he know what I'm going through? Cats have an amazing ability to detect when their humans are happy or sad.

The phone rings and I check the caller ID. The name of an agency I found in the Yellow Pages displays on the tiny screen.

"Hi, this is Susan from The Write Stuff," a cheery voice says. "Is this Cheryl?"

"It is."

"I'm calling about a project you might be interested in. A project manager at Microsoft is looking for an indexer. I see that you have indexing experience on your résumé."

"I do." My heart pounds faster.

"I don't have a lot of information yet, except it's a contract for six months to start. Most of the assignments we have at Microsoft extend. Would you like me to send your résumé to him?"

"Yes, I'm interested." I'm trying to speak calmly and professionally, but my mind is turning cartwheels. What if I don't get the job? What if I don't have enough experience? And if I do get it…what will it be like to work again? Will it help with Tom's edginess?

"Great! I will send it to him today and follow up with you when I hear from him."

"Do you mind my asking what happens after that? I'm new to contracting."

"Not at all. If he's interested, he will ask me to send you to Microsoft for an interview. He will make a decision after interviewing a few candidates. If you're hired, we'll have you come to our office to fill out the paperwork and we'll schedule a start date."

As soon as we hang up, I say, "Hey, Tiger, guess what? I got a job lead!"

I peek through the doorway and see Tiger frozen on the windowsill, staring at the squirrel.

I dunk the mophead into the bucket of water, wring out as much water as I can, and swish and swirl the mop across the floor. What if this contract will be mine?

You've got it, my inner voice says. I've named her Charlotte after the wise spider in E.B. White's famous story, *Charlotte's Web*. The spider's quick thinking of weaving complimentary words in her web saved a pig from becoming Thanksgiving dinner. I've admired her, although she's a fictional character, from the time Miss Atkins, my sixth-grade teacher, read that book to the class. Every day after lunch, Miss Atkins read to us for an hour before we resumed our lessons.

My first encounter with inner voice Charlotte was at the age of ten, when my grandfather was admitted to the hospital after a doctor's appointment earlier the same day. An uneasy feeling nagged at me and triggered thoughts that he'd never return home. He died three weeks later. Four years later, I began having dreams about finding my grandmother in distress somewhere and I couldn't help her. A month after those dreams started, she died suddenly from a heart attack.

Both experiences were unnerving, but Charlotte's revelations weren't always tragic. When Tom and I started dating, she quickly encouraged me to take the plunge. I was wary at first because of my bad experiences with men. My first and only boyfriend before Tom dumped me to date a fourteen-year-old, who soon became pregnant with his child. During a second date with another man, he invited me to his apartment after dinner for coffee and spent the next forty-five minutes lecturing me about the importance of wives submitting to their husbands. I refused to see him after that. The other guys who scheduled dates stood me up. But Tom was always a gentleman and never broke a commitment. Charlotte reminded me every chance she could with, *He's the one.*

I learned through these experiences and others that Charlotte is always right, but there are still times I either don't believe her or don't take her advice, and that gets me into trouble. Today is one of these days. I've been out of work long enough to be skeptical of her reassurance that I've got this contract at Microsoft. How can she know I'll be hired? I don't want to get my hopes up only to be disappointed if the contract falls through.

Despite my struggles believing Charlotte today, I can't wait to tell Tom about the lead when he returns home from his sales route. He needs to hear some good news. Sharing bad news or no news every day is tiring for me, so surely hearing it is tiring for him, too.

I hear a thump against the glass in the living room and turn around to see Tiger land on the floor in front of the bookshelf on all four feet. He freezes for a few seconds with a stunned look on his face, then shakes himself from head to tail and strolls into the bedroom.

I chuckle, hoping Tiger doesn't hear me. He forgot about the window again when he lunged at the squirrel.

Silly cat. He'll never learn. I hope I'm better at seeing the clear boundaries in my life.

Tom arrives home at three-thirty, his usual time. His eyes look weary and his shoulders droop when he walks through the door from our enclosed back porch into the kitchen. I'm at the sink, washing the dishes I used to prepare dinner.

I kiss him on the cheek. "How was your day?" I ask. "You look tired."

He frowns, then kisses me on the forehead. "It was okay," he says in a sad voice.

"It doesn't sound like it was okay."

We go to the living room and sit on the couch, facing each other. "George called me. He was in a bad mood."

"Again? He seems to be in bad moods a lot lately."

"Yeah, he's always complaining. Let's talk about something else."

"I have some good news. I got a call today about a contract at Microsoft. The recruiter said that it starts at six months but will probably extend. She sent my résumé to the hiring manager."

"That's nice," Tom says in a monotone. Usually he's more excited about news like this.

"Are you sure everything is okay?" I ask.

"It's fine," he replies in the same monotone.

His voice doesn't convince me that everything is "fine." Maybe a tasty meal will help.

"I'm baking a pork roast with the orange-raspberry glaze you like for dinner tonight," I say. "It'll be ready in a half hour."

"That sounds good, but I'm not hungry. I'll have some later."

Tom never turns down food.

"Are you sure you're okay?"

He nods, but his face looks worried.

"Let's go for a drive tonight," he says. "I want to check the cereal aisle at the Albertsons in Magnolia."

Maybe a drive will make him feel better, but I wonder why he wants to go to a store in his territory so late in the day. Why didn't he do it earlier?

Tom changes his mind about skipping dinner after I pull the pork roast out of the oven, but he's still distracted. We eat in silence. Usually we talk about what happened during the day or make plans for the weekend.

The silence continues while Tom clears the table and I wash the dishes. He dries them with a towel and puts them away.

As soon as we're done, he asks, "Are you ready?"

I nod.

"Let's go."

He seems to be in a hurry. None of this makes sense to me, and I wonder whether something is seriously wrong.

I become more confused when we leave. Instead of taking the direct route from West Seattle to the Magnolia neighborhood, Tom roams a few back streets along the way.

Isn't Tom in a hurry to go to that store? If not, why?

Tom is looking in the rearview mirror more often than usual. He continues focusing on the mirror until he parks the car in the Albertsons lot.

"Stay here," he says. "I'll be back."

Tom strolls to the store and enters through the automatic doors at a casual pace. While I wait for him to return in the dark, empty parking lot, so many questions fly around in my head that I can't answer: What's happening? Why is Tom acting this way? Why was he in a hurry after we washed the dishes tonight but took his time to drive here? Why did he meander through West Seattle before heading over here? Why didn't he rush into the store? Is he telling me everything about his problems at work? Has George threatened to fire Tom because Tom isn't meeting his expectations?

Tom is one of the top salespeople in the Northwest, so I don't understand why George would be unhappy about his performance. I don't know if this is the real reason Tom is distracted and worried. I can only guess, but I don't have any answers. I wish I did.

I feel helpless waiting in the dark, empty parking lot. If there's anything I can do, I don't know what it could be. The more I dwell on my confusion, the more frightened I become.

Tom returns to the car fifteen minutes later with a worried look on his face. He's quiet while he drives out of the parking lot and turns onto the main road.

I don't say anything. I decide it's better to watch him and hopefully I can figure out what's going on. If I talk to him, he probably won't tell me anything. Whatever he's going through, he doesn't want me to know about it. But if he doesn't want me to know, why did he ask me to go on this drive with him? Maybe he wants me to be near him, to keep him company.

As soon as we're on the main road, Tom shifts his focus to the rearview mirror. "We're being followed," he says.

I turn around and see four cars with their lights shining behind us. Yes, they're following us, but this is the only way to reach the closest highway through Seattle.

"Don't look," Tom says. "They might see you."

"How can they see me in the dark?"

Tom doesn't answer.

I turn around and start monitoring the mirror on the passenger door. The four cars stay behind us.

Tom maintains a close watch in the rearview mirror, fear gripping his face. He turns left at the next intersection. All the cars behind us pass, continuing their journeys toward the exit.

"Where are we going?" I ask.

Tom doesn't respond. He's watching the rearview mirror. No cars are behind us now.

All the roads we follow in this residential area are dark and empty, except for the occasional streetlight shining on the sidewalks or reflecting in puddles. Most of the lights in the houses are off because it's late.

I'm scared. It's hard for me to think. Even if I could think, I wouldn't know what to do.

Twenty minutes later, Tom returns to the main road and resumes our journey home. The worried look fades from his face, but he's still quiet. I think about asking him if he's okay but decide to wait until he's ready to talk. I don't know how he'll react.

As soon as we're home, Tom sits at the small teak desk in the corner of our kitchen and dials into the company's email server from the modem in his laptop. The modem hums, splutters, and screams while it connects. It's silent while Tom downloads his messages, uploads replies to messages he received earlier, and logs off.

I sit on the couch and hope that Tom will talk to me after he finishes reading his new messages. I want to know what's going on but don't want to ask. Judging by my observations tonight, he won't talk to me if I start asking questions. I don't know if he'll get angry if I persist. I feel so helpless because I don't understand why Tom is behaving this way. This is not the same Tom I've known for so long. I don't know where this new person came from.

Tiger jumps on the couch and curls into a ball next to me. I rub his head between his ears, and he starts purring softly. The more I rub, the louder he purrs. The sound comforts me.

Tom turns off the laptop, closes the lid, and goes to the bedroom. I hear him crawl into bed in the dark room. Usually we kiss and say *good-night* before going to bed.

He forgot about me. This hurts.

I stay on the couch, my thoughts a jumbled mess of confusion and fear, and rub Tiger.

Cheryl Landes

Night Shift at the Ski Area

Massachusetts, January 2005

Across the hall from my cubicle, I see giant fluffy flakes falling outside the windows. At least another foot of snow has accumulated since I arrived at the office this morning. It's now three-forty in the afternoon, and I just finished writing the last paragraph for the manual that's due today. I save the chapter, compile a PDF for the administrative assistant to print for the training next week, back up the files on the network, and shut down my computer.

I leave here by four o'clock to make my shift at the restaurant on time. The skiing will be great tonight—perfect for working up some hearty appetites and hopefully some hearty tips. I'd really love to sleep in a comfortable bed in a warm room at the Motel 6 tonight.

Where will Tom be tonight? I ask myself this question a lot. No one has heard from him since he disappeared. This isn't the first time he disappeared, but it has been the longest. I stopped trying to file missing person reports after the first time he disappeared because the woman at the front desk of the local precinct didn't finish the paperwork after I told her about his paranoia.

"Usually in cases like these, they'll return in a few days," she said. She didn't clarify what cases she was talking about, but I knew she was referring to "people who are mentally ill."

How does *she* know what Tom will do? He doesn't trust anyone because paranoia has consumed his life. Is this why he disappeared? I don't know the answer to that question. I can only guess that Tom is so afraid of those evil, imaginary people following him twenty-four seven that he believes he must disappear to survive. I can't imagine what it's like to be scared like that constantly. I feel sorry for him.

I think about Tom's parents. They died two months apart after losing battles with long-term health problems more than a year ago. I'm sad they're gone because they were like parents to me, too, but I'm glad they don't know what's happening to Tom and me now. They would be devastated, just like I am.

The dining room is packed when I arrive for my shift. I peek out the windows that overlook the ski area between serving customers. The hill is covered with skiers enjoying the real snowpack. In Massachusetts, ski areas make snow when there isn't enough to keep the lifts running. It's a new concept for me, because in the Pacific Northwest, the ski areas rarely make snow. Mother Nature takes care of it.

The stream of customers continues until we close, and many tip generously. When we cash out, I wonder how much I made. Despite how busy we were tonight, everything went smoothly. No customers complained, which is always a good sign. Everyone was in a good mood, probably from the freshly fallen snow. Even the bartender seemed less jaded than usual.

When the manager finishes balancing the tills, he hands a stack of bills to me. I hold my breath while I count the money and think I might faint when I finish. I count again just to make sure. Three hundred dollars—my best night ever! I can pay off one bill and spend two nights at the Motel 6. I can't wait to check in.

Although I'm excited about my mother lode tonight, I don't let my emotions show, so people don't know what I'm going through. It's how I was raised. "Never give up," Grandma said often. So did Mom. When we faced challenges, we remained calm and moved forward. Grandpa spoke only when he had something important to say. Everyone respected his wisdom.

We never asked for help, either. "You don't want people to feel sorry for you," Grandma said. "You've got to be strong and take care of yourself."

Being homeless is embarrassing and humiliating. I didn't choose to be here. I don't want to be here, so I'm working as hard as I can to get back on my feet. I'm making progress, but I have a long way to go.

I don't want to think about sleeping in my car again after my two nights at the Motel 6. For now, I will enjoy the comfort of a warm room, soft bed, and not having to shower at the office. Maybe we'll be blessed with more big snow nights before the end of the season and the customers will be generous again.

When I drive from the restaurant to Leominster, I wonder where Tom is tonight. *Please lead him to a warm, comfortable, safe place*, I pray.

The Black Box

Seattle, February 1996

I'm sitting at the end of our couch sipping a cup of coffee and watching Tiger sleep at the top of the cat tree next to the picture window in the corner at the opposite end of our living room. I can't stop thinking about that scary drive in the Magnolia neighborhood two weeks ago. Tom hasn't talked about it since; it's as if he forgot about it. I debate whether I should ask him about it but decide it's best to try to forget about it, too. Maybe Tom overreacted to the stressful phone conversation with George earlier that day, but if he did, this is unusual behavior.

Why doesn't Tom talk to me about what's happening with George? He knows I would never tell anyone about our conversations related to his job. It's not healthy to keep that stress locked inside.

I jump when the phone rings and almost spill my coffee.

"Hey, Cheryl. It's Susan from The Write Stuff again. I'm calling because Microsoft wants you to come in for an interview for the indexing contract."

My heart begins racing. "That's fantastic!"

Hopefully the volume of my voice didn't cause Susan to become deaf temporarily. Apparently it didn't, because she quickly replies with, "Are you available Tuesday at two o' clock?"

"Yes. I'm looking forward to it!"

Susan gives me the interviewer's name and directions to his office. "This is a new position for indexing clip art, so Bert will have a lot of questions about your process. Good luck! Call me after the interview to let me know how it went."

After we hang up, I begin to panic. I've never indexed a piece of clip art. What if Bert figures this out during the interview? I can't let him. I need this job. It would help reduce Tom's stress and mine.

I log onto our computer. With less than four days to prepare, I must make the most of my time. I'm a stellar researcher, thanks to my training in journalism. I've got this!

You've got this! Charlotte echoes in the back of my mind.

Three hours later, I finish a draft of my indexing process and start editing it. Tiger jumps on the desk and walks across the keyboard. He turns around and stops in front of me, blocking my view of the computer screen, then sits and stares at me with his big green eyes.

"Are you telling me it's time for a break?"

His eyes are fixed on mine. He'll sit here until I either move him or give him some attention.

"Okay, let's play." I pick him up and carry him into the living room. I look for his favorite toy but can't find it.

"Hang on. I'll be right back."

I return to the office, grab a sheet of scrap paper, and scrunch it into a ball.

"Here you go!" I throw the paper wad through the doorway. It flies over the low-pile beige carpet across the living room and lands in front of the gray couch. Tiger runs after it and catches it in his mouth. He struts over to me, tail pointed high, and drops the paper wad between my feet.

I move in front of the cherry entertainment cabinet opposite the couch, drop to my knees, and throw the paper wad again. This time, it lands on the couch. Tiger jumps on the couch, picks up the paper wad with his mouth, and repeats his proud strut, which ends with him dropping his prize in front of my knees.

We repeat the cycle. Sometimes he cuffs the paper wad back and forth between his paws before returning it to me. I laugh at his antics and reward him with head and chin rubs.

I hear the back door open and close and footsteps climb the stairway on the enclosed back porch. The steps continue through the kitchen, then Tom emerges through the entryway into the living room. His shoulders droop and he's frowning. He sighs after he sits on the couch. Tiger jumps on the couch with the paper wad in his mouth and drops it in Tom's lap. Tom briefly scratches Tiger between the ears, then stares out the window.

I join them, then place my hand on Tom's shoulder and look

into his eyes.

"Looks like you had a rough day," I say.

Tom's tired glassy eyes scan my face. "I had my performance evaluation today," he says. "It wasn't good."

"How is that possible? You exceeded your sales goals this year—by a lot." Tom's parents taught him the value of hard work, just like my grandparents and Mom did, which has resulted in high performance marks, several awards, and generous annual bonuses during the past eight years.

"I know, but George wants me to sell more," Tom says. "He's never happy with my work."

I reach for Tom's hand and hold it gently. "I'm so sorry he treats you this way."

Tom gazes at the paper wad. His voice shakes when he says, "After he finished the evaluation, I refused to sign it. I asked to be transferred out of his district."

"Did he approve it?"

"I don't know. He ended the conversation and I left."

Tom sighs and looks at the window. I rest my head on his shoulder, and he wraps his arm around me while we watch the raindrops glide down the glass.

Since Tom started reporting to George, George has been tough on him. I wonder if this is George's way of getting his salespeople to produce more. Maybe there's a personality conflict. Or maybe both. One time when Tom opened up a little about George, he said that George isn't treating his other salespeople the same way, although they aren't selling as much as Tom. Does George know that Tom is making him look good as a manager? Surely he does. Who wouldn't want someone like Tom on their team?

I can't imagine how Tom feels right now. He loves his job and works hard but gets a bad performance review in return. What a gut punch! I can understand why he refused to sign the review and asked for a transfer. But what happens if George doesn't approve the transfer? Could he fire Tom? He could make Tom's working life unbearable to force Tom to quit.

Will my news console Tom at a time like this? It's time to try.

I gently squeeze Tom's hand. "I have some good news. The recruiter called and said the hiring manager at Microsoft wants to interview me for the indexing contract. It's at two o'clock on Tuesday."

Tom wraps his arm around me tighter, still focused on the window. "I'm happy for you," he says.

We continue watching the raindrops.

When I awake the next morning, Tiger is stretched out on his side in Tom's spot, sleeping soundly. I listen for sounds in the house, but it's quiet.

I walk into the bathroom and look out the window. The car isn't in the carport.

Where did Tom go, and why didn't he tell me where he's going? On Saturday, we run errands together. Could he be checking on some of the stores in his territory today? Does he feel like he needs to work weekends now to appease George?

I look under the desk, where Tom keeps his briefcase. It's still there.

Maybe he wants to be alone for a while. He needs some time to think about what happened yesterday.

I start a pot of coffee. While it brews, I shower, dress, and print out a copy of the notes for my interview. I'll make breakfast when Tom returns. He'll probably be hungry by then.

When Tom returns home a half hour later, I'm sitting at our oval maple dining table at the end of the living room, sipping a cup of coffee and editing the printout. I can see Tom clearly through the kitchen doorway. He's carrying a plain paper bag, which he places on the counter by the stove. He pulls out a large black box with an antenna attached to one end.

"What's that?" I ask.

"Shhh," he replies.

He extends the antenna and turns a knob on the box. The box hisses while he slowly moves the antenna like a wand over the kitchen walls, ceilings, and floor.

I start to get up to take a closer look at the box.

"Stay there," he says, slightly louder than a whisper.

I sit again, watching him as long as I can see him.

He slowly moves from the kitchen to the bedroom. A few minutes later, I hear the hissing in the office. Then he's in the living room, scanning the tip of the antenna along the ceiling and walls. He monitors something on the side of the box while he moves the antenna. From my angle, it looks like a small screen, but I can't see what's on it.

What is he looking for?

Tom eases closer to the table. My heart beats faster, and I wonder whether that antenna can detect my pulse through the static. Tom ignores me while he moves the antenna along the ceiling above the table and tilts the box closer to his chest, blocking the screen from my view.

Did he do this intentionally? Why isn't he telling me what he's doing? I don't understand what he's doing, why he's doing it, and what he hopes to find.

I think about the drive in the Magnolia neighborhood again. Tom thought someone was following us that night. Is this related to his behavior today?

Tom carries the box to the back porch, and I hear him descending the stairs into the basement. The hissing volume lowers, then stops.

I hear the back porch door close and get up to look outside. Tom backs the car into the alley and drives away.

This is scary. I feel like I'm in a strange movie, but the story is real. What is happening to my husband? Why is he behaving this way?

I return to the table, but I can't focus on editing the printout anymore. I sip my cold coffee and watch Tiger lying on top of the bookshelf, surveying the world through the window. My mind searches for answers about Tom's unusual behavior but comes up empty. I don't know what to do, and that scares me even more.

Why isn't Charlotte giving me any answers at a time like this? Is she upset at me because I'm wary of her certainty about my landing the contract at Microsoft? I could use her advice right now. Or maybe it's because I'm too scared to listen to her if she recommended a clear solution.

Tom returns an hour later. Now he's carrying a small black box with a knob on one end. He places the box on top of the refrigerator and turns the knob. White noise instantly fills the air.

I go to the kitchen to take a closer look at the box. When I start to pick it up, Tom says, "Don't touch it."

"What is it?" I ask.

"It blocks our conversations," he says. "No one can hear us now."

"But no one is listening to us."

Tom stares at the box.

Tom's Layoff

Seattle, December 1997

Today is my work-at-home day. My manager at Microsoft lets me work at home twice a week. It's nice to take breaks from the three-hour, round-trip bus commute. I get more done when I'm at home because I don't have to attend meetings.

My clip art indexing contract has been extended a few times. I've worked for this team for almost two years, but it's coming to an end. New Year's Eve is my last day. On January 6, I'll start indexing encyclopedia articles for another team for six months, maybe longer.

My business has been growing, too. Publishers began contacting me a month after my contract started at Microsoft, and now I have steady indexing work from a few. I've also finished some small technical writing projects and published Pacific Northwest travel articles in a few regional magazines.

I've made a few friends at Microsoft, too. I spend the most time with Betty and Lily. We met about three months after I started the clip art indexing contract, when we all worked for the same team, and quickly became friends. Now we eat lunch together in a cafeteria or café on campus and, when we don't have looming deadlines, take short mid-afternoon walks along the trails on campus.

George approved Tom's transfer a week after that terrible performance evaluation. Jill, Tom's new manager, treats everyone on her team fairly and respects them. Since Tom joined her team, his sales numbers have soared, and he has received more awards. I'm so proud of him.

The black box still sits on top of the refrigerator, but Tom doesn't use it anymore. After he bought it at the spy shop (I found the receipt while cleaning one day), he wouldn't talk to me in the house unless it was turned on. He believed the house was bugged. When I asked him who would do this and why, he never answered.

As time passes, I've noticed a pattern in Tom's behavior: The more stress he's under, the more he's convinced someone is snooping on us at home or following him at work. This must be Tom's way of handling stress, but it still seems unusual. I've never known anyone who reacts to stress this way.

Since Tom started reporting to Jill, his pleasant, patient demeanor has returned. He's the man I fell in love with. I'm happy he's back and he can continue working a job he loves with less stress. I missed him so much.

It's two o'clock, and I'm almost finished indexing the latest batch of clip art, a collection of fruits and vegetables. Tom should be home by the time I'm done. We're going out to dinner tonight at the Coho Café, our favorite restaurant in the neighborhood. My stomach growls from writing food keywords and thoughts of eating perfectly grilled salmon with fresh asparagus spears and homemade rice pilaf with slivered almonds. Maybe the chef will have the chocolate mousse on the menu tonight. It's Tom's favorite dessert, but I love it, too.

At two-thirty, I hear the back porch door open and close, and footsteps on the stairs. Tom is home early. When he appears in the office, his eyes are red and glassy, and his cheeks are wet.

Oh, dear, he has been crying. Why was he crying? I've never seen him cry.

My heart breaks for him, even though I don't know why he's so sad. I stand, place my hands on his shoulders, and gaze into his eyes. "What's going on?" I ask.

He hesitates, struggling to fight back the tears.

"They're laying me off," he says in a trembling voice. "New Year's Eve is my last day."

I don't know what to say. I'm too shocked to think of any comforting words, so I hug him instead.

Tom pulls me closer. His tears land in my hair and on my shirt. We hold each other for a long time. I feel Tom's chest shake while the tears flow and he struggles to compose himself.

When he releases me, he says, "I'll be back," and heads to the back door.

"Where are you going?" I ask, but he's already outside.

I rush to the bathroom window, which has a view of the carport, to watch him drive away while hoping he doesn't have an accident. He's too distraught to be behind the wheel.

I return to the desk and try to concentrate on writing keywords for the rest of the images. This batch is due today, so I must push through it. It's hard to focus on fruits and vegetables with my thoughts about Tom's layoff swirling in my mind. I worry that he will have a hard time recovering from this, because I've read reports from researchers about how a man's perception of his job differs from a woman. Women usually don't define themselves by their jobs, but men do. When most men lose their jobs, they lose their identities. Tom is like that. He has been a salesperson since he graduated from college.

Tom returns home two hours later, back to his usual self. I'm still in the office, wrapping up the project. He grabs a chair from the table, carries it into the office, and sits next to me.

"How are you?" I ask.

"I'm fine now," Tom says. He watches me attach the keyword spreadsheet to an email and send it to the project coordinator.

"Where did you go?"

"I called Mom and Don. Then I drove around the neighborhood."

I'm glad he called at least one of his three older brothers.

"How did they react?"

"They were shocked."

"You know your mother will worry about you non-stop now."

"She worries about everything."

"That's what mothers do, I suppose."

Tom nods. I shut down the computer.

"How hungry are you?" he asks.

"I'm hungry but not starving. What do you have in mind?"

"Let's look at the lights before dinner."

We're silent during the short drive to the base of the bluff. Tom parks the car at a viewpoint with a breathtaking panorama of Elliott Bay and Seattle's skyline. The colors from the setting sun reflect in the water and on the buildings. When darkness arrives, lights from the office towers, ferries, and ships flicker like stars.

This is our favorite place to sit and talk. Over the years, we've talked about almost everything here, from life's challenges to our dreams. The beautiful scenery inspires us. We never grow tired of it.

We sit in the car and soak in the view for a long time before Tom breaks the silence.

"The company laid off the entire sales force. They've decided to farm out the work to a broker."

"Won't they lose market share?"

"They will, but they're focused on reducing overhead. They've watched all our competitors use brokers and decided it's more cost-effective than keeping a sales staff."

"That doesn't sound like a very good business plan."

"It isn't. The reason my sales were so high is because I had good relationships with the store managers in my territory. They liked me and trusted me. Brokers represent products from different companies, so they have competing interests."

We watch a ferry glide across the bay toward Bainbridge Island. The reflections from the lights dance on the ripples in the water.

"Have you thought about what you'll do next?" I ask.

"I have. I'm not sure I want to stay in sales anymore. I'm thinking about moving into finance."

Tom and I met when we were studying for our second bachelor's degrees. I was a transfer student from Eastern Oregon University in La Grande, where I majored in a general studies program and minored in history and psychology. My ultimate goal was a journalism degree, so while I was at Eastern, I worked with an advisor at the University of Oregon to ensure my credits would transfer. Two-thirds of the course requirements at the University of Oregon were outside my major; the rest were in journalism. By the time I finished the transferable credits for my journalism degree, I had enough to get the bachelor's in general studies from Eastern.

Tom received his first bachelor's degree in general science from the University of Oregon, seven years before we met. He returned from his hometown of Coos Bay, Oregon, to study finance at the business school the same year I moved to Eugene. After he graduated, he didn't pursue a job in finance because he didn't want to leave the Pacific Northwest. All the entry-level finance jobs are in the Northeast.

"That means a move to New York City," I say. "Your dream was to move to Seattle after you graduated. Are you sure you want to leave here?"

"I've been researching positions here. Most of them require at least five years of experience. If I could break in in New York and work there for five years, then I'd be able to move back here and get a job. We could stay here permanently."

Tom and I have never spent any time in New York City, but judging from what I've seen and heard about the culture there, it's a high-energy place. How well can Tom handle the stress there? I'm not sure how well I can manage it, either, but I don't want to discourage him. A career change would be good for him.

We both love Seattle—the laid-back lifestyle, the beautiful scenery, the bountiful outdoor activities, and the climate. It will be hard to leave, but we can manage it temporarily.

But can I maintain my career momentum after such a big move? It was hard to get started in Seattle, but now everything is going well. I have steady work from the Microsoft contracts and am getting more indexing projects from publishers. Will that continue if I uproot? If Tom takes a break to study for his tests, I can support both of us in Seattle but not in New York City. The cost of living is much higher there. I know about this from conversations with colleagues who moved here from New York.

Should I mention this now? We've both faced so much today. It doesn't feel like the right time. Tom supported me through my struggles to get back on my feet. I don't want him to believe I'm not supporting him, but we need to talk about this.

"I need to get some certifications before I start looking," Tom says. "The CFP (Certified Financial Planner) is top priority. The Series 7 would help, too."

"You could study here and take the exams before you leave."

"There's a testing site in Tacoma."

I decide to say something. "I need to figure out what to do with my career, too. I'm not sure whether I can be as successful in the Northeast."

"Why not? The biggest publishing companies in the country are there."

"That's true, but most of my work comes from high-tech. New York doesn't have giant high-tech companies like Microsoft. And the publishing companies out there are very competitive. Would they even look at my experience?"

Tom gently squeezes my hand. "By the time we move out there, you'll have so much work that you won't have to worry. You can do your work from anywhere as long as we have a computer and an Internet connection."

"That's true, but if other high-tech companies are like Microsoft, they'll want me to work onsite. I'm fortunate that my current manager lets me work from home two days a week. Most managers don't allow it."

"Everything will be okay. We're a team. We can make this work."

I lay my head on Tom's shoulder and stare at the lights across the bay. He's right; we've been through tough times and together, we've come through stronger than ever. But this is different. It's the biggest step we've ever taken. It seems like the best thing to do, but I worry about the stress and uncertainty. Is my uneasiness Charlotte's way of warning me that something bad will happen if we move?

I want to support Tom, but what happens if this doesn't work out? We won't know until we move forward—one step at a time.

The Cat in the Birdbath
Seattle, March 1998

I'm riding home on the city bus after another day at my latest contract at Microsoft. I'm indexing encyclopedia articles and pictures for eight months at Encarta. My new manager and the indexers on the team are fun to work with, and the hours fly every day.

It has been three months since Tom was laid off from his job, and he seems happier and more relaxed. He has started studying for the first test in the CFP series.

I've noticed that Tom isn't paranoid anymore, either. Is it because he's no longer stressed from his sales job? It's nice to see him back to his old self. I hope this career change will work out for him. I want him to be happy in his career like I am in mine, but now I'm not sure what will happen with my career. I don't like the uncertainty, but I'm trying to keep it from getting in my way. I'm planning ahead by marketing to more publishers and other companies that will allow me to work remotely. I have a few publishing clients already that aren't in New York. If more publishers continue to hire me, I can maintain a steady income without the Microsoft contracts. Maybe by the time we leave Seattle, I can convince Microsoft to allow me to telecommute from the Northeast, but that's probably a long shot. I want to make this big move work for both of us.

When I arrive at home, Tom is sitting at one end of the dining table, his thick hardback books and binders of study materials spread out in front of him. One of the binders is open. He's reading the pages and pauses off and on to write notes in a spiral notebook.

I kiss him on the cheek, then sit in a chair at the side of the table. He looks at me and smiles, his hazel eyes sparkling.

I smile back. "How's it going?" I ask.

"Good," he says. "I've read the first half of the study guide for the first exam. I'll have to review it a few more times."

He pauses while he closes the spiral notebook and places the pen on top of it. "I scheduled the exam for June. That's the earliest I could sign up at the testing site in Tacoma."

"Great!" I'm happy he's moving forward so quickly, but at the same time, I'm afraid of him moving so quickly. Am I really ready for this?

Tom places a bookmark in the binder and closes it. He folds his arms and leans forward, resting them on the edge of the table, and looks at me with worried eyes. My heart skips a beat while I wonder what's on his mind.

"I saw the neighbor's cat sleeping in our birdbath again today," he says. "He spends a lot of time there lately."

He's worried about another cat. I haven't seen this side of Tom for a long time—focusing on an animal instead of himself. His love of animals is another thing that attracted me to him. This is another sign that Tom has returned to his old self, and I'm relieved.

"I haven't noticed," I say. "Usually, he's roaming around in the alley or on the sidewalk in front of the house. Maybe he's hanging out in the birdbath to avoid those boys who torment him so much. They like to chase him. If they catch him, they pull his tail. Their parents let them run wild. Aren't they worried a car will hit them? There's a lot of traffic in this neighborhood."

The brown and black short-haired tabby cat lives three houses south of us, on the same street. He's outside weekdays and goes home after his humans return from work. We never see him on the weekends.

"Did you notice he's losing a lot of weight?" Tom asks.

"I haven't," I say. I haven't seen him since my new contract started because I work onsite full-time now.

Then it dawns on me why he's probably losing weight.

"Didn't the neighbors move three months ago?" I ask.

"They did," Tom says.

"Oh, no! They left the cat here! How can anyone do that to their pet?"

"Let's take him in," Tom says. "He needs a home."

"How will Tiger handle that? I don't know if he'll be happy

about it. He's had us to himself for the past eight years. But I don't want the alley cat to starve to death. He needs a home, and he seems like a sweet boy."

"Tiger will get used to it. We'll ease him into it. They'll keep each other company."

I stand. "Is the cat out there now?"

"He was a few minutes before you came home. Let's check."

We go to the back porch and look out the window. The cat is curled in a ball, sleeping in the middle of the birdbath.

"Let's leave some food in the carport for him," Tom says. He grabs the bag of cat food from the shelf on the back porch. I follow him into the kitchen.

"We don't have any more pet food bowls, but there are some aluminum pie pans in the drawer under the stove," I say. "We can fill one with food and the other with water."

I pull out two pie pans and hand one to Tom. He pours the food to the brim while I fill the other pie pan with water. He carries the pans outside while I watch from the back porch and places them in a corner of the carport where we can see them from the house. The cat runs away when he sees Tom in the carport.

"I hope he finds the food," Tom says when he returns.

"He will," I reply. "He's scared. He'll probably wait to return after dark. We can check on him in the morning."

As soon as Tom awakes the next morning, he goes outside to check on the cat and returns quickly with his report: "I didn't see him, but half the food is gone."

"That's good news about the food," I say. "He'll probably be back later today. Maybe you'll see him again. When he's comfortable being around us, we can bring him inside. We'll have to figure out how to introduce him to Tiger."

Tom nods and smiles. "It probably will take some time before he trusts us, but at least he knows where to get food now."

I'm happy to see Tom upbeat today. He should have a productive day studying for his exam. I remember how hard he worked to prepare for tests in college, and he usually fared well. The CFP exams will be more challenging than any test he took in college, so I hope he passes on the first try. I don't know how failing a test will affect him. At the same time, I'm hoping I don't fail in my career with this big move.

The Hotel Suite

Massachusetts, February 2005

It's ten o'clock in the morning. I'm sitting at the desk in my office cubicle, editing a sales bulletin for the release of a product upgrade. I'm struggling to stay awake because I couldn't sleep well in my car last night. Although I have a thick cushion in the back of my SUV, pillows, some blankets, and a comforter, I couldn't get comfortable after spending two nights at the Motel 6 in Leominster.

I glance across the hall, where floor-to-ceiling windows rise behind a row of cubicles. Fluffy snowflakes are falling again. It will be another busy night at the ski area, so maybe I can earn enough tips to pay down another bill and squeeze in one more night at the Motel 6.

My computer chimes, alerting me to new messages in my inbox. As I scan the list, one catches my attention from Tom's email address. The subject line reads, "Call me." This is the first time I've heard from him in weeks.

I open the message.

Hi, Cheryl.
I need help typing a paper for a class. I will pay you. Call me when you get this message.
Tom

No "Love, Tom." Just "Tom," a single word that speaks volumes about how much our relationship has changed. He's slipping farther away, despite his reaching out for help, and my heart breaks even more.

I stare at the message, trying to gather my thoughts on what to say when I call. Apparently he's still taking classes in the business management certificate program at the Harvard Extension School.

He should have graduated by now. I wonder where he's staying and how he can afford to pay the rent. He has been unemployed for more than seven years, and when we were together, no one wanted to hire him because he had been out of the workforce for so long. With his worsening paranoia, he probably couldn't hold a job for long if anyone took a chance on him.

Calling Tom is an excuse to take a break. Well, maybe it really isn't an excuse. I don't know. I want to talk to him because I want to know he's okay, but I don't want to talk to him because I never know what to expect. It's painful to hear his paranoia and his blame. On the practical side, I can grab another cup of coffee from the kitchen on the way back to my desk. Maybe the caffeine will jolt me awake. The first two cups haven't helped so far.

Am I the only one who multitasks like this? It's such a sad statement on my life. Not sad; it's downright depressing how much my world has changed.

I slip on my coat, grab my flip phone, and walk to the car. It's the best place to talk to Tom. I don't want anyone to overhear our conversation.

When Tom answers, his voice sounds like his pleasant self from the early days of our relationship, but he doesn't ask how I am.

"I have a paper that's due on Friday and wonder if you could type it for me," he says. "I will pay you."

"Where have you been?" I ask.

"Here and there. I'm in Boston now."

"Why didn't you call and tell me where you are? I thought something happened to you."

Tom doesn't reply.

By now, I should be accustomed to not hearing from Tom for long periods of time. I'm not. I don't know if I ever will be.

"Have you talked to Don?" I ask. "Does he know where you are?"

"No," Tom says. "Too many people are following me."

Here we go again. The last thing I want to do is talk about those imaginary people spying on Tom twenty-four-seven.

"I can't meet you tonight because I'm working at the ski area," I say. "I'm available tomorrow night."

"Sounds good."

"I can come over after work. Where are you staying?"

"Call me when you're off work tomorrow, and I'll tell you where we'll meet."

"Why don't you tell me now so I don't have to call again? If you're in Boston, you know it's a two-hour commute from Acton during rush hour." Tom knows I don't like driving in Boston, and parking is expensive. When I go there, I drive to the Alewife T station in Cambridge and ride the subway train.

"I can't tell you where I am now, other than Boston. Call me tomorrow."

I want to say something, but my words will not make a difference. I'm spending time helping him, but he doesn't want to help me.

"I have to go," Tom says. "I'll talk to you tomorrow." I hear the click at the end of the line.

I close my phone and drop it on the front passenger seat, grab the top of the steering wheel, and rest my forehead on top of my hands. My heart is racing. I'm angry. I don't want to be in this situation. I want the happy life we once had, but it's drifting farther away, out of my reach.

Surely deep down, Tom knows I still love him. Why can't he see how much this is hurting me, how it has turned our lives upside down? Why doesn't he get help so we can mend our relationship and clean up our financial mess? Will he ever be able to see through his paranoia and understand those people are not real?

Sadly, nothing will change unless he gets counseling and treatment and sticks with it. But he doesn't trust anyone enough to ask for help. I tried to convince him to get counseling before our lives moved in different directions, but he wouldn't. He said, "I don't have the problem. You do."

Tom doesn't know I'm living in my car now. I will tell him when we meet tomorrow night. That's why I'm going. If I tell him how hard I'm struggling, maybe he will seek help. I'm trying to be hopeful, but I'm running out of options.

When I leave the office at four o'clock the next day, I call Tom from the car. "Meet me at the McDonald's across the street from the Boston Common," he says.

"I don't know how long it will take to get there," I say. "It's rush hour now."

By the time I arrive at the Park Street station two and a half hours later and climb the long stairway that exits onto the Boston

Common, I'm exhausted. I would love to go to bed in a warm, cozy room and get a good night's sleep, but I continue trudging through the falling snow and frigid wind to the intersection. Flakes land on my hood and shoulders, and the wind stings my cheeks and nose while I cross Tremont Street. I watch my steps on the pavement and sidewalk to shield my face in the scarf wrapped around my neck as much as possible.

At McDonald's, Tom sits at a table next to the window, watching the cars and people bundled in thick winter coats and scarves pass. From a distance, he looks like his old self dressed in business casual: a pair of khaki pants, a long-sleeved light blue sweater over a blue button-down shirt and black snow boots. The boots look new. His charcoal wool coat is draped over the back of the chair.

I sit in the chair across the table. He smiles at me. It's the same smile that charmed me when we first met.

"Do you want anything?" he asks.

Such a loaded question. There are so many things I want, but all he wants to know is whether I want a drink and sandwich.

"I could use a cup of coffee," I reply. "It has been a long day."

"I'll treat," he says.

While we place the order and Tom pays, I wonder where the money came from.

We grab our drinks, my large regular coffee with half and half and a large Dr. Pepper for Tom. "Are you ready?" he asks. "It's a short walk."

We walk three blocks against the biting wind. Then Tom stops and turns toward a tall building with a Hyatt Regency sign at the entrance.

He looks at me and smiles. "This is where I'm staying," he says.

I glare at him. How can he smile at a time like this? I want to punch something—anything—but it would make a scene.

We're silent while we enter the hotel, walk through the lobby, and take the elevator to his room. When he opens the door and we step inside, I'm stunned. Straight ahead at the end of a hallway, I see a large room with a king bed and a flat-screen TV perched on a long dresser across from the bed. On the left side of the hallway, we pass the entrance to a large bathroom. On the other side of the bathroom, there's an open living area with a couch, two chairs, a coffee table, and another flat-screen TV. On the right side of the hallway, across from the living room, I see a large workstation along the wall, where Tom's laptop waits for me.

Tom is staying in a suite while I'm living in my car. I'm so angry, I can't speak.

He places the cup of Dr. Pepper next to a yellow legal pad on the coffee table and tears a few handwritten pages off the pad. We return to the workstation, where he pulls out the black vinyl swivel chair and motions for me to sit there. He hands the pages to me and looks over my shoulder while I thumb through the pages.

I turn and look up at him, my eyes wide. I can feel my face flush from the anger boiling inside me. Words finally surface.

"This place must cost at least two-fifty, three hundred a night," I say. "How can you afford this?"

Tom responds with a blank expression on his face. His voice is flat when he says, "I'm almost finished writing my paper. I will write the rest while you type these pages."

"You didn't answer my question," I say. "How can you afford to stay here?"

I know the answer now but want to hear it from him. He's tapping into his 401(k), his two-hundred-fifty-thousand-dollar 401(k). After we moved to New York City, we drained our savings, thousands of dollars in a money market fund and four mutual funds, so he could take classes at New York University (NYU) and enroll in professional development workshops sponsored by financial organizations. He finished one certificate program at NYU but the rest of the classes he completed didn't count toward any degrees or certificates. With all the money we spent, he could have had a Master of Business Administration (MBA) degree by now. I enabled him until I forced him to move to Massachusetts almost two years ago. Why did I allow this to go on for so long? I could have stopped the financial bleeding but not his paranoia.

The neutral expression on his face tells me I will never receive an answer. I search for any signs of emotion in his eyes but can't find any. Although I'm hot from anger, a shiver runs down my spine.

"I have been living in my car since January because I can't pay rent anymore," I say, my voice shaking. "We have more bills than I have income. I'm working two jobs and I'm exhausted. I can't keep up this pace. I need your help!"

Tom looks away and strolls toward the couch.

"Did you hear anything I said?"

Tom sits on the couch, his back facing me, picks up the pen on the coffee table. "Start typing," he says. "I'll finish some more pages soon."

I glare at the back of his head. My voice cracks when I say, "Why aren't you listening to me?" Tears well in my eyes and spill onto my cheeks.

Tom starts writing on the legal pad.

I turn around to hide my tears and pull a tissue from a box on the desk to dry my face. When I compose myself, I open Tom's laptop and start typing the paper. I'd rather walk away, but I already made a commitment. While my fingers sail across the keyboard and I fight back more tears, I promise myself that this is the last paper I'll type for him. It's time to take care of myself.

The CFP Exam

Seattle, July-August 1998

I'm sitting at the dining room table, nursing a cup of coffee and staring out the window. It's a cloudy Saturday morning, but I can see the sun's rays trying to break through the trees behind the neighbors' houses across the street. Tiger is asleep on top of the cat tree, and the alley cat we adopted is curled up at the end of the couch with one eye open and the other closed. We named the alley cat TC, short for "tabby cat."

Tom is in Tacoma this morning to take the first test in the CFP series. The test started at ten o'clock, ten minutes ago, I'm wondering how he's doing and silently wish him well. He has studied hard for this test. Hopefully he passes it on the first try.

Tiger doesn't like sharing his humans with another cat. He often growls and hisses at TC, but TC never fights back, cowers, or leaves. Instead, TC stands firmly on all four paws and stares at Tiger with an expression that appears to ask, "What's wrong with you?" Tiger doesn't know how to react, so he turns around and walks away.

Tiger and TC could become best buddies if Tiger would allow it. Since TC joined our little family four months ago, I've noticed he loves all creatures. He made friends with a squirrel that hangs out in our yard. Before TC became an indoor cat, they chased each other around the yard, and often we saw them side by side, sharing the cat food in the pie tin in the carport. Our next-door neighbor is a foster dog parent, and any dog she cares for becomes friends with TC. Some are reluctant at first, but TC's charm eventually wins them over. He never seems offended when other creatures don't like him.

Tom seems to be drawn to TC more than Tiger. I wonder if it's because of TC's struggles outside after the neighbors, his previous humans, abandoned him. Or maybe it's because of TC's easy-going nature. TC doesn't have any notions of how the world should be like Tiger does. He rolls with the flow like Tom.

Maybe TC's arrival is good timing. Maybe he's here to help me learn that I need to stop worrying so much about what will happen. I've been stressed about our future move to New York City. I'm torn between staying in Seattle and going to an unfamiliar place. I want to support Tom in his career change, but I don't want to leave our comfortable life in Seattle. If I follow TC's lead, I should simply enjoy every second and look forward to where every moment leads. The outcome will probably be better if I maintain a positive attitude.

When Tom returns home four hours later, I'm sitting on the couch reading a book. He kisses the top of my head and sits next to me. I stop reading and turn to face him. He smiles.

"How did it go?" I ask.

"It seemed to go well," Tom says. "I think I will pass."

"When will you get the results?"

"It should be a couple of weeks. They'll mail the results to me."

A month later on my way home from work, I stop at Mailboxes Etc. to check the mail. While thumbing through the stack from our box, I find an envelope from the CFP Board. I'm tempted to open it, but that wouldn't be fair to Tom. If this is the test results, he should see them first.

When I arrive at home, I kiss Tom's cheek and hand the mail to him. "It looks like your test results arrived today," I say.

Tom pulls the envelope from the stack and slides the flap open with his finger. He pulls out the letter, unfolds it, and reads it. His smile fades into a frown.

"What is it?" I ask.

Tom stares at the letter, then shifts his gaze to me. His eyes are glassy.

"I didn't pass," he says.

"How is that possible? You studied hard. You were ready."

Tom looks at the letter again. "I missed passing it by a few points."

"How many points are a few?"

"One hundred twenty-five."

"That sounds like a lot of points."

Tom glances up at me, then looks at the letter again. "Not the way the scores are calculated," he says.

"How are they calculated?" I ask.

Tom hesitates, then replies, "It's a complicated system."

"Can you ask them to double-check the score?"

"I can, but they'll charge a fee."

"How much?"

"I'm not sure."

"I think you should check. It would be worth it."

Tom slowly folds the letter, inserts it into the envelope, and places it on the table. He rests his hands on top of the letter, lacing his fingers. I lay my hands on top of his to reassure him. We look at each other, and he smiles to hide his sadness.

My worst fears seem to be coming true. I'm worried about how Tom is affected from failing this test. I'm afraid he will not ask for the score to be re-evaluated, and if the score is still not in his favor, I wonder if he will take the test again. He encourages me to never give up, like the drawing taped to the file cabinet in our home office where the frog grips the stork's neck while the stork tries to swallow it, but I wonder how persistent he will be in his career-change journey. He has a tendency to procrastinate.

Our routine continues throughout the summer: I'm traveling back and forth to work at Microsoft Monday through Friday, while Tom continues studying for the CFP exam. We run errands on the weekends and take long walks in our neighborhood.

Tom stops talking to me about how he's feeling and how his studying is going. When I come home after work every day, I see him sitting at the end of the dining room table with his open textbooks and study workbook binders spread across the table while he reads and takes notes. Often when I arrive, he acts like I'm not there. It's as if he's in his own world and he doesn't want to share it with me.

When he wants to talk, he won't start until he turns on the black box on top of the refrigerator. The white noise streaming from the box fills the air. His fear of people following him has returned and sometimes he talks about them during our conversations, which usually go like this:

"I saw the same car go by again today. The driver was staring at the house."

"What did the car look like?"

"It's an old car. I see it at the same time every day, one-thirty in the afternoon. It's always heading south, toward the West Seattle Junction."

"What color is it? What type of car is it?"

"It's an old gold car. Probably made in the seventies. I don't know what type it is. Maybe a Chevy."

"Do you recognize the driver?"

"I can't see him."

This puzzles me because Tom always identifies the driver as a man. If he can tell that the driver is male, why can't he describe him? I've never seen a car like the one he describes in the neighborhood, but I haven't consciously looked for specific cars in the middle of the day.

"Have you tried to get the license plate?"

"No. The car passes by too fast."

"If you're concerned about this man, you should get the license plate so we can report it to the police. I don't know what they could do because he's only driving down our street. Maybe the person has a history of casing other people's houses."

Tom lowers his eyes and frowns.

"Can you do that the next time you see it?"

Tom nods, eyes still lowered.

That white noise doesn't drown our conversations unless we're standing next to the black box. The sound is annoying to me, but it comforts Tom. If someone were listening in, they could hear every word we say.

I start watching for the car when I'm at home. After lunch, I sit at the end of the couch closest to the window with a book and a cup of coffee. Usually I sit on this side of the couch anyway, so although Tom can see me while he's studying at the dining table, he doesn't notice anything unusual. We both love to read books and often read while relaxing on the couch.

While I read, I glance out the window whenever a car passes. No cars match the old, gold seventies-style Chevy Tom described. And most of the time, no cars pass our house at exactly one-thirty in the afternoon.

I don't know what to think about this. If I talk to Tom about it, he could say he only sees the car when I'm not at home. No one would know when I'm not at home unless they constantly watch our house. Whenever I go anywhere alone, I walk or take the bus. But there's no reason for anyone to watch our house. Who cares about what we're doing?

I think about Tom's fears of being followed before his layoff and wonder whether there's a connection. More than six months have passed since his job ended. No one he worked with would care about what he's doing now. He was never close to his coworkers, except for one part-time person who reported to him for four years, but even this was just a cordial working relationship. George cut that person's job two years before Tom's layoff, and they never stayed connected after that.

The only people who care about Tom are me and our families and friends. They wouldn't spy on him. Neither would I, but I want to understand what's happening and why. I don't understand why Tom would tell me about this car if it doesn't exist.

I've asked Tom a few times when he plans to retake the exam. "It's on my to-do list," he replies.

"When is the next test scheduled?" I ask.

"Soon," he says, but he never shares a date.

Tom hasn't said whether he asked the CFP Board to re-evaluate his score from the first exam. Despite his vague comment about the scoring system, missing a passing score by one hundred twenty-five points still seems high to me.

To satisfy my curiosity, I do some research during a lunch break at my desk at Microsoft. I enter "certified financial planner test scoring system" into the search field in the Internet Explorer browser. The first hit leads me to a CFP Board page that explains how the testing process works. There are one hundred seventy questions, and each question counts as one point. The board provides two results: a preliminary score immediately after the exam and the official results, which are mailed four weeks after the exam. The official results report has a summary of the student's strengths and weaknesses in "Principal Knowledge Topics." Students can retake the exam if they don't pass.

I can't find any information about score re-evaluations, but there's a link to a page with some exam statistics. I click the link and discover the last test had a sixty percent passing rate.

Since Tom missed passing the test by one hundred twenty-five points, that means only forty-five answers were correct. Now

I understand why he doesn't want to talk about the exam. He feels humiliated from the results.

Why wasn't he honest with me about his test results? He would have known as soon as the test ended. Did he hope his score would be different when he received the official results in the mail—enough to pass? That would be quite a leap, based on what I'm reading on the screen.

Maybe Tom downplayed the results because he thought I would see him as inadequate. He has now suffered two losses in less than a year: a job he loved and failing an important test. In the meantime, my career has taken off. Some husbands have trouble handling their wives excelling at their careers while they feel like they're being left behind. Surely Tom knows I would never view him as an inferior person. I know he can have another successful career because I have faith in him.

But his reactions concern me. No matter how I try to rationalize this, Tom was not truthful about the test. We've always been honest with each other, but now my trust in him has been broken. It feels like a stake was driven into the heart of our relationship.

My half-eaten lunch next to my keyboard waits for me to finish it. I'm glad I bought a chef's salad at the cafeteria, because a hot lunch would have been cold by now.

While I'm at the CFP Board website, I look for the exam dates. The exams are held three times a year over an eight-day period in March, July, and November. The deadline to register for the November exam is in October. Tom has plenty of time to prepare for the next test, but will he be ready?

I debate whether I should talk to Tom. I think about his Chevy sightings, the car and driver I never see. He's paranoid again, so if I talk to him, he'll probably believe I'm spying on him. He might stop talking to me at all, and that would fracture our relationship even more. We've suffered enough damage already. Our team spirit is unraveling.

My Scouting Trip

New York City, November 1998

I'm sitting in coach on a red-eye flight, trying to sleep on the way to New York City for a four-day weekend. That's the most time I can take off from work for now. In September, I started a new contract at Microsoft Windows NT/2000, where the deadlines are tighter than my previous projects at Encarta.

Being in a window seat lets me prop the tiny pillow the flight attendant gave to me on the wall of the plane and lean against it, but I still can't get comfortable. I'm a side sleeper, so leaning back against the pillow on the back of the seat keeps me awake.

I might have slept lightly for about twenty minutes during this flight. It's hard to tell because I've lost track of time.

My mind drifts to Tom's solo trip to New York City three weeks ago, when he spent a week "getting my bearings," as he described it. Every day, he called me with a new report. Every time he called, he couldn't contain his excitement. Everything to him was shiny and new, even the historic sites he visited like the Statue of Liberty and Ellis Island. When we talked, he reminded me of a kid who received everything he wanted for Christmas.

His paranoia stopped during that trip and didn't return after he came home. The people and cars following him are gone. No one is bugging our house and tapping our phone.

Tom's reports about New York City give me hope that maybe my views about the city aren't true. Maybe our future there will be happy and full of opportunities.

I try to stretch my legs under the seat in front of me, but there isn't much room. I rest my feet on my backpack stowed under the seat in front of me. It's comfortable enough for now.

My thoughts wander to Tom retaking the CFP exam. He said he registered for the test this month, but he hasn't shared the date. I recall his dishonesty about his score for the last test and wonder whether he really signed up.

Tom talked me into taking our trips to New York City. "We should check it out to help us get ready for the move," he said.

"But we aren't moving until you pass your first CFP exam," I replied. "That's what we agreed to."

"I know, but we don't know what it's like out there," he said.

When Tom suggested we visit New York City, he played into my motto of always being prepared. Although I believe we aren't ready yet, he knew I'd support his idea of exploratory trips. But as soon as I said "yes" to Tom, Charlotte began repeating, *Don't do it!* She's nagging at me now, and the volume of her warnings increases the longer I ignore her.

My feet are falling asleep on top of my backpack, so I place them flat on the floor. I'd stand, except I'd wake the passenger in the middle seat. This flight is packed. If only the rest of my body would sleep, but Charlotte won't let it. She's as determined to make me listen to her advice as I am to pretend she isn't awake in my mind.

At five o'clock today, I'm attending a workshop at NYU about how to become a freelancer for the big publishing houses in Manhattan. I found it in the catalog Tom brought home from his trip. Hopefully, the two instructors will share some good tips for getting some indexing and editing projects there. I now have a healthy publisher client base for indexing books, but none are in New York City.

When we land at LaGuardia and I exit through the gate, the charged atmosphere in the terminal hits me without warning. Crowds of people are everywhere, and everyone is in a hurry. I feel the tension in the air and Charlotte stops badgering me. Apparently, she has decided to let me figure this out on my own.

I push my way through the crowds to Ground Transportation. As soon as I step outside, a nippy breeze tingles my face. I follow the signs to the taxis, a walk that seems to go on forever. When I arrive at the taxi stand, a long line of people wait for a ride while a sea of yellow cars wait in a parking lot behind the taxi stand. At the front of the line, a dark-skinned woman with short black hair, dressed in a black pantsuit, blows a whistle to alert the next taxi in the queue to move forward. As soon as the taxi loads the next passenger and drives off, she repeats the cycle.

I've never seen anything like this. At Sea-Tac Airport, a line of orange, green, yellow, black, and white cabs waits for passengers. The drivers and passengers take turns in an orderly, friendly fashion. No one needs to direct them.

When Tom talked about the taxi service here, he said, "I took a taxi from the airport to the hotel." He didn't describe this scene. During a phone call two days after he arrived, he said he discovered a shuttle bus that takes passengers from LaGuardia to the subway in Queens, but he didn't tell me where to catch it. I opted for a taxi out of fear of getting lost if I search for that bus.

I work my way to the back of the line, which moves fast despite its length. When my turn comes, the woman opens the back door on the passenger side, and the trunk lid swings open as if someone cast a magic spell on it. I load my suitcase in the trunk, close the lid, and climb into the back seat.

After I shut the door and drop my backpack on the seat, I look up and see the expressionless driver staring at me through a square opening in the plexiglass between the front and back seats. She's a young woman, probably in her early thirties, with light brown skin and black hair pulled into a curly ponytail. It takes a few seconds for me to realize she's waiting for me to tell her where I want to go. Why doesn't she just ask me?

"Hi. I'm going to Chelsea," I say, and read the name and address of the bed and breakfast. She turns on the meter, shifts the car into drive, and speeds to the airport exit.

She rushes to the Queensboro Bridge and crosses into Manhattan. From there, we sit in traffic more than we move, so any time she finds a sliver of an opening between cars, she weaves in. One time when I'm distracted from watching the sights, I slide all the way across the black vinyl seat when she swerves into a space. After that, I hold on tight in case it happens again. My heart races and at times, it feels like it wants to escape from my chest.

Tom didn't talk about what it was like riding in a taxi here, either. "It's faster to travel by subway because they don't get stuck in traffic," he said. Now I'm wondering how much he omitted from his daily reports. We usually travel together, except to his former employer's annual sales meetings and my technical writing conferences, and he shared many more details in those trip reports.

The bed and breakfast in Chelsea is a narrow five-story building with a brick exterior. The driver double-parks in front of the building and pushes a button to open the trunk. I hand the fare and tip to her through the plexiglass opening. She counts it and stuffs it into her money bag.

"Thank you. Have a nice day!" I say.

She grips the steering wheel and stares through the windshield. I imagine her on a racetrack, lined up in position, waiting for the green flag to wave.

In Seattle, the cab drivers would have thanked me and wished me a nice day as soon as I paid them. Maybe in New York City, they're in too much of a hurry to talk. Whatever the reason, I believe her behavior is rude.

"They're in a rush," Tom said when he described the behavior of the people he interacted with here. Surely he noticed the rudeness during the week he was here. I remember our fifth anniversary trip to London, where he overreacted to the innkeeper opening the door unannounced when we were taking a nap. Then there was the worker in the Tube who responded in a curt voice after we got turned around and asked him for directions. The man answered our question and we easily found the platform to our connection, but Tom took his grumpiness personally. "He didn't need to talk to me like that!" Tom growled while we rushed to the train. "I didn't do anything to set him off!"

I reminded Tom that "he's under a lot of stress because the conductors are on strike. People get mad at him because of the delays, but it isn't his fault."

"You're defending him. You should be defending me!"

Now I'm wondering whether Tom noticed other behaviors in New Yorkers, whether he ignored them, or whether he didn't tell me because he didn't want to discourage me from taking this trip.

I pull my suitcase from the trunk and close it. As soon as the driver hears the lid latch, she speeds off.

The entrance to the bed and breakfast is down a stairway of four steps, which leads to a long narrow lobby with light olive walls and a round walnut coffee table next to a dark green, low-back couch and matching chairs. A granite fireplace is built into the back wall, and a mirror with a silver frame hangs over the fireplace.

The registration clerk, a woman with curly shoulder-length dark brown hair, sits behind a granite counter at the left side of the lobby. She checks me into a room on the second floor. "The bathroom is at the end of the hallway on your floor," she says. "It has a shower." She speaks so fast, I have to concentrate to understand every word.

She points to an uncovered patio next to the lobby with five round glass tables with cast-iron legs. There's barely enough room between them for people to sit. "Breakfast is served in the courtyard from seven to nine," she says. "The elevator is behind you."

If this is New York City's version of a courtyard, what does a yard look like here?

A short man in a bellman's uniform stands at one side of the elevator. He's so still, he could be mistaken for a statue. When I approach, he reaches for my suitcase. "I will take your bag to your room," he says at the same rapid-fire pace as the clerk in an accent I don't recognize. It takes a few seconds for my brain to process what he said.

"Thank you for the offer, but I'm fine," I say.

"It's our policy. I will store it until you settle in your room." He reaches for the handle on my suitcase while locking his dark brown eyes onto mine as if he's challenging me. Before he can grab the handle, I back up just out of his reach.

"I need my suitcase," I say. "There's no reason I can't take it to my room now."

I step up to the elevator panel and reach toward the UP button. The bellman cuts in and pushes the button before I make contact.

He glares at me. "*I* operate the elevator," he says.

I return his glare. My hand grips the suitcase handle tighter, and I press the suitcase against my leg.

The elevator doors open. The bellman enters, and I reluctantly follow him. If I'd seen a set of stairs, I would have taken them, because this guy is scaring me.

Would the bellman have been this aggressive if Tom were with me? I doubt it because Tom is taller and bigger than he is. Now I'm regretting that Tom and I didn't travel together this time. He could have waited until I could take time off. I want to know about Tom's reactions to the city first-hand, by observing him instead of relying on his reports. In my short time here, I've already discovered he omitted a lot of information. What else will I learn? Did Tom think I wouldn't notice the details he didn't share? He knows me better than that.

The bellman pushes the button to the second floor before I clear the doors. I stand across from him, watching him with my suitcase pinned between me and the wall. If he tries anything, I can hit him with my backpack. It's heavy enough to send a message.

When the elevator starts moving, we both stare at the row of numbered lights above the door until we reach the second floor. As soon as the doors open, I grab my suitcase, rush into the hallway, and look over my shoulder to see if he's following me. He stays in the elevator.

When the doors close and the car descends, I stop, take a deep breath, and look around the narrow hallway with walls painted in light olive green and a carpet in a black-and-white wavy pattern. At the end of the hall, I see the bathroom door, its color matching the walls and framing a window of milky glass on the top half. The doors for each room are painted white with silver numbers. My room is near the opposite end of the hall, which ends with a small window revealing a view of the red brick building across the street.

The room is small, clean, and inviting, with a twin bed covered in a flower print bedspread and pillows with matching shams leaning against a white wooden headboard, a nightstand with a tiny electric globe lamp, and a Victorian-style chair in the corner by a narrow floor-to-ceiling window framed with lacy curtains. A white bath towel, hand towel, and washcloth are folded neatly on the foot of the bed. Above the bed hangs a print matching the flowers on the bedspread in a wooden frame that reminds me of driftwood on the beach. Light gray walls complete the décor.

I place my suitcase next to the nightstand and sit on the bed, staring at the building across the street. The mattress cradles my bottom. It's soft but not too soft. I should sleep well tonight.

Although I'm tired, I'm wide awake, and my neck and shoulder muscles are tense. I arrived in the city only three hours ago, and I'm stressed already. Will I feel like this when we're actually living here? Or will it be worse?

I close my eyes, take deep breaths, and focus on the sounds outside. It's quieter than I expected. Sometimes I hear people talking, dogs barking, or passing cars. I expected to hear non-stop horn-

The Best I Can Do

honking, like in the movies and TV shows set in the city. I'm glad to have this time to relax before deciding what to do next.

My workshop starts in a few hours, so I should have enough time to take the subway to the Macy's flagship store at Herald Square. I'm curious about it after years of watching the Thanksgiving Day parade on TV.

Tom gave me an extra subway map from his trip. I pull it from my backpack, unfold it, and plot my route. It's a short walk to the closest stop. I'll have plenty of time to browse the store before the workshop.

I remove my toothbrush and toothpaste from the suitcase, and grab the washcloth and hand towel to freshen up in the bathroom. It's a tiny space that's functional and efficient. There's no bathtub, only a walk-in shower.

On the way back to my room, I look around for an exit sign that leads to a stairwell but don't see any. I hope I don't run into that bellman when I ride the elevator again.

Timidly I press the DOWN button and hold my breath while the elevator rises to the second floor and the doors open. No one is inside. I exhale and hold tightly onto the rail while the elevator descends, and hope the bellman doesn't appear in the lobby and lecture me about operating the elevator myself. Fortunately, when the doors open on the first floor and I walk into the lobby, he's gone. The clerk behind the counter doesn't look up when I leave the building.

It's a pleasant walk through the neighborhood. The sun breaks through the clouds on this crisp November day with a gentle breeze. I pass brick buildings with restaurants, shops, and offices on the ground floor and apartments above. A block away, I see rows of brownstones with empty ceramic pots of different shapes and sizes arranged neatly on the stairway landings. I imagine flowers growing in these pots in the spring and summer, adding splashes of color and natural beauty to the neighborhood. Maybe I could live here.

Occasionally people pass me at a fast clip; some are walking their dogs. A few smile at me quickly when our eyes make contact. I think about what it would be like to walk along these sidewalks with Tom.

The crowds appear again when I descend the stairway to the 14th Street station. Lines of people push their way through the turnstiles, and the platforms are packed. They squeeze into every car on the train until the doors barely shut. I join them and grab a handrail.

When the train leaves the station, I spread my feet a few inches apart to anchor myself while the cars rock along the tracks and navigate the curves on the tracks.

Ten minutes later, we arrive at 34th Street–Penn station. When I emerge into daylight, I notice Macy's across the street. From my angle, the building stretches along the entire block, but I can't see where it ends. I've never seen a department store this big.

The closest entrance is to a hallway with a short stairway stretching to the back of the building on the right. The landing at the top of the stairway stops at a row of doors. I think about the game show, *Let's Make a Deal*, and wonder which door I should pick. I choose the first door on the right, which leads into the fragrance department, my least favorite place. The faster I can pass through it, the better, but there's a problem: I don't see an exit other than the door I just walked through.

While I'm looking around the room figuring out what to do, a woman on my left dressed in a black suit and white blouse spots me from behind a glass counter filled with perfume bottles. Short curly brown hair frames her face covered in a thick layer of makeup.

I try to break eye contact with her, but it's too late. She grabs a half-full spritzer on the counter and walks briskly toward me. Before I can escape through the entrance, she stops directly in front of me and points the nozzle at me.

"This is our latest fragrance," she says in a cheery, harried voice. "Would you like to try it?"

"No, thank you," I say, and rush toward the entrance. She follows me, steps in front of me, and points the nozzle at me again. She stops so fast, I almost collide with her.

"Why don't you try it?" she asks.

"I can't wear perfume," I say. "The strong scent triggers migraines." Perfume, cigarette smoke, and drinking or eating anything containing alcohol launches migraines that can last two days or more. My migraine medication doesn't faze them. All I can do is lie still in a dark room until the pain subsides.

"This won't hurt you," she says while waving the spritzer in front of me. "You'll love it!" Obviously, she's never had a migraine.

"No, I won't!" I step around her and walk as fast as I can toward the entrance while she follows me, waving the bottle in the air.

"C'mon, try it!"

"Get away from me!"

I run for the exit, and she follows me. As soon as I'm outside, she disappears. She probably returned to her post to wait for her next victim.

I lean against the wall to catch my breath, wait for my pulse to stop racing, and think about what to do. If I go inside again, I must pass the entrance to the fragrance department to enter another doorway. Chances are high she'll see me again, and I don't want to deal with it, so I decide to walk back to the bed and breakfast. The two-mile walk will be good exercise, will clear my head, and will give me a closer look at a few neighborhoods. I'm trying to give the city a chance, but my experiences so far aren't encouraging.

The walk is refreshing, but my thoughts quickly return to our plans to move here. Tom is calling me after the workshop tonight, and I don't know what to say. I don't want to discourage him. He has supported me through career transitions and starting my own business. We had a few bumps, but we made it through.

During my walk, Charlotte returns, repeating her warning, *Don't do it*, faster and faster. My pace quickens to the rhythm of her voice. I try to distract myself by focusing on the sights along my route, but she refuses to stop.

Charlotte is telling me what I already know: I really don't want to do this, but I can't listen to her. I don't want to be responsible for shattering Tom's dreams. Somehow I have to make this work.

Within minutes after I return from the workshop later that evening, the phone on the nightstand rings. It's Tom.

"How did it go?" he asks in a cheerful voice.

"It was a good workshop," I say. "Two editors from the big publishing houses gave a lot of advice about how to break in as a freelancer. I'm contacting them after I come home."

"That's good news," Tom says. "Did you do anything else today?"

"I took the subway to Macy's and walked back to the B and B. I didn't have time to do anything else before the workshop. I want to go to the Statue of Liberty and Ellis Island tomorrow."

Okay, it isn't the full truth, but he hasn't been honest with me about what this place is like, either.

"Make some time to take the ferry to Staten Island," he says. "It's free, and the views of the Statue of Liberty are better."

"I will," I say in my most pleasant voice.

After a short pause, I say, "Let's talk some more later. I'm fading. I couldn't sleep well on the plane last night." I'm not in the mood to talk anymore tonight.

"I need to study another hour or two anyway," Tom says. "I'll try to call tomorrow or Saturday. I love you."

"Love you, too," I say while in my mind, I want to yell at him with, *Are you out of your mind? How in the world do you expect us to live here? This is out of our league!*

After we hang up, I sigh with relief. It's better to talk about my impressions of New York after I've had a good night's sleep. Or maybe after I'm home. Or maybe never. Maybe it's my turn to withhold information, but I'm already feeling guilty for what I've excluded so far.

Charlotte hasn't given me any advice about this. Will she? She might not because I've been trying my hardest to ignore her today.

The next three days are better, but I can't stop feeling the tension. That might be a different tactic from Charlotte because I haven't been listening to her warnings. In the meantime, I visit the Statue of Liberty and Ellis Island. I take the elevators to the top of the Empire State Building and World Trade Center after dark to see the city lights. I ride the ferry to Staten Island, walk along the Promenade, and return to Manhattan.

Tom was right about the views of the Statue of Liberty being better from the Staten Island Ferry, and the ferry wasn't crowded during my midday trip.

During these three days, I also learn how people cope with the crowds and stress. It's a part of life. They accept it and move on. I'll need to remind myself about this constantly after we settle here.

And then, Charlotte repeats, *Don't do it!*

Will she ever stop?

The Holidays

Seattle, November 1998-January 1999

When I return from New York City, Tom picks me up at Sea-Tac. He waits for me at baggage claim and gives me a big hug when I arrive.

"Let's look at the lights on the way home," he says. He picks up my suitcase and carries it to the car.

By the time we arrive in West Seattle, the sun is setting. We park in our usual spot on Harbor Avenue and walk hand-in-hand to an old pier that has been renovated into a park. We stand at the railing and watch the sun slide behind the Olympic Mountains. The lower it goes, the brighter the stripes of purple, red, and orange become above the mountain silhouette.

After the sun sets, we sit on a bench on the east side of the park, where there's a sweeping view of downtown Seattle. Rich colors from the afterglow reflect on the glass skyscrapers and in the water. The colors fade to navy blue, then black, while more lights in the offices shine, twinkle, and reflect in Elliott Bay. A horn blast warns everyone that the ferry is leaving the dock.

Tom wraps his arm around me and pulls me closer. I rest my head on his shoulder.

"I signed up for the next test," he says. "It's two weeks from Thursday."

"I'm glad," I say. "How do you feel?"

"I feel like I'm ready. I will pass this time."

I'm relieved he hasn't given up and hope he passes this time.

Tom looks into my eyes. "I've been thinking while you were gone," he said. "Maybe we should move to New York City in January."

I pull away and sit up, facing him. "I can't leave now. I committed to another year at Microsoft. I have ten months left. And you know they often extend my contracts."

"You can come when you finish your contract."

"Maintaining an apartment out there and renting our house here will be expensive. Can we manage that? I don't want to tap into our savings."

"We saved the money from my unemployment. We planned to use it for this."

"Yes, but it won't last long. We don't know how fast you'll get a job."

"The economy is booming. It shouldn't take long for me to find a job."

"We should wait. Remember, we said we would move after you pass the first CFP exam? I'm okay with you moving ahead of me—after you pass the exam. We'll manage to cover expenses here and in New York until you get a job."

After I utter those words, Charlotte's voice returns, stronger than ever. *Don't do it! You'll regret this!*

I close my eyes and rub my temples in hopes Charlotte will leave. Tom puts his hands on my shoulders.

"Are you all right?" he asks.

I stop rubbing and look up at him. "I'm fine…just recovering from the flight."

The morning of the CFP exam, I awake at five o'clock, my usual time when I'm commuting to the Eastside. Tom is sleeping on his side, his back facing me.

I grab his shoulder and shake him. He shoots up, bleary-eyed with an irritated look on his face.

"What?" he demands.

"You need to get ready for your test today," I say. "If you don't leave soon, you'll be late."

I shouldn't have to remind Tom about this. He knows what traffic is like at this time of day.

Tom rubs his eyes. "My test is at one o'clock today."

"What time will you be home?"

Tom stretches his arms and yawns. "I'll let you know."

"Please do." I kiss him. "Good luck!"

Tom slides under the covers and rolls on his side.

During the bus ride to work, my mind is restless. The book I'm reading is from one of my favorite authors, Lilian Jackson Braun of *The Cat Who...* cozy mystery series, but James Qwilleran and Koko and Yum Yum, his Siamese cats, can't pull my thoughts away from Tom's behavior this morning.

My uneasiness continues during my walk from the bus stop to the office building where I work on the Microsoft campus. Something doesn't feel right. Is Charlotte trying to tell me something?

I start wondering whether Tom will go to Tacoma today and feel guilty for thinking this way. Whenever he makes a commitment, he never backs out.

As soon as I log onto my computer, I pull up the CFP Board website to verify the dates of the exam. This is the week they're offered, but I can't find the times listed. When Tom took the last exam in June, he said he had to arrive at the testing site by eight o'clock that morning. I assumed that meant the test started at that time, so if he arrives in the afternoon today, will they allow him to take it? My uneasiness returns and lingers the rest of my shift.

When I return home from work, Tom is sitting at the end of the dining room table reading pages in his study binder. He watches me shed my backpack and jacket, lean the backpack against the wall behind the table, and drape my jacket on the back of the chair next to him. I sit in the same chair.

"I didn't expect you to be home so soon," I say.

"I didn't go," Tom says.

"You...*what*?"

"I didn't go." He looks down, focusing on a page in the binder.

"Why?"

"That car has been circling the block all day."

He's referring to the old gold Chevy again.

"I didn't see it on my way home," I say.

"It's out there. Every time I look out the window, I see it."

"Why would that stop you from taking the test?"

Tom flips a page in the binder, then looks up at me with narrowed eyes. "Don't you get it? They're interfering with my plans!"

"Who's interfering? You're here all day, every day, with Tiger and TC. They wouldn't bother you unless they jump on the table. They're asleep most of the day. When they aren't, they're watching the birds and squirrels. And I'm at work. I never call you from work, unless it's important, because I don't want to disturb you."

Tom crosses his arms on the table and leans toward me. "I think you're interfering."

I lean back in my chair and stare at him, dumbfounded. It feels like someone punched me in the stomach. My cheeks flush from the hurt and anger brewing inside me.

"You know I'd never do that," I say. "Why would you even think I would? I'm supporting you through this career change. I want you to succeed."

"Why don't you see that car, but I see it all the time? You must know who it is and what they're doing."

"How can I know? The reason I don't see that car and driver is because they don't exist!"

Tom leans back in his chair and crosses his arms across his chest. He looks down at me as if he's a judge on a bench, delivering a sentence. "Why don't you want me to go New York in January?" he asks.

"Why are you in such a rush? We agreed you would pass the first test in your CFP exam before moving out there. Have you forgotten about that?"

"Plans change. I need to go now."

"Why? I don't understand. Give me a good reason because I think it's too early. How will you get a job if you don't have proof that you're working on your CFP certification? The best way to do that is to pass the first test before you leave. It shows commitment."

Tom's judgmental stare unnerves me. He has never looked at me like this. It hurts to be blamed for something I haven't done, something I'd never do. And now he wants to turn our lives upside down without a good reason. It doesn't make sense. The Tom I met and fell in love with is a rational person. He always takes a lot of time to weigh the advantages and disadvantages when he's faced with a tough decision. Now he's being impulsive when we're at a crossroads that will affect our lives and maybe our marriage. This is not the time to react hastily to an urge he isn't communicating to me. Why is he doing this?

I've got to find a way to reason with him. There's too much at stake for both of us.

"One thing I learned during my short trip to New York is that people aren't convinced easily," I say. "They want proof. Solid proof."

Tom leans forward, his arms still crossed. His piercing eyes jab my soul.

"You don't like New York, do you?"

"I didn't say that. I'm just making an observation."

Tom breaks eye contact and flips another page in the binder. "I don't want to talk about this anymore," he says. "Let's order pizza for dinner tonight."

Tom closes the binder, sits on the couch in front of the dining room table, and turns on the TV. I stay at the table and watch the news anchors on KIRO Channel 7 over the back of the couch, trying to recover from the conversation. Those depressing reports they're reading from the teleprompter aren't helping.

During the commercial break, Tom turns around and stares at me. "Well…when are you ordering the pizza?" he asks.

I call in the order and go into our home office to check messages and resume work on an index for a publishing client. Maybe writing index entries will help me forget about what just happened, but I can't ignore it forever. Charlotte won't let me.

For the next week, Tom and I don't talk much. When we do, it's about the weather or another topic that isn't emotionally charged, but the air in our house remains full of tension. Even the cats feel it. Usually Tiger likes to sleep next to me, but not anymore. In the mornings, I find him and TC sleeping on opposite ends of the couch. Tom and I stopped taking our long walks in the neighborhood and driving to the viewpoint to enjoy the sunset and city lights. I miss those moments.

A few days before Thanksgiving, Tom starts relaxing again. We celebrate the holidays the same way every year and always look forward to it. On Thanksgiving morning, we get up early to watch the Macy's Thanksgiving Day Parade and cook a turkey dinner with all the trimmings. But this year, it's hard for me to enjoy the parade because my memory of the Spritzer Lady dominates my thoughts. Tom doesn't know about her, and I've decided to keep it that way.

The day after Thanksgiving, we buy a spruce tree at Ace Hardware near the West Seattle Junction, set it up next to the brick fireplace in our living room, and decorate it. We always go to Ace Hardware because the trees are fresh and they last longer. One of the workers there said the trees come from a farm in Hood River, Oregon. The scent of spruce in the house relaxes and comforts me. Decorating the tree and the rest of the house is our favorite part of the holiday season, and this year, despite the tension, Tom has returned to his childlike manner that's prominent throughout late November through the New Year—the thrill of the lights, decorations, and cheer of the season. For a few weeks, the world feels normal again.

During the Christmas holidays, we spend a week in Coos Bay, Oregon, visiting Tom's parents Theresa (whose nickname is "Tess") and Al, his brother Don, and Don's wife, Nancy. His other two older brothers, Sam and Ron, live in California and Nova Scotia, respectively. They rarely return to Coos Bay for the holidays. Instead, they celebrate with their wives' families and call us on Christmas Day to wish everyone a happy holiday. We don't spend the holidays with my mother, because she travels constantly with her partner, a long-haul truck driver. She calls me when they're at a place with cell reception. My father was never in my life because the relationship between him and Mom ended before I was born.

Throughout the holidays, Tom doesn't talk about anyone following him, and he has forgotten about the old gold Chevy circling our neighborhood. We don't talk about New York City, either. I hope his urge about moving there in January has subsided, and he concluded that our original plan is the best option.

Tom's family doesn't know about his behavior. That side of him never surfaces when we're visiting Coos Bay, not even when I'm alone with him. I wonder whether Tom's being home makes him feel safe. I've thought about sharing Tom's unusual behavior with his family, but would they believe me? It's still hard for me to believe, so why would they have any reason to believe me? Would they think I have an ulterior motive by telling them? I feel close to them, and they treat me like part of the family, so I don't want to shatter that relationship.

When we return home from Coos Bay after the holidays, Tom doesn't talk about New York for a few days. When he does, his paranoia returns, worse than ever. Now, he says more than one car is casing the neighborhood, but he no longer describes them. He believes the house is bugged again, and he's convinced I'm somehow involved in a plot to interfere with his plans for his career change and his life.

His constant fear and accusations wear me down, and I finally agree to him flying to New York again and looking for an apartment.

"I will book a flight for you," I say.

"No," Tom says. "*I* will. I don't want anyone knowing my schedule."

What a blow. I haven't done anything to risk his trust in me, but he doesn't trust me. I don't understand how or why this happened. Here I am, supporting both of us, soon on opposite sides of the country, and he doesn't want me to know what he's doing. How can we manage our finances this way? We don't have unlimited funds and I can work only a finite number of hours. He needs to find a job as fast as he can after he settles in New York to support himself and ease my load.

Charlotte returns from her vacation, and her voice inside me is stronger and louder than ever. Over and over she says, *Don't do it! You'll regret it!*

I try to reason with her. *Can't you see how tired I am? I can't fight Tom on this anymore. I need to let him go.*

It doesn't work. She changes the words, but the message is the same. *You're making a mistake. Please don't do this! I'm trying to protect you.*

Charlotte has good intentions, but I've convinced myself that things are different this time. Despite Tom's behavior, I still have faith in him to move forward, get his CFP certification, and succeed at his career change. I shouldn't trust him, especially after his lies about his CFP exam and repeating the test. I don't understand why he's in a hurry to go to New York now, but I'm trusting there's a good reason. I wish he would tell me, but his paranoia won't let him.

Maybe I am making a mistake like Charlotte says. Maybe I will regret this. But for now, I'm taking the ride.

The Move to New York

Seattle and Staten Island, February-December 1999

Weeks pass. It's now the last day of February, and I'm starting to believe that Tom has changed his mind about moving. I want to believe he forgot about it. Last month, Tom was in a hurry to fly to New York and look for an apartment. This month, he doesn't talk about it. The change puzzles me.

Maybe Tom decided to attempt the CFP exam again in March in Tacoma. Every weekday when I return home from Microsoft, he's sitting at the end of the dining room table reading the study binder and his finance textbooks, but he never talks about retaking the test. I've stopped asking because he accuses me of interfering again. My heart and soul ache every time I hear this.

Today when I come home from work, Tom is sitting on the couch, watching the evening news. I sit next to him.

"Are you taking a break from studying today?" I ask.

Tom nods. "Let's go for a drive," he says.

Instead of driving to our usual spot, Tom heads toward downtown Seattle. He stops at Kerry Park, about halfway up the steep Queen Anne Hill, where there's a panoramic view of the Space Needle in the foreground with the skyscrapers of downtown Seattle clustered close behind. Mount Rainier rises above the Kingdome and the baseball stadium called Safeco Field, which opened last year. We see our neighborhood, a forested peninsula dotted with houses and condominium and apartment buildings across Elliott Bay. It's a clear day today, rare for February, and a beautiful sunset is on the way.

Usually when we go on a drive, Tom prefers a quiet spot to talk, so it's strange he chose Kerry Park. It's always busy there on a nice day like this. The park will be packed by the time the sun sets behind the Olympics.

He finds a parking spot at the edge of the park, and we walk to the railing to enjoy the view. We silently watch the colors change on the buildings and in the sky while the sun slips behind the horizon. Then we return to the car.

Tom drives back to West Seattle and parks at our usual spot. By the time we arrive, it's dark, and the lights from downtown are reflecting in the bay. We stay in the car and focus on the view for a long time.

Tom shatters the silence with, "I booked a flight today."

It's happening, I think. I'm not feeling any shock or surprise; my mind simply registers this fact. *Tom booked a flight to New York City today.* I watch the lights twinkle but can see Tom studying my face in my peripheral vision.

"When are you leaving?" I ask.

"In two weeks."

"How long will you be gone?"

"A week."

I nod, my eyes still glued to the city lights.

The silence returns. We watch the view from the car for fifteen minutes, then return home.

During his trip to New York, Tom calls me once with news that he found a studio apartment on Staten Island. He signed a lease and paid a deposit to hold the apartment.

"When are you telling your family?" I ask.

"When I'm back," Tom says.

When Tom returns home, he spends three days packing a few boxes to ship to Staten Island, then drives to Coos Bay for two weeks. After he returns, he books another flight to New York. Before he leaves, I call Sleepy's on Staten Island to order a twin bed so he doesn't have to sleep on the floor. Tom overhears me on the phone and rushes into the kitchen.

"What are you doing?" he yells behind me.

I ask the clerk at the end of the line to hold and place my hand over the mouthpiece. By then, Tom is standing next to me.

"Why are you so upset?" I ask.

"I don't want you calling anyone from the house! Someone will hear you."

"The only people who will hear me are you, the person I'm talking to on the phone, and me. No one is spying on us."

"You want them to know what I'm doing!" Tom's red face glares at me.

"No one cares what we're doing. If you want a bed, I need to finish this call."

Tom turns on the black box on top of the refrigerator and disappears into the bedroom. I continue placing the order with the clerk and hope she didn't overhear my exchange with Tom and the static streaming from the box. She doesn't say anything about it, but I'm still embarrassed. Tom is acting like a spoiled four-year-old.

After Tom settles on Staten Island, he returns to his old self. When he calls me, he's excited and happy about his career change. He signs up for the next CFP exam in Manhattan in June and starts taking workshops hosted by professional organizations in finance.

During one of our conversations a month later, he asks me to fly there for a long weekend so he can show me around the neighborhood.

I fly there two weeks later and meet Tom at the Whitehall Ferry Terminal, where we board the ferry to Staten Island. During the trip, we stand on the top deck and admire the Statue of Liberty while the ferry passes it.

The apartment is seven blocks from the St. George Ferry Terminal, on top of a steep hill with a view of the harbor and the skyscrapers of Lower Manhattan five miles away. The complex is an old military barracks that has been renovated into apartments. The white five-story stone buildings look like giant rectangular blocks neatly arranged in a U-shape with square corners surrounding a well-groomed grassy courtyard with a sidewalk cutting the lawn in half. The complex is surrounded by a black cast-iron picket fence that's a few inches taller than me with gates on the north and south sides. The gates are locked.

Tom pulls a card key from his pocket and taps it on a reader next to the gate. I hear a click, and he pulls the gate open and waits for me to pass through. He follows close behind.

His apartment is on the second floor, overlooking the courtyard. It's much bigger than I expected. Based on what I've heard about apartments in New York City, I assumed it would be a tiny room with a cramped bathroom, but the apartment is about the same size as most studio apartments in Seattle. Gray carpet covers the floor and the walls are painted in a cream color. The twin bed I ordered from Sleepy's and the boxes we shipped from Seattle are the only items in the apartment.

"They have studios and one- and two-bedroom apartments," Tom says. "We can upgrade to a bigger apartment when you move here."

We rent a car and drive around the island. When we return, we walk through the neighborhood. It's much quieter here compared to Manhattan, and most of the buildings aren't squeezed into small spaces. People here are still in a hurry but not as much as in Manhattan. I also notice many parks and green spaces with trails attracting walkers, joggers, and dogwalkers.

As the weekend continues, I begin to relax. Maybe I will like living here, but I'm not looking forward to it. And Charlotte stops delivering warnings. Maybe she decided things will be okay after all.

Tom is relaxed, too. He isn't talking about people following him or bugging his apartment.

When I return to Seattle, I notice that the black box on top of the refrigerator is gone. Did Tom take it with him? I didn't see him pack it, but he could have while I was at work. I didn't see it in his apartment on Staten Island, either. I wonder whether I will ever see it again and hope I don't.

The months pass. Tom returns to Seattle in May to pack more items in the car and drives cross-country. I continue my busy pace for Microsoft and my other clients.

We hire a business coach who has extensive experience in finance. She helps Tom rewrite his résumé to target it toward an entry-level position in finance and guides him on how to interview for openings. A month later, he starts getting a few interviews at some small and mid-sized firms, but no one offers him a job.

Then a large company in Lower Manhattan invites him to an interview. The first interview turns into two, three, four, and eventually twelve. Twelve interviews or more are common at the finance companies in New York, according to Tom's business coach, because they're focused on making sure their new hires are the right fit for the company's culture. She said one of the biggest firms in the city would schedule up to sixty interviews before making a decision.

I can't imagine going through that many interviews for one job. The most interviews I've ever encountered were three, but two are the most common in the tech industry—even for contract work.

After the twelfth interview, Tom never hears from the company again. He asks his business coach about it, and she says sometimes companies take extra time when they're close to making a decision. She isn't concerned because she's familiar with the company and some of her clients were hired there. She advises Tom to continue following up.

Tom accepts her advice. He checks in with the company several times during the next month, but no one replies.

The ghosting from the company devastates Tom. I can tell during our phone conversations because he stops talking about his job search. I try to stay upbeat, but it doesn't help.

"When are you retaking the CFP exam?" I ask during one of our conversations.

He doesn't answer.

His lack of response tells me he skipped the test in June or never signed up. He stops talking about the business coach, so I assume he isn't using her services anymore. I confirm this when I receive the next batches of bank and credit card statements, because I don't want to ask him directly. I'm afraid he will accuse me of interfering and my emotional wounds will open again. As long as I can keep myself busy, I don't have to think about them.

In August, Tom signs a lease on a two-bedroom apartment in the same complex on Staten Island. When I ask him why he didn't wait for me to sign this lease like we did on the house lease in Seattle, he says he listed me as a tenant. My role as a team member is withering. Resentment creeps in because it feels like the only reason I exist is to make money. I don't want to feel this way. I started my business to have flexibility and financial stability so I could enjoy my life and spend more time with Tom pursuing the things we love together. It hasn't turned out this way and I wonder if it will ever change.

Throughout the summer, my routine is mostly the same: Get up, feed Tiger and TC, refresh their water dish, clean the litter box, go to Microsoft, come home, check messages, take care of Tiger and TC's needs again, eat dinner, give them some more attention, work on another client's project, and go to bed. Tom and I take turns calling each other. Some nights when I call him, he doesn't want to talk because he believes someone is listening on the line. I never know when he will act this way, and it frustrates me.

Betty, Lily, and I still meet for a late lunch or early dinner in a central location as often as we can. It's more challenging now because of the distance and the traffic. Betty occasionally works short contracts at Microsoft, ranging from three to six months, but usually she's on assignments at other companies on the Eastside. Lily found a steady full-time job at a company on the south end of Seattle.

Betty and Lily know about Tom's layoff and career change, but I've never told them about his unusual new behaviors. It's because I'm still trying to make sense of this. When I've thought about opening up about it, I change my mind. These stories are too bizarre and embarrassing to talk about, even with the two people who are my closest friends.

In September, I take two weeks off to pack the belongings we want to keep and drive them to Staten Island in a rented moving truck. Tom flies home to help me.

We take Tiger with us because a twenty-pound cat is too big to fly in coach and he wouldn't like riding in the cargo hold. I ask Connie, our catsitter, to check on TC while I'm gone. Tiger loves road trips, so we release him from his carrier and let him hang out in the cab with us. Sometimes he naps on the seat between us. Other times, he sits on my lap and watches the world pass by. The rest of the time, he curls up and sleeps under the seat behind my legs.

The trip starts well. Tom is happy and excited during the first day's drive from Seattle to Haugan, Montana, where we spend the night at the Silver Dollar Inn. We eat dinner at the restaurant there and admire the massive collection of silver dollars on display.

But Tom's mood changes the next day, several hours after we're on the road again. Near the Montana-Wyoming border, he starts glancing at the rear-view mirror more often. When I notice, I look at the mirror connected to the passenger door but see nothing behind us.

"What's going on?" I ask him.

"We're being followed," he says.

I look at the mirror again. Still nothing. Our truck is the only vehicle on the road.

"Who's following us?" I ask. "No one is on this road, except us. How could anyone be following us?"

"Someone is tracking the truck."

"How is that possible? No one knows where we are."

"Someone planted a bug on the truck when it was parked at the hotel last night."

"Why would someone do that? No one cares about what we're doing."

"You told someone at the restaurant where we're going."

What is he talking about? We were together everywhere we went last night, except for going to the bathroom in our hotel room before bed and taking showers this morning. If I could have contacted someone from the bathroom, why would I? None of this makes sense.

"How could I do that?" I ask Tom.

He doesn't answer. He stares at the road and continues his constant glimpses in the rearview mirror. The tension is thick in the air. We don't talk again until it's time to find a place to stop for lunch, and then, the topic is only about what we want to eat.

Tiger, who sat on my lap watching the view before this conversation started, senses the tension, too. He jumps off my lap and hides under the seat. He doesn't come out until we park at a hotel for the night.

The next day in South Dakota, we take a side trip through the Badlands. We stop at a viewpoint near the end of the loop and when we get out of the truck, Tom leaves his clip-on sunglasses on the passenger side of the seat. I don't see them when I climb back into the truck after our walk. When I sit, I feel something move underneath me and hear a crunch. My weight crushes the clip, and it falls off.

Tom picks up the pieces, throws them on the dashboard, and faces me, his eyes blazing.

"Why did you do that?!" he yells. "I can't drive without those glasses!"

It's the first time in our marriage that I've seen him so angry and it unnerves me. I'm on the verge of tears. It takes a lot to make me cry.

"I didn't see them," I reply in a shaky voice. "Why did you leave them on the passenger side? You always put them on the dashboard so something like this won't happen."

"You need to pay attention!"

Tears stream down my face. I look away and try to compose

myself.

"Why are you crying? Crying won't fix my glasses."

I look at Tom as the tears continue to fall. "Why are you making such a big deal out of this? It was an accident."

"It was not an accident. You did it on purpose!"

"We can get another pair at Wall Drug. They're up the road. You said you wanted to stop there."

"And you believe that will fix the problem? You did this to interfere with the trip."

"No. It was an accident. Why can't you see this? Why do you blame me for interfering with your life when you know I'd never do it? What happened to us being a team?"

Tom looks away, turns the key in the ignition, and the truck sputters to life.

Wall, South Dakota, is a classic tourist trap in the middle of nowhere. It's surrounded by grasslands as far as the eye can see. We park in a lot a couple of blocks away, which is almost full, and stroll to the heart of town.

The town is one street lined with buildings in the false front style typical of the pioneer Western towns. Cars fill every parking spot on both sides of the street. Wall Drug takes up one side of the street; the entrance is in the middle of the walkway.

Inside Wall Drug, there's a long hallway flanked with doors to different rooms filled with merchandise for sale. I look at the signs above each door to find a pharmacy and find it about halfway down on the left. The pharmacy is a long narrow room, half the width of the others along the hallway, with shelves filled with first-aid items, over-the-counter medication, and health and beauty aids. The pharmacy is in the back in another room separated by a glass window with an opening to conduct transactions. I find the sunglasses in a round standalone display in a corner in front of the pharmacy. The clip-ons are at the top of the display.

I grab two pairs of the clip-ons before Tom catches up with me.

"Why are you buying two?" he asks.

"I want to have a backup in case you leave them on the seat again and I accidentally sit on them." I don't want to hear him blaming me again about something that's his fault.

"I want a cup of that free water," he says. "Where is it?" He turns around and walks back to the hallway.

I pay for the clip-ons and meet Tom in the hallway. We follow it to an exit into an outdoor courtyard surrounded by a tall, weathered picket fence. A few steps away, another door leads into another room. We peek inside; it's the Wall Drug café.

What a maze. It's as complicated as Tom's unpredictable behavior these past two days.

"Let's grab some lunch before we hit the road again," Tom says.

I think about how quickly Tom's mood has changed. About an hour ago, he was yelling at me because I sat on his clip-ons and broke them during our stop in the Badlands, and now he's talking about lunch as if nothing happened. How can he shift emotional gears so fast when I'm still hurt from the way he treated me?

Before we arrived in South Dakota, we took turns driving. After our break at Wall Drug, Tom drives the rest of the way. Our conversations dwindle to decisions on where to eat and sleep. Tiger senses the tension and spends most of his time under the seat behind my feet.

The new apartment is on the bottom two stories in the corner of a building facing St. Mark's Place. There's beige, low-pile carpet throughout, except in the kitchen and bathrooms. Two bedrooms and a full bath are on the bottom floor, and a living room, kitchen, and half bath are on the second floor. A carpeted stairway between the master bedroom and full bath connects the two floors and exits in the living room. The color of the linoleum in the kitchen and bathrooms matches the carpet. The kitchen is big enough for one person to work in. Through the small kitchen window and north-facing living room windows, I see the deep blue water in New York Harbor and the tops of the skyscrapers in Lower Manhattan. St. Peter's Catholic Church, an ornate tan stone building with a giant round stained glass window above the entrance, is across the street. The shape of the stained glass window reminds me of a flower.

Before we unload the truck, I make a bed for Tiger on the downstairs bathroom floor by piling soft blankets in the corner by the bathtub. He's under the seat in the cab when I return to retrieve him. I ease him out and gently pick him up, cuddling him in my folded arms with one hand under his feet to make him feel secure while carrying him to the bathroom. When I gently place him on top of the blankets, the pile molds to his body while he sinks. He freezes into a ball and looks up at me as if he's asking, "What's going on now?" After a week of so many changes in scenery, I understand why he has a curious look on his face.

"We're in our new home now," I say. His big green eyes continue staring into mine. "I know it's a lot to take in. I'll bring your litter box, food, and water in here so you can relax. When we're finished unloading, you can explore the apartment. You'll have a lot of room to roam around."

I rub his head between his ears, and he closes his eyes, squeezing them tightly.

"That feels good, doesn't it?"

A soft purr builds in his throat.

"I'll be back. Don't worry; everything is okay." As soon as I say that, I wish I could convince myself that everything will really be okay.

After I finish setting up Tiger's space, I resume helping Tom unload the boxes. Although it takes only four more hours to carry and sort the boxes by floor, everything seems to move in slow motion. We mostly work in silence, because any time I talk, Tom shushes me.

"I don't want you telling anyone what we're doing," he says.

"Tom, no one is listening to us."

But I know what he means. He believes someone bugged our apartment. How can someone bug an apartment, even if they wanted to, in such a short time when they don't even know where we are?

I've never felt so tired in my life. The physical and emotional aspects of many quick changes and Tom's accusations overwhelm me. His makes me feel guilty, but I don't understand why I'm feeling guilty when I haven't done anything to feel guilty about.

Back and forth we walk from the truck parked in a driveway at the side of the apartment building, pushing hand trucks piled with boxes through the dark hallway into our apartment. When we need to leave any boxes upstairs, we take the elevator. Sometimes I take a break and stare out one of the living room windows, catching glimpses of the container ships waiting for a dock to open in the port on the west side of the harbor in Elizabeth, New Jersey. North of me, the bright orange Staten Island Ferry sails to and from the Whitehall Terminal in Manhattan. I also see the Statue of Liberty to the north, her outstretched arm holding a lighted torch to welcome anyone who enters the harbor. From this distance, she looks like a small green doll standing in the water.

The view draws me in. I want to stay here and watch the boats in the water instead of finishing the dreadful task of unloading the truck. Maybe it's my way of holding on to our connection to Seattle. I think about the beautiful panoramic views of Elliott Bay, the skyscrapers, and mountains from our neighborhood in West Seattle. Although this view of New York Harbor is vastly different, there will be a view of the lights in Manhattan tonight, five miles away as a bird flies. Although I haven't seen it yet, I imagine the night view as a faded galaxy that's out of my reach, just like our home in Seattle.

But the moving needs to end and we need to unpack and put everything away. We have only three more days before I fly back to Seattle to finish the final weeks of my contract at Microsoft. I need to clean the house before shutting off the utilities and returning the keys to the landlord. There's furniture we couldn't move that needs a home. I'll donate it to the Salvation Army or anyone else who'll take it. It's in good condition, so it will find another person or family who needs it quickly. Tom will stay behind on Staten Island with Tiger and continue looking for a job. That is, I hope Tom will continue looking for work. After the ghosting from his last set of interviews, he seems to have given up. Now I'm beginning to believe our move is a mistake, but it's too late to stop it. Why didn't I listen to Charlotte?

As soon as I return to the mostly empty house in Seattle, TC runs to me, meowing. Usually he isn't a chatterbox like Tiger, but he certainly has something to say now. He stops at my feet and I pick him up and rub the top of his head with my chin. That's his favorite thing. He rubs back, pushing harder against my chin the longer we're in contact.

My end date for my Microsoft contract approaches, but the project isn't finished. We've had several delays because of unexpected last-minute changes in the product, which affects the documentation. The writers have to update it, which means the other indexer on the team and I need to update the index when they're finished. This time, most of the documentation has been affected, so the other indexer and I are working overtime to finish.

Because of the changes, I've had to request two extensions on our lease and change the departure on my plane ticket. When the end date changes a third time and I contact the airline again, the booking agent says I can't extend the ticket again. Either I fly or forfeit the ticket without a refund.

I ask my manager at Microsoft if I can finish my work remotely, because I can't stay any longer. She reluctantly agrees because she can't find another indexer on short notice. When I share the news with Tom, he doesn't react. He wants me to come to New York, so why is he behaving this way?

Then I start contacting agencies in New York and sending résumés. The recruiters don't want to talk on the phone; they prefer scheduling in-person appointments after I settle there. I add the task to my to-do list.

On a sunny fall morning, I call a cab to take TC and me to Sea-Tac. I ask the driver to stop at the landlord's home on the way. He isn't at home, so I drop our house keys into the mail slot. TC lies on his stomach in his carrier in the middle of the back seat, front paws tucked against his chest, and stares at the seat in front of us. I sit next to him with my arm wrapped over his carrier and watch the scenery pass one last time while fighting the urge to cry.

Goodbye, Seattle. I wish I didn't have to leave. I hope to see you again someday.

We board the plane and find my seat. I slip TC's carrier under the seat in front of me and settle in. TC looks at me with his big green eyes, which appear to ask, "Where are we now?"

I poke my index finger through the bars on the carrier door and rub between his ears. He tilts his chin slightly and closes his eyes. "We're on a plane, flying to New York. We're going to our new home."

TC soaks in the attention. A flight attendant asks everyone to fasten their seatbelts.

I lean back, strap myself in, then lean over to see TC's face. "Sorry to stop, sweetie, but we're taking off now."

TC curls into a ball while we taxi the runway. I wonder how he'll react when we take off. As far as I know, this is his first flight.

He's quiet during takeoff, except for shifting for a more comfortable position. He falls asleep as soon as we're airborne and wakes up two hours later when we land in Phoenix, where we'll make our connection to Newark, New Jersey. When we walk through the airport, people take a second look and smile when they notice TC in his carrier. A five-year-old girl sees him and tugs on her mother's hand to come closer.

When they stop, the girl looks at her mother and asks, "Can I pet the kitty?"

"Ask the nice lady," her mother says.

I smile at the girl and her mother. "It's okay. He loves attention, especially rubbing between the ears. He won't bite and scratch."

The girl cautiously reaches through the carrier door with her index finger and stops while TC sniffs the tip. He leans forward and she stretches her finger to the top of his head. When she touches it, she pulls back quickly, tucking her hands against her chest and giggling. TC watches her with wide eyes. I wonder if he's asking why she stopped giving him attention so soon.

I smile, thinking about how TC's charm works everywhere. It never dawned on me that he could cast his spell on everyone in a crowded airport.

The flight from Phoenix to Newark is uneventful. TC falls asleep again after we take off. When we land, the pilot announces that we have to wait ten minutes for a gate to clear. Ten minutes turn into forty-five. The passengers are getting restless, but TC is patient, except for a couple of meows that seem to ask, *When are we getting outta here?!* I think some of the passengers who are complaining a lot could learn a lesson from him. So can I.

Tom picks us up at the airport. He's in a good mood and isn't talking about anyone following him. I've stopped wondering whether they'll ever completely fade away. Now I brace myself for when Tom believes they're back. I'm on a roller coaster with his mood swings, from what was once his usual mellow demeanor to panic and blame.

When we arrive at the apartment, Tiger is happy to see me until he notices TC in the carrier. Instead of greeting TC, he runs into the master bedroom. TC acts like nothing happened.

My Dot-Com Retreat
New York City, January 2000-February 2001

After settling on Staten Island, I finish the project for Microsoft a week earlier than scheduled and begin looking for a local steady technical writing contract. Although I still have work with my publishing clients, it comes and goes.

My first three appointments with agencies are today in Manhattan. It's a nippy day, with a mix of sun and clouds, when I board the Staten Island Ferry. A thin layer of fog hugs the water, which gives the Statue of Liberty and the skyscrapers in Lower Manhattan the appearance of floating on a cloud. On the Verrazzano Bridge side, the fog looks like it's trying to escape under the bridge.

The first agency's office is a six-block walk from the ferry terminal, on the twenty-fifth floor. When I arrive, the receptionist greets me and asks whether I want anything to drink. I ask for a cup of coffee and sip it while waiting for the recruiter. Less than five minutes later, she appears through a side door and escorts me to a conference room.

We sit across from each other at one end of a long table, and she pulls my résumé from a manila folder. She scans it, lays it at the side of her tablet, and looks up at me.

"Your experience is impressive," she says. "I see you have a programming background. Tell me about it."

I'm confused. Where does she see that I have programming experience?

"My background is in technical writing, not programming," I say. "I work with programmers. I write instructions on how to use the products they create."

She holds up my résumé, scans it again, then looks at me.

"We have some openings for junior programmers in Jersey City," she says. "If you're interested, I will send your résumé to the hiring managers."

I don't understand why she's trying to pigeon-hole me into a programming position.

"Thank you for the offer, but I'm not qualified," I say. "I'm not a programmer. I'm looking for technical writing work. If these companies are hiring programmers, surely they're looking for technical writers, too. They need someone to write instructions on how to use their products."

She glances at my résumé again. "We need programmers. Your résumé shows that you have programming experience."

"If you're looking at the programming languages I listed in the skills section of my résumé, it clearly states that I have a basic knowledge of BASIC and C. That means I know enough about those languages to talk to programmers about them. It doesn't mean that I can write programs in those languages. Nowhere on my résumé do I list experience working as a programmer."

"We don't have any openings for writers," she says.

Then why did she call me for an interview? She has no clue about what I do, and I can't think of a better way to explain. Where does she think product manuals come from?

"I will keep your résumé on file," she says.

"I'd appreciate that," I say, knowing I'd never hear from her again. What a waste of time!

My next two appointments follow the same script with different recruiters at different agencies. It's enough to convince me that my strategy is the wrong approach in this new world. I will have to figure out another way to crack the technical writing job market here or return to secretarial work. My income as a secretary won't support both of us. If Tom had a job, we could manage, but I don't want to be a secretary again. I want to stay in the career I love.

I need to find more work fast because our bills are growing. Tom keeps signing up for classes and charging them on the credit cards. He never tells me when he's doing it. I don't know until the charges show up on the statements. We depleted a chunk of our savings to move and now have to tap into it to cover the rent. It's dwindling much faster than we built it up and I'm afraid we will drain it in less than a year at the rate we're going. We can't continue this pace. We're not independently wealthy.

I decide to confront Tom about this one night after he returns from a workshop in Manhattan. I'm in the master bedroom, sitting on the bed and watching TV when he walks in.

"Have you taken a look at our credit card statements lately?" I ask him when he sits on the bed.

"No. Why?"

"We need to slow down our spending."

"I need to study for my certifications."

"From what I'm seeing, you're just taking a bunch of workshops. I can't tell how these are related to your certifications. You won't even tell me what you're doing but I'm expected to support both of us."

"You agreed to do this."

"We agreed we would both work while you're going through this career change, remember? We're spending money faster than it's coming in."

"I can't find a job with those people following me around. You're interfering, just like they are."

No matter how much I pour my heart and soul into keeping the team spirit alive and well, he bashes me with blame. And now I'm trying to tell him it's important to get our finances under control. Of all people, he should know better. The anger rises inside me.

"You've been here for almost a year," I say. "You should've had a job by now."

"I need to pass the first CFP exam before I can get a job."

"You can't pass if you don't retake it! I never see you studying for it anymore. Where are those study guides?"

"I still have them."

"Where are they?"

Tom stares at the TV.

"When are you retaking the first exam? The next one is in March. You can sign up at the site in Manhattan."

Tom whirls toward me, his eyes blazing. "How do you know where the test is?"

"It's on the website," I say.

"I knew you were interfering!"

"It's a public website. Anyone can find it. Why would I interfere? I gave up a lot in Seattle to come here."

"I don't want to talk about Seattle anymore."

"Have you ever thought that I came here to support you? That I have faith in you? Have you ever thought about how much it hurts me to hear you blame me for interfering with your life when I'd never do that?"

Tom stands and glares at me. "This conversation is over!" He climbs the stairs to the living room. The floor creaks from his footsteps until he sits at the dining table.

I wonder whether he unpacked his books yet and remember we stored the boxes in the closet in the second bedroom, which we're using as an office. I sneak across the hall into the office, quietly slide the closet door open, and scan the labels on the boxes. The CFP study guide box is on top of one of the stacks, and it's open. I look inside. The books and study binder are stacked neatly with the binder in the bottom of the box and the smaller books on top.

My heart sinks. I conclude that Tom has lost interest in retaking the exam because he's afraid he'll fail again. He's blaming me for interfering to avoid admitting he's scared. That's probably why he believes those other people are following him and listening in on our conversations. It's a way he can cope, but it's a strange way for anyone to handle their struggles. I've never known anyone else who has done this. Until now, he was never the type of person to give up.

Nothing else makes sense to me, and I don't know what to do.

I search the online job boards and apply for any technical writing openings with qualifications that mostly match my experience. It's tough to find openings with enough hits because most of the positions are in finance and these companies want writers with at least five years of full-time experience in the field. The only expertise I have in financial writing is typing and editing Tom's papers during college and watching Tom's favorite finance shows on PBS. He doesn't watch those shows anymore.

The holidays come and go. They're different this year. We don't watch the Macy's parade and cook our traditional Thanksgiving dinner. Instead, we order takeout at a small Chinese restaurant a block away. Our only Christmas decoration is a three-foot-tall tree with LED lights that change colors—a purchase from a Duane Reade in midtown Manhattan for twelve bucks. We don't exchange gifts, and Christmas dinner is takeout again from the Chinese restaurant. Tom calls his parents and Don to wish them a happy Thanksgiving and Christmas, but he won't let me talk to them. He talks to them as if nothing unusual is going on. My mind reminiscences about celebrating the holidays in Coos Bay while my heart misses those special times.

I don't call Mom because I don't know what to say to her, and Tom would scrutinize every word. She can tell when something is wrong by listening to my voice. I've never figured out how she can do that. I haven't given our new phone number to her yet, because I'm afraid if she calls, Tom will claim she's snooping on us. After the holidays, I will write a letter to her with an update about what is going well—if I can think of something. Otherwise, it will be a short letter.

Here we are, living in the largest, most crowded city in the country, where we're the most isolated we've ever been during our marriage. Staten Island's population is the same as Portland, Oregon. Add the residents of all five boroughs, and the total comes to eight million people. Eight million…

On New Year's Eve, we go to bed early. We could have watched the fireworks over the harbor from our living room windows. I don't have any energy after another stressful day. We should have been celebrating the crossover into a new millennium instead of fighting Tom's invisible tormentors.

A week later, I'm dusting while Tom sits at the end of the dining table in the living room reading *The New York Times*. The phone rings. I look at the caller ID, which displays a number from an area code I don't recognize.

I answer to a cheery voice with a sweet Southern accent. "Good morning! I'm Bob Jameson from Jameson and Associates, calling from sunny Raleigh-Durham in North Carolina. How are you today?"

His friendly tone lifts my spirits, although I don't recognize his name or the company. My voice sounds the happiest it has been for weeks when I reply, "I'm fine. Thank you for asking. May I help you?"

"Yes. I received your résumé from Monster-dot-com for a job opening in New York City. Do you have a minute to talk about it?"

"Sure." I wonder why a recruiter from North Carolina would be working with a company in New York City. All the recruiters I worked with in Seattle focused on placements in the metro area.

"It's a great start-up," he says before revealing the company name. I don't recognize it.

"They were in Melbourne, Australia, but they moved to Wall Street a year ago to be close to the funding sources. They're at the very end of Wall Street. Can't get any closer than that to the money! Yep, they really thought that through. Anyway, they're growing fast and now they need a technical writer."

"I'd like to hear more about it."

"They make software that people use on the Internet. Their customers don't have to install anything. They log onto a website with a username and password and use the software from there."

I'd never heard of a product like this. It's an interesting concept.

"What does the software do?" I ask.

"People can build their own websites from the web," Bob says.

"How peachy keen is that?"

"Sounds like cutting-edge technology."

"Sure is! They're looking for someone with a wide range of experience like yours because you'll do more than technical writing. People who work at start-ups wear a lot of hats. That's why your résumé jumped out at me."

Bob pauses when a muffled voice with a strong Southern accent speaks in the background. "Hold on a minute," he says. "I'll be right back."

"Okay."

Tom lowers the paper a couple of inches, revealing his forehead and gold wire-framed glasses. "Who's that?"

I cover the mouthpiece with my hand. "It's a recruiter from North Carolina."

Tom shrugs his shoulders and tilts the paper to its original position. The pages hide the upper half of his body, except for his hands holding the paper open.

Why did he react like that? This is not the man I married! Where did he go?

When Bob returns, he says, "It's a fun group to work with. The management and most of the employees are from Melbourne. The hiring manager is a buddy of mine. You'll like him."

My mind wanders to the Missouri Ozarks, on the fringes of Southern Country, where I grew up. I remember everyone being friendly in the South and they can become friends with anybody if they want to. That doesn't necessarily mean they're best buddies with everybody, although often they say they are. But I must believe that Bob is being honest with me if I want to be hired for this job.

"I'd like to meet him," I say.

"Great! I'll send your résumé over today. I'll call you as soon as I hear from him. While you're waiting to hear from me, check out their website." He gives the address to me, and I write it on a notepad by the phone.

Tom folds the newspaper and lays it on the table after I hang up. "Why is a recruiter calling you from North Carolina?"

I sit across from Tom. "He has an opening in Manhattan, on Wall Street. A start-up needs a technical writer. He's sending my résumé to the hiring manager today."

Tom gets up and jogs down the stairs.

"Where are you going?"

Before I finish my question, the door at the entrance to our apartment opens and closes. There's no point in following him. He'll blame me for interfering again.

He returns five minutes later, holding the apartment keys in his hand.

"Where did you go?" I ask.

"I checked the mail," he says.

"Where is it?

"There wasn't any today." He turns around and goes downstairs. The bathroom door closes, and soon the shower is running. I wish that shower would wash away Tom's paranoia and my pain.

Bob calls back early Monday morning, soon after Tom leaves for another workshop in Manhattan.

"Hey, I have great news!" Bob sings over the line. "They want you to come in for an interview this week!"

"Wow, that was fast," I say.

"As I said, they're in a hurry to find someone. Speaking of that, what are you doing tomorrow?"

"I don't have anything scheduled."

"Could you meet them at ten o'clock?"

"I'll be there."

"Great! I will let them know." He gives me the names of the people I will meet, directions, and where to check in when I arrive.

The office is easy to find. After I leave the ferry on the Manhattan side, I walk five blocks down South Street, and the building is on the left at the intersection of Wall Street. I think about what the commute would be like every day, especially not having to ride a packed subway during rush hours. I love the ferry rides across the harbor, and I never tire of the view of the Statue of Liberty along the way. She's a stable force in my life, her presence always reassuring me that there is hope.

Alan, my main contact, greets me in the lobby with a big smile and hearty handshake. He's my height, with a skinny build and curly, shaggy gray hair. His Australian accent is strong and charming, perfect for his role as the "Marketing Guy," as he calls himself. Bob said his title is "Marketing Director."

"Let's go to the conference room," Alan says. "Everyone is waiting for us there."

When we arrive, he opens the door into a small room with a small rectangular table and chairs for everyone in our meeting. The rest of the room is packed with storage boxes. There's enough space for someone to walk around the table.

"Pardon the mess," he says. "The conference room doubles as a storage room for now. We'll have more space soon from our latest round of funding. We got it yesterday."

He introduces me to the other men in the room: Peter, the Chief Information Officer, and Gordon, the lead programmer. Peter is a tall, husky man and completely bald. He might have been a football player in a former life. Gordon is tall and thin, with short, neatly trimmed salt and pepper hair—more pepper than salt. He wears glasses with brown plastic frames.

"Gordon wrote the original code for our product," Alan says.

Peter, Gordon, and I shake hands. The interview starts, but it doesn't feel like an interview. It reminds me of friendly everyday chat at the local watering hole, except no one is nursing a pint. They weave their questions about my experience into our conversation.

The time flies, and the longer our conversation continues, the more we're laughing and joking. At the end of the hour, Alan says, "We want to hire you. Are you interested?"

Peter and Gordon nod and watch me as if they're waiting for me to open an envelope and announce the grand prize winner of a contest.

I wasn't expecting them to offer a job so soon. I assumed they'd leave and talk about what they heard before springing a decision on me. No one at an American-run company moves this fast. I'm overjoyed but try to contain my excitement. I don't know why I'm worried about this because they seem to be the type of people who wouldn't care if I got up and danced all over the room—if there were enough space. Who knows, they might have joined me.

"Yes," I say. "I'm looking forward to working with you." I smile and so do they.

"Great!" Alan says. "I'll take you to our HR person. She'll give you the paperwork to fill out."

When I shared the news with Tom that night, he smiled. At least I got a smile out of him. What's happening to the man I married?

I start the following Monday and settle in quickly. This office is a world completely different from the harried pace outside. Everyone is friendly and works well together. We soon move into a larger office space that covers the top two floors of the same twelve-story building. The walls, painted the color of a ripe orange, match the company's logo. Lots of natural light shines through the large picture windows with views of the skyscrapers in the neighborhood. The shiny silver ductwork is exposed under the ceiling, an interior design trend in the early 2000s. Our workstations are state-of-the-art—L-shaped tables with low-cut, glazed glass partitions with a wavy design that allows us to look directly at the others working in our area. Each workstation has a pedestal, a fancy name for a three-drawer cabinet with wheels where we can store supplies. The bottom drawer is large enough to hold files.

Our workstations are laid out so that two people face each other. The person across from me is one of the junior programmers. His wife, another junior programmer, also works here. When we take breaks, we talk about traveling, and they ask me a lot of questions about Seattle, where they've never been. They've traveled to places I've never been all over the world, and I dream of my own adventures someday.

The Australian work culture is much different than the American version. Everyone works hard eight hours a day and has fun doing it. At the end of the day, they go somewhere to have fun—dining at their favorite restaurants, having a drink or two, hanging out with friends, or all of the above. They rarely work weekends, either. Their mastery of work-life balance makes them more productive. We accomplished more in less time than at any American company I've worked for.

I look forward to coming to work every day. It's an escape from the stress at home. Tom spends more time obsessing over the people following him, even when he's sitting at home all day. He's convinced they've installed bugs in our phone and cameras in every room of our apartment, so it's harder to have any meaningful conversations with him. I miss our old conversations.

One night when I return home from work, I go to our office to leave my backpack under the desk, its usual spot. After I push the door a few inches, it stops. I try pushing it again, but it won't move. I look down and spot the problem—a shoestring tied around the doorknob and looped around the latch in the doorframe. I find the knot in the shoestring and, after a lot of effort, untie it.

I sense someone behind me and turn around to see Tom looking at the shoestring in my hand. His angry eyes shift to my face.

"What are you doing?" he yells.

"Putting my backpack away like I always do after work," I say. "Why is a shoestring tied around the doorknob?"

"Someone broke in today and took some stuff out of the office," he says.

"How is that even possible? You were here all day."

"Not all day. I walked over to the Chinese restaurant to buy some wings for lunch."

"You're telling me that someone snuck in here while you were out for maybe ten minutes and took stuff. No one can get in here that fast. Security wouldn't let them through the gate! They scrutinize anyone who doesn't have a gate key."

"How do you know that?"

"C'mon, Tom, you've seen and heard it. We both have. Remember last weekend when we returned from a walk and Security was grilling a man who forgot his key?"

I look around the office and in the closet. Tom stands in the doorway and watches me.

"I don't see anything that's missing," I say. "What do you think is missing?"

Tom watches me but doesn't reply.

I look around the office again. "Everything in here is the same as when I left for work this morning. What's missing?"

Tom continues watching me.

I look into his eyes. "Nothing is missing. No one was here today, other than you."

"You told them when to come in."

"That's impossible! I have no idea what you're doing when I'm gone."

"I don't believe you. You're trying to disrupt my life. I don't want you in this office anymore."

"Why? I have to work on my indexing projects in here. Have you forgotten that I still have publishing clients? We need all the money I can make. Without it, I can't keep up with the bills. Do you realize that we're close to our credit limit on every card we have? I've begged you to cut spending, but you aren't."

"I need these classes to get a job."

"What you need to do is look for a job. I need your help! I can't do this alone."

"I don't want to talk about this anymore." He retreats upstairs.

I leave my backpack under the desk, look for the shoe with a missing shoestring, and thread the string to its original position. Our argument exhausted me. I have to finish another index tonight and need to muster enough energy to do it. I'd love to go for a walk, but if I leave now, Tom will believe I'm out talking to someone about his whereabouts. Instead, I go upstairs, make a cup of instant coffee, and carry it to my desk. Hopefully it gives me enough energy to finish this project.

Tom's mood usually softens when he's in a class or workshop. Maybe it's his way to escape. If it is, I wish he'd find a cheaper option.

Sometimes when he's in Manhattan for an all-day class, he calls and asks me to join him for lunch at the Au Bon Pain. Occasionally at the end of my workday, he'll meet me in the lobby and we'll walk to Fine and Schapiro, a favorite restaurant in the shops at the bottom of the World Trade Center. I treasure these moments, because Tom is back to the person I fell in love with, but I'm still frustrated and angry that he refuses to look for work.

The roller coaster of emotions grows longer and bumpier. My next unpleasant surprise comes one day when I meet him for lunch at the Au Bon Pain, where he shares a memory I've never heard over soup, sandwiches, and sodas.

"When I was in high school, Mom tried to matchmake me with

someone," he says.

"Really?" I ask. All the stories I've heard from Tom and Tess about his high school days led me to believe that Tom had no interest in girls. Football was his life. He played tackle on the varsity team. Tess even said I was the first and only woman he'd been interested in.

"Yeah, she was the daughter of the Bowmans."

"Who are the Bowmans? I never met anyone by that name when I lived in Coos Bay. They never came to the Dairy Queen."

I lived in Coos Bay for two years during my late teens, when Mom and my second stepfather moved there from the Ozarks after my grandparents died. I didn't know Tom when I lived there. We met in Eugene four years later after I transferred from Eastern Oregon University to the University of Oregon to finish my journalism degree. Tom was working on his second bachelor's degree at the business school, majoring in finance. He was a regular customer at the 7-Eleven where I worked swing shift and alternated grave on the weekends.

I learned later that the Dairy Queen where I worked is three blocks from the house where Tom grew up. His parents lived there until their poor health led them to separate assisted living centers. After they left, Don renovated the bottom floor of the house into his law office and now practices there. The top floor of the house and an extension on one side are segmented into one-bedroom apartments.

"They're a prominent logging family in Coos Bay," Tom says.

Coos Bay's main industries are logging, fishing, and tourism.

"What happened?" I ask.

Tom laughs. "Nothing. I wasn't interested. Mom kept trying but finally gave up." He laughs again while watching me.

I stare at him. Where did this absurd story come from? Tess knows her four sons would never tolerate her meddling in their romantic lives. She doesn't care about social status, either.

We finish our lunch in silence. Tom leaves for his workshop, and I return to the office and try to forget about his tale.

Escapes

New York City, March 2001

If hell is like my life right now, I never want to go there. The nonstop pace of the city and Tom's never-ending paranoia have pushed me into survival mode. I'm amazed I can sleep at night with the adrenaline constantly rushing through my body. Probably it's because I'm so exhausted at the end of every day, my system forces me to shut down. No matter how much sleep I get, I never wake up feeling like I've had a good night's rest. I don't know how much longer I can cope, but I don't know how to jump off this strange merry-go-round.

The dot-com is where I escape. I can spend those forty hours every week being myself, away from the nightmare my life has become. I've thought about calling Don several times and telling him the real story of our lives here, but when I gather enough courage, I convince myself that he won't believe me. Why should he?

I'd never talk to Tom's parents about this. Al would probably take the news in stride; he never lets things get to him, but it would be hard for him to hear me talk about his youngest son this way. He might not understand everything I say anyway, because his hearing is mostly gone from years of not wearing hearing protection in his woodshop.

Tess is a compulsive worrier. News like this would push her deeper into depression and might further damage her health. From the bits and pieces of news I've gathered during Tom's occasional phone conversations with Don, Don doesn't know how much longer she'll last. I often wonder how these updates are affecting Tom. He doesn't talk about them.

Now when Tom's paranoia is at its worst, he combines the

usual vague claims of people following him with stories about the Bowmans. One night when we go for a walk two blocks away to enjoy an unobstructed view of New York Harbor, he adds to the story he shared at the Au Bon Pain:

"They were friends with George. Every year I went to the regional sales meetings, they were there. They'd meet with George in the bar and have drinks. The daughter was always with her father and her father wouldn't stop trying to set her up with me."

Only the company's sales employees and managers were allowed to attend these meetings because they were held at expensive resorts. George was a mid-level manager, so it would have been impossible to get an exception approved for the Bowmans to travel there if he knew them.

"Why did you wait until now to tell me about this?" I ask.

"You would have told them."

"Why do you say that? I don't know who these people are. I've never met them. I never heard of them until you started talking about them. If this family is as well-known as you say they are, I would have heard of them or at least met some of them. Social status doesn't stop people from getting their favorite ice cream treats at the Dairy Queen."

"I don't believe you. You won't stop interfering in my business."

"We're married. We live in the same place. I work in an office five days a week and on side projects at home. You have every day to yourself. You don't tell me what you're doing. You won't look for a job. We came here for your career change, but I'm carrying the burden. Why have you given up?"

Tom turns away and stares at the lights twinkling from the skyscrapers in Lower Manhattan.

"Tom, I'm exhausted. I need your help. We're heading into a financial crisis. You should know, for God's sake, because you have a finance degree! You can help me stop the bleeding by getting a job. I made a commitment to you before we left Seattle. It's time for you to keep yours."

Tom watches a ferry cross the harbor. A light catches my eye, the torch the Statue of Liberty never stops holding high in the air. I think of the famous line, "Give me your tired, your weary…" I want her to take me in her arms and comfort me. I need a change. It's time to take action.

The Best I Can Do

I start walking toward the ferry terminal.

Tom spins around and glares at me. "Where are you going?"

"I'm done. I can't take this anymore." I continue walking toward the ferry terminal. Tom watches but doesn't follow me.

My pace quickens the closer I come to the ferry terminal's side entrance. I walk through the door, pass the concession stands that are now closed, and enter the vast waiting room. I sit on a hard wooden bench near the dock, waiting for the next ferry to Manhattan and pondering what I'll do when I reach the other side. I don't want to do this, but I can't turn around now.

After I board the ferry, I climb the stairs to the top deck and look at the subway map mounted in a glass case between the entrances to the bathrooms. There's a YMCA across from Central Park on the Upper West Side. It's a good place to start. Maybe they'll have some rooms where I can spend the night.

Almost halfway through the thirty-five-minute journey across the harbor, I walk outside and stand at the railing midship on the port side. Directly ahead of me, I watch the Statue of Liberty, her green body and robes shining bright from the spotlights at the base. The golden flame from her torch glows in the dark sky.

"Thank you for comforting me," I whisper.

An hour later, I'm standing outside the YMCA, a tall brick building with an arched entrance. I take a deep breath and walk into the lobby. The layout is simple: walls painted white, high ceilings with fluorescent lights, a floor covered in tan linoleum with a hexagon pattern, and a wooden circular counter. There aren't any chairs, except for the one used by the man sitting behind the counter.

I walk up to the counter. The thin, tan-skinned man has short black hair and wears a black T-shirt with "YMCA" in white letters and blue jeans. He's reading a paperback pressed open against the desktop. His brown eyes look at me over spectacles framed in black plastic.

"Do you have any rooms available for one person?"

"It's eighty-five dollars a night."

"I'd like one for tonight."

He takes his time bookmarking his spot and closing the paperback. Then he pulls a registration card from a slot in front of him. He places the card on the counter and hands a pen to me.

"Fill this out."

When I'm finished, I pay in cash. He hands a key to me and points at the number on the key ring. "You're on the fifth floor, near the end of the hallway facing Central Park. Have a nice night."

The elevator opens onto a floor with rows of doors stretching the length of the hallway on both sides. There's a window at the end of the hallway looking out into the darkness. I find my room number and have to jiggle the key in the knob a few times to release the lock.

The room has a twin bed with a cast-iron frame shaped like the beds from the forties, a wooden nightstand, and a digital clock. A thin tan blanket and white bedspread cover the white sheets. Fluorescent lights shine from the high ceilings. I look for a switch to turn them off, but there isn't one. I'm not good at sleeping with the lights on and hope that because I'm so tired tonight, maybe my body will adjust.

Somehow I fall asleep but not for long. I feel the springs through the thin mattress, and every time I move, they squeak. My thoughts return to my argument with Tom at the viewpoint tonight, and I hope with my walking away, something stirs inside him to break the paranoia spell and bring him back to the person he once was—the loving, responsible person who respects his wife as a partner, a human being. I've forgotten what that feels like.

Eventually I fall asleep for an hour. When I awake, the green numbers on the digital clock read *5:30*. I think about what I need to do today. I won't miss work, but I need to find a change of clothes and decide where I'll sleep tonight. I have enough cash to spend another night at the YMCA. I don't want to charge any more money on the credit cards.

I freshen up in the shared bathroom. Because I took my backpack on our walk last night, I have a comb, toothbrush, and toothpaste. While I'm in the bathroom, I stand in front of the mirror and straighten my wrinkled clothes as much as possible, then take the elevator downstairs and check out.

I ride the subway to the closest stop for the Kmart on Houston Street and buy two pullover tops, small packages of underwear and socks, and two pairs of slacks. From there, I walk the remaining half mile to the office and change in the bathroom before settling at my desk. I hide the bag from Kmart in the bottom drawer of the pedestal.

It's hard to concentrate on work today. My mind dwells on Tom's behavior. Something is horribly wrong, but I don't know what it is or how to fix it. Even if I could, I don't know how it would happen because Tom has lost interest in everything, except his obsession over being followed and now, the Bowmans.

All day, I keep to myself by sitting at my desk and trying to focus on writing. When I can't concentrate, I pretend to work on my computer. If I look busy, I don't have to talk to anyone. I'm afraid if I do, I'll shatter into a million pieces.

At the end of the day, I skip dinner and take the subway back to the YMCA. The same man helps me check in and assigns the same room to me. As soon as I lie on the squeaky bed, I fall asleep until five o'clock the next morning.

When I check out, a manager is on duty. Maybe he can help me find another place to stay tonight.

"I was wondering if you know if there are any shelters for women around here," I say when I hand the keys to him. "I had to leave my husband, and I ran out of money last night. I don't have anywhere else to go."

"I'm so sorry," he says. "I don't have any information, but we have a counselor here who can help you. He isn't here now. He can call you when he comes in at eleven."

"I don't have a cell phone," I say. "I can give you my work number, but I can't talk freely there."

"That's okay. When he calls, he will ask you 'yes' or 'no' questions so no one can hear what you're talking about."

I hand my business card to him. "Thank you. I appreciate your help."

The counselor calls me a few minutes after eleven. "You don't have to talk. Just listen," he says. "We have a women's shelter outside the city, and you're welcome to stay there until you can get back on your feet. When you get off work tonight, take the seven train to the end of the line. That's the Flushing-Main Street Station in Queens. Someone will meet you there and take you to the shelter."

"Okay," I say. "I'm not sure how long it will take."

"That's okay. They'll wait for you."

A few hours later, Tom calls me. His voice is back to his old self. "How are you doing?" he asks.

"I'm okay." I'm trying not to sound tired and I don't want to convey any enthusiasm from his call.

"We need to talk," he says. "Meet me at the Au Bon Pain after work tonight. I will wait for you there."

"All right," I say. At least I can hear him out before going to Queens, but I'm not expecting anything to change. Deep down, I'm not sure whether this is a good idea. Maybe Charlotte is telling me not to go.

At Au Bon Pain, Tom smiles at me and stands when I arrive at the table he saved for us. He pulls the empty chair from the table and motions for me to sit. He helps me slide the chair closer to the table, then returns to his seat, reaches for both of my hands, squeezes them gently, then looks into my eyes.

"I miss you," he says. "I want you to come home."

I pull my hands away. "I can't."

"Why?"

"I can't live the way we are anymore."

"I'm sorry if I've hurt you. Please give me a chance."

I remember similar conversations with Mom and Bubby, my stepfather. He could be the sweetest man in the world, but whenever he got mad, he was violent. We never knew what would set him off. Mom left him several times, but Bubby always found her and talked her into coming home. Things would improve for a while, but when his anger returned, he was more violent than ever.

When Julie turned thirteen, she ran away from home, and a year later, I devised an elaborate, successful escape plan. I was eighteen then, and there was nothing Bubby could do to stop me. Mom's opportunity finally came when Julie's husband intervened. It took sixteen years for Mom to break free. Many women in situations like Mom's never escape. They die trying.

Tom never physically abuses me, but often his words cross over into the verbal abuse category. It's a different type of beating, except the cuts and bruises linger inside.

Do I give Tom another chance? I don't want to fall into the same trap Mom did. On one hand, I won't feel guilty if I give him another chance. At least I will know that I tried. On the other hand, if things get worse, I can't cave in. I must remain strong and protect myself.

"I will," I say.

Tom reaches for my hands and gently squeezes them. "Let's go home," he says.

During our walk to the ferry terminal, Tom holds my hand the entire way. He doesn't let go when we board the ferry. After we climb the stairs to the top deck, he wraps his arm around my shoulders while we stand at the railing on the starboard side, watching the Statue of Liberty pass. The light from her torch is bright as usual, but tonight, I'm not finding comfort in her. The feeling from Tom gently holding my hand and wrapping his arm around me doesn't reassure me, either. I'm restless, fearing what could happen next, but I stand still while the uneasiness in my gut quietly rumbles and the Statue of Liberty fades from view.

Tom returns to his old self and starts looking for work again. I'm happy to have my real husband again, but this shift reminds me of the back-and-forth with Mom and Bubby. Every time she left, he was sweet to her after he successfully begged her to return. He would treat her like a queen for a few weeks, then become more violent than before she left. No one was spared from his beatings and verbal abuse.

My experiences with Mom and Bubby's relationship make me wonder how long Tom can maintain his current behavior. I hope it's permanently, but Charlotte says *it's only temporary*. She won't tell me when it will change.

After I return home from work a week later, Tom announces, "I applied for a sales position at a food company in Connecticut. The office is close to a Metro North stop."

I'm relieved and confident they'll hire him because he worked for a competitor.

The company calls him for an interview. He takes the train to Connecticut early that morning and returns late in the evening. He's beaming when he walks into the bedroom, where I'm lying in bed watching the news.

Tom kisses my forehead and I look into his sparkling eyes. "It went well," he says. "I think they'll give me an offer."

I smile at him. "I hope they do. You deserve it." We deserve it. I deserve a break in easing the financial burden.

A week later, he receives a thanks-but-no-thanks email. The company found someone with more recent experience. Tom has been out of the workforce so long that even a competitor won't hire him. His successful track record in sales doesn't matter anymore.

Tom continues to apply for sales jobs but doesn't receive any more calls for interviews. He doesn't seem discouraged, and I hope this continues. Surely someone will hire him.

Three weeks later, I go upstairs to refresh the cats' food and water dishes. Tiger is hunched over the water bowl, resting his chin in the water. I kneel next to him and stroke his back. His weary green eyes look up at me but the rest of his body doesn't move. His mouth is open in the water but he isn't drinking.

"Tiger, what's wrong?" I ask.

Tiger looks down at the water dish but still doesn't move.

I call the vet and describe Tiger's symptoms.

"Bring him in now," the receptionist says. "We can squeeze him in."

"I'm on the way."

Tom is still asleep when I return to the bedroom. I shake him awake.

"Something is wrong with Tiger," I say. "I called the vet, and they can see him now."

"I'll go with you," Tom says.

"I'll put Tiger in his carrier while you get dressed."

Usually Tiger fights me when I try to put him in the carrier, but today, he doesn't care. He's definitely not feeling well.

"Hang on, sweetie," I say. "Everything will be okay."

He lays his head on his front paws and closes his eyes.

When we arrive at the animal clinic, Tom waits in the reception area and I carry Tiger to the exam room. The vet checks Tiger's vitals, draws blood, and takes the test tubes to the onsite lab. We wait for the results in the exam room. Tiger hunches on the exam table, looking disoriented. I stand next to him and stroke his back to comfort him.

"Everything looks good," the vet says when he returns, "except Tiger's glucose reading is at four hundred fifty. He has diabetes."

"I thought only humans can get diabetes," I say. "Is this common in cats?"

"It is," the vet says. "Usually we see symptoms in older males."

Tiger is twelve years old—a senior cat.

"We need to lower Tiger's glucose levels," the vet says. "To do this, he needs insulin. I'd like you to start with three units, twice a day, and schedule a follow-up in a week to check his glucose again. I'd also like to put him on a special diet. It's a dry prescription cat food we have for sale here."

He hands two prescriptions to me, one for a vial of insulin and the other for a box of syringes.

"How do I give a shot to a cat?" I ask. "Tiger will fight me, and he will win."

"He won't feel it," the vet says. "My assistant will give him a shot before you leave, so she can show you how to do it. Call us if anything changes. Wait here for my assistant."

The assistant shows me how to draw the insulin into the syringe and measure the number of units Tiger needs. When she gives the shot to him, she pinches the scruff of his neck, where mama cats pick up and carry their kittens, inserts the needle through the skin, and injects the insulin. Tiger doesn't flinch.

"He can't feel it because there's so much skin there," the assistant says. "The pinch distracts him. You don't have to pinch him hard—just enough to grab enough skin for the injection."

By the time we return home, Tiger is feeling better. When I release him from the carrier, he jumps on the bed and falls asleep. The insulin is working.

Later that day, I try my first shot. I expect a fight, because nothing ever goes as well at home with a cat as it does at the vet's office, but Tiger surprises me. He sits still while I grab the skin on the back of his neck. When I poke the needle through his skin, it feels like I'm puncturing a sheet of vellum.

Tiger's diagnosis brings two problems, one new and one old with a twist. First, I can't separate his prescription food from the regular cat food. When I try, TC believes Tiger is getting something special, so he refuses to eat the regular cat food. Finally, I ask the vet if I can give the prescription food to TC, too, and the vet says it's okay.

The second problem concerns Tom. The people are following him again, and he claims someone is contaminating him with a "colorless, odorless substance."

One night when I return home from work, I go upstairs to give Tiger his shot. I pull the handle on the refrigerator door, and the door won't budge. I try again. No response. I look down, where the resistance is coming from, and discover a heavy-duty chain wrapped around the refrigerator and through the door handle with a padlock securing it in place.

I search for Tom. He isn't upstairs. I find him downstairs in the office, surfing the Internet.

"Why is there a lock and chain around the refrigerator door?" I ask.

"It's there for protection," Tom says.

"Protection from what?"

"Contamination. Someone contaminated me again today."

"That's ridiculous! No one would come in here and do that. We aren't living in a spy movie!"

Tom continues surfing.

"Will you give me the key, please? I need to give Tiger his shot and cook dinner."

"You're not cooking anymore."

"What? Are you serious?"

"You're not cooking anymore, because I don't want you to contaminate my food."

"Why would I do anything like that? We can't afford to eat out all the time!"

Tom gets up and climbs the stairs. I follow him. He removes the padlock and watches me draw Tiger's dose of insulin into the syringe and place the vial back on the shelf inside the refrigerator door. He closes the refrigerator and secures the chain.

"You don't expect me to go through this twice a day, do you?"

"You're not using the refrigerator unless I'm here!"

"If Tiger doesn't get his insulin, he could die! Don't you understand that? This isn't a game."

"Then why are you playing games with me?"

"No one is playing games with you."

Tom drops the padlock key in his pocket and returns downstairs. I stand in the kitchen, bewildered at Tom's new fantasy. If he wants to act this way, then I won't cook dinner. I won't buy takeout, either. A few days without dinner will make him change his mind.

Another Layoff

New York City, May 2001

Why has the copy machine been running all morning? It's nine-thirty, and I'm sitting at my desk, kitty-corner from the machine, hearing the hum and pulsating of the printing and a click when another piece of paper spits out into the tray. The stack of copies has grown to almost twelve inches in the last half hour. I'm thinking about asking the administrative assistant who's making so many copies and where the pile should go.

The Human Resources Officer rounds the corner, checks the status on the small copier screen, and lifts the stack from the tray. She walks away. The machine continues to hum and spit out more pages.

A half hour later, the machine stops. Silence at last!

A chime from my computer alerts me to new messages in my inbox. The first message in the list displays a red exclamation point at the left of the subject line, meaning it's urgent. It's from the Human Resources Officer: "Mandatory meeting at noon today."

I double-click the message to open it.

"Steve will be speaking to everyone at noon today in the main conference room. Everyone must attend. We will order pizza for lunch."

Steve is our CEO. A shiver trickles down my spine. He's rarely in the office, so this can't be good news.

When the dot-com received its last round of funding three months ago, our last CEO was fired and Steve took his place. We learned that Steve is the lead investor, and he wants to be closer to operations to make sure we have a clear mission. The last CEO changed the company's mission daily, after he read one report after another about the latest trends during his commutes to the office. His inspiration from the business media always prompted quick strategy meetings with marketing and sales. I'm invited because I help marketing write promotional materials.

After a few weeks of this, our best sales rep got fed up and spoke out during a brainstorming session. "I don't know what to tell my prospects anymore because our message changes every day. I need clear direction. Without it, I don't know how to sell our products."

I heard the anger and frustration in his voice and understood why he felt this way. After years of Tom working in sales, I saw how the best reps operate. They're like missiles—give them a target to achieve, and they're instantly locked on. Nothing will stop them until they strike successfully.

"We must keep up with the trends!" the CEO replied. "If you're unable and unwilling to do it, then it's time to submit your resignation."

The sales rep was silent for the rest of the meeting. The next day, he was gone. The administrative assistant told me he was fired.

Charlotte's voice awakens and breaks through my memories. *Something bad is about to happen*, she says. *Be prepared.*

First the copy machine. Now her. I'm not in the mood today.

That's all you're telling me? That's not helpful! Why tell me anything?

That's all you need to know for now, she replies in her calm, steady tone. Nothing rattles her. She's like a reporter who speaks the facts only when she knows the timing is right.

A bigger shiver crawls down my spine and my hands feel clammy.

At lunch, everyone reluctantly strolls into the conference room. Some sit in a chair; others sit on the windowsill or lean against the wall. When the pizza arrives, no one digs in. Usually the programmers rush to the table first and fill their plates with three or four slices. Finally one of them steps forward and everyone else slowly falls in line.

We eat in silence. When we're done, Steve steps inside and closes the door. He's slightly shorter than I am, with thick gray hair and a short gray beard, neatly trimmed around his cheeks and chin. He's dressed in business casual, with a powder blue button-down shirt under a blue sweater vest, khaki slacks, and beige canvas loafers. He takes a deep breath and slides his hands into his pants pockets. Everyone's eyes are focused on him.

I bow my head, close my eyes, and imagine I'm walking through a beautiful Douglas fir forest in my old neighborhood in West Seattle, where the breeze from Puget Sound gently strokes my skin. I want to go home.

Steve's voice invades my thoughts. "I have some sad news," he says, "and I don't want to prolong it any longer. As you might have heard, the investors are tightening the reins on funding start-up companies. They expect us to produce, which means we must show a profit. Although our revenue has increased substantially during the past three months, we are still far below projections."

Steve pulls his hands from his pockets, folds his arms across his chest, and walks to the window of the conference room. He looks at the view of Lower Manhattan for a minute, as if he's seeking answers from the dark office towers staring back at him in front of a gray sky. The sun struggles to break through the clouds and finally gives up.

He turns around to face the still, silent audience and clasps his hands behind his back. Our eyes are fixed on him, waiting for him to deliver the rest of his news.

"When we met with the investors again last month, we presented strong evidence that we could continue this positive trend, but they were not convinced. As a result, they will no longer fund us. We contacted other firms that invest in start-up companies, but they will not support us, either."

He pauses and looks around the room. No one moves. No one speaks. Although I expected this to happen with the recent layoffs, it's still hard to believe. Forty of our seventy employees were laid off or fired during the past four months.

"Now, we're out of money," Steve says. "Therefore, effective at five o'clock today, we must close permanently and file for bankruptcy. Please be assured that you will be paid through today. I am taking care of it personally. Your checks will be ready to pick up on Monday."

We stare at him in shock. Then a few people bow their heads, staring at their shoes or the carpet. Others gaze at the cold leftover pizza on the conference room table.

I'm among the people whose gaze is fixed on Steve. The first thought that pops in my mind comes from my public relations classes in journalism school: *Bad news is always delivered on Friday. It's done to ease the sting over the weekend. People will forget by Monday.*

No one will forget this. They just lost their jobs. We're among the last start-up companies from the dot-com boom to close in Manhattan so for many of us, it will be hard to find another high-tech job in the city.

The Human Resources Officer breaks our trances with, "We have packets with information on how to file for unemployment and apply for COBRA. They're on the table next to my office."

I dread telling Tom about this. I can't anticipate how he will react because his behavior grows more unpredictable every day. I wish I knew what is wrong with him and could find a way to help him, but I don't know where to turn. Even if I did, who would believe the bizarre stories I'd tell them?

I go to the bathroom to be alone for a while. I lean on the sink and stare into the mirror, gathering words in my mind to break the news to Tom tonight.

Celeste, the marketing manager, walks into the bathroom, stands next to me, and gazes at my reflection in the mirror. Her lemon-yellow pantsuit and ivory blouse complement her blue-gray eyes and shoulder-length, curly ash blonde hair.

"That was quite a shock, wasn't it?" she asks.

"It was," I say, looking back at her reflection. "What are you going to do?"

"I don't know. It's hard to find work in my field here. Too much competition."

"I'm in the same boat. The only full-time technical writing work left is in finance, and no one will hire me because I don't have the experience they want."

Tears build in my eyes and a couple spill onto my cheek. I lower my head to try to hide them. Celeste notices and rests her hand on my shoulder.

"I'm sorry," I say, staring at the sink. "I'm worried. No, I'm scared. My husband is in school. He hasn't worked for four years, and I don't know what I will do. He won't be happy when I tell him about this."

Celeste wraps her arm around my shoulders while my tears escape the well.

… The Best I Can Do

Interviews

New York City and Massachusetts, May-June 2001

The ferry ride home from the office went too fast after that fateful meeting in Manhattan. I stand at my usual spot on the upper deck, watching the view and trying to compose myself. The clouds parted after I left the office, and now the warmth from the sun's rays comfort my skin. The water is a deeper blue than I've noticed since making these trips back and forth every weekday for almost a year and a half. Even the Statue of Liberty's copper robes are a deeper shade of green.

Everything will be all right, Charlotte says, but I'm not so sure. I don't want to share this news with Tom, but it's better to get it over with. He'll probably blame me for the company closing. My logic doesn't make sense, but nothing is logical anymore when it comes to Tom's perspectives.

After leaving the ferry terminal, I walk the seven blocks to our apartment. The view along the Promenade is equally beautiful with the sapphire water lapping the shore from the wakes of the boat traffic and the skyline of Manhattan rising in the distance. The bright orange ferry reflects in the water when it departs the terminal for its return trip to Lower Manhattan. I stop to savor the view before climbing the steep hill from the police precinct to our apartment building. Hopefully the workout will provide more energy for my task.

When I arrive at our apartment, Tom is sitting at the end of the dining table in our living room, reading a book. He looks up when he hears me climb the stairs and lays the book open, face down, on the table.

"You're home early," he says. He doesn't notice that I was crying, or if he does, he keeps his observation to himself.

I sit in a chair at the side of the table facing the view of the harbor, then look directly into Tom's eyes. "The company closed today," I say.

"What?" Tom asks, leaning forward in his chair.

"They ran out of funding, so now they're closing and filing for bankruptcy. Today was our last day."

Tom leans back in his chair. "Everything seemed to be going so well."

"There were signs—layoffs and budget cuts. Six months ago, we were up to seventy people, but by last month, we were down to thirty. That's the same number of people who was there when I started."

Tom looks through the window facing the harbor and I do, too. I'm bracing myself for him to blame me for something, but he seems to be back to himself this afternoon. I can't let down my guard because I never know when his mood will shift.

He turns toward me, still leaning back in his chair and examining my face with his eyes. "This isn't a good time for this to happen," he says.

"There's never a good time for a layoff," I say. "We have to be careful with our finances. I can draw unemployment, but it won't cover the rent."

I stop short of saying Tom needs to find a job—any job that will help me cover the expenses of living in one of the priciest cities in the country—but I'm too tired to fight today. I want his mostly mellow mood to last as long as possible.

"I'm going downstairs to search the job boards," I say.

Tom nods.

When I'm at the edge of the stairwell, I glance over my shoulder and see Tom reading his book as if nothing happened. I wonder if the magnitude of my job loss has sunk in but doubt it has. His reaction makes me feel isolated and unloved.

My search results display a long list of writing jobs in the finance industry. I apply for a few where I have enough qualifications to be considered, then search for jobs at companies from the Mid-Atlantic to New England. I'm tempted to apply for some contracts in Seattle, but if I get one and return, I'll never come back to New York. I wish Tom would admit it's time to go home.

A week later, a recruiter calls from an agency where I worked in

Seattle. "I have a short contract for Microsoft," she says. "They need someone to index a programming book."

"I'm no longer in Seattle," I say, "so I can't work onsite full-time."

"That's why I called you," the recruiter says. "You can work on this project from anywhere."

I accept the contract, and she sends the files via file transfer protocol (FTP) within the hour. Four weeks later, I finish the index and submit the final versions of the files to Microsoft.

A few days later, a call comes from a company in Newton, Massachusetts, for an opening I'd forgotten I'd applied for. Yvette, the Human Resources Coordinator, has a pleasant, youthful voice.

"We received your résumé for our technical writer opening from Monster-dot-com, and we'd like you to come in for an interview. Are you still looking?"

"Yes," I reply.

"I noticed that you're living in New York," she says. "In case you're not aware, we are not providing relocation expenses."

"I am. If I'm hired, I'm willing to relocate at my own expense." Hopefully she hears the seriousness and commitment in my voice.

"All right. Would you be able to come to the office on Tuesday morning at ten o'clock?"

"I'm available."

"Great! Please plan to be here all day. You will be speaking with seven members of our marketing and engineering teams. I will email a list of their names and titles."

The company is ten miles west of Boston. I research the closest hotels to the office and transportation options. The least expensive option is to take Amtrak from Penn Station to Boston and connect to the T, Boston's subway system. The closest stop on the T is a ten-minute ride from the office. I find a Holiday Inn near the T, a short taxi ride to the office.

I make the reservations before telling Tom what I'm doing. It's time for me to take charge. I've been waiting for him to do something for too long. He has no interest in getting a job, in helping me refloat our sinking ship.

Despite all the changes in our lives during the past four years, Tom has not grayed or wrinkled. I'm now completely gray and hide the evidence with hair color that matches my natural dark brown locks as closely as possible. Some lines are forming across my forehead that are visible when I raise my eyebrows.

It's too early to be completely gray; I'm only forty-one. Premature graying runs in my family—I remember Grandma telling me that my great-grandfather was completely gray by the time he turned twenty-one—but despite getting my first two gray hairs at seventeen, I believe the stress accelerated the process.

Remaining hopeful can be good and bad at the same time. It's nice to be hopeful, but at what cost? My hanging onto hope for so long has dragged us down emotionally and financially. Probably it's more accurate to say it has drug *me* down. Tom doesn't seem to understand how his actions are affecting me, and he still hasn't faced the reality of our financial situation. He has stopped signing up for workshops at the financial institutions, but he's still taking one or two classes every semester at NYU.

Maybe my hope is changing with this upcoming interview in another state. If I get this job, I can stop the financial bleeding. We can move to Massachusetts and start over. We've never been there, and I'm hoping a new environment will be good for both of us.

I go upstairs, where Tom sits at the table with the pages of *The New York Times* spread open. "We need to talk," I say. "Let's go for a walk."

"What about?" Tom says, staring at the pages.

"I have an interview near Boston on Tuesday morning. I'm taking the train there on Monday. I'll be back on Tuesday night."

Tom looks at me with furled eyebrows. "What happened to looking for a job here?"

"I have been looking but no one responds to my applications. All the jobs are in finance. They won't hire me because I don't have a background in finance writing."

"That's an excuse. You don't want to live here anymore. You never wanted to live here."

"You don't know how hard I've tried to make this move work. You don't even want to understand. All you want to do is go to school and blame me for interfering with your life. We can't even enjoy a good home-cooked meal anymore because of that lock and chain around the refrigerator."

"I'm being contaminated with an odorless, colorless substance. You're not cooking because you'll contaminate me."

"That's ridiculous, and you know it! You started complaining about that after I started giving insulin shots to Tiger, and I don't understand why. Tiger needs those shots to keep his glucose levels under control. He's diabetic, remember?"

My boycott of buying takeout for dinner didn't change Tom's mind on removing the lock and chain around the refrigerator, but it forced him to prepare our meals. He's a good cook, which is another trait that attracted me to him so long ago. His mother taught him. In happier times, we took turns cooking meals or cooked together. We'd try new recipes and experiment with new techniques, like drying fruit and meat and creating our own chocolate candies. That chocolate candy-making journey started after we met a chocolate maker from Tacoma at her booth at the Washington State Fair in Puyallup, sampled her handiwork, and took a flyer home that advertised her classes. Then we signed up for an introductory class and were hooked by its end. We took more classes, where we learned how to make candy in molds with colorful designs, truffles, chocolate-covered cherries, and other treats. We bought molds and supplies and made treats for family and friends for Christmas and other special occasions. They loved it.

But now, Tom isn't cooking like he used to. Meals consist of mostly frozen entrees or the occasional sandwiches. He's never been a breakfast person, but I must eat something first thing in the morning or I don't function well for the rest of the day. I've managed to make toast with peanut butter and a cup of instant Folgers coffee for my breakfast without his interference. I'm a coffee-with-cream person who now simulates the flavor with powdered creamer and pretend I'm enjoying it with half and half, but the taste isn't the same. Tom doesn't like coffee, except for the aroma.

What's odd about the refrigerator is the lock and chain restricts access to only the refrigerator. I can still open the freezer on top if I want, but I don't. Tom would notice if I add, move, or remove anything in there, which would trigger more blame about my involvement in the "attacks" on him. I don't understand why he's obsessed over anyone using the refrigerator but not the freezer. Like most aspects of Tom's behavior, there's no logic behind his reasoning or actions. What is this that I'm dealing with?

Fortunately, Tiger hasn't needed insulin shots for a couple of weeks. His latest tests show his glucose levels have leveled off. We still go to the vet twice a month for blood tests because the vet says his levels could spike again—despite him continuing the special food diet. Tom hasn't gone to any of Tiger's checkups since the emergency visit where Tiger was diagnosed.

Tom breaks into my thoughts with, "I don't want you to go to Boston."

Anger flares inside me, but the only word that passes my lips is, "Why?"

Tom starts reading the paper again.

"What's wrong with going to Boston?" I ask. "You don't know anything about Boston. You've never been there."

Tom flips the page and continues reading.

"Silence won't change my mind," I say, glaring at him. "I'm going. I can't find work here, so it's time to go somewhere else."

Tom's eyes continue focusing on the newspaper.

"I don't care what you think about my job search," I say in a shaky voice. "I know how hard I've tried, and that's all that matters. If you really care, you'd keep your end of the bargain and find a job so we can get out of our financial mess. You can't go to school forever."

Tom looks up at me. "I need those classes!"

"No you don't. You need a job! I don't care what kind of job it is, as long as it helps me pay the bills."

Tom flips another page and starts reading again.

There's no use trying to talk to him anymore. I return to the office downstairs. On the way, Charlotte says again, *Everything will be all right*. I want to scream at her and say, *What gives you the right to say that at a time like this?* But I feel an odd peaceful presence washing away my anger and replacing it with hope and an eagerness for my trip.

Maybe everything will be all right. Maybe Charlotte is telling me I'll get this job and start a new chapter in my life.

Throughout my trip, Charlotte continues reminding me that *everything will be okay*. Her words comfort me, but I don't know if she's referring to the interview, Tom's mood, or something else.

From the moment I arrive at the office in Newton, everyone I encounter makes me feel welcome and comfortable. Yvette escorts me to a conference room, where the interviews start with Matt, the hiring manager and the Director of Marketing, a thin man slightly taller than me with short light brown hair. His interview doesn't feel like an interview, except for sitting inside a conference room. It's like we're meeting for dinner and having a casual conversation. Matt asks about my experience occasionally, but it's clear he read my résumé thoroughly. He doesn't ask for writing samples, so I offer to show my portfolio to him.

He looks at the binder briefly before opening it, then thumbs through it. "This is a nice presentation," he says. "I've never seen a portfolio like this."

I thank him.

"I will take a look at this and return it to you before you leave today," he says.

"I made extra copies," I say. "This one is for you. You can keep it."

The day continues the same with the other six managers and engineers who interviewed me. When one person leaves, Matt or Yvette stops by to check on whether I need anything before the next person arrives. By noon, I've talked to four people, including Matt, and we stop for a lunch break. Yvette orders sandwiches from the café downstairs, and when they arrive, Matt and I eat in the conference room. We chat about our families and what life is like in New England.

After lunch, I talk to the last three people on the list, and the tone is the same. When we're finished, Matt returns.

"How do you feel?" he asks. "I know it's a long day, but we wanted to make the best use of your time because you've traveled so far."

"I appreciate your thoughtfulness," I say. "I enjoyed my conversations with everyone. I think this position will be a good fit for me."

"Are you sure you want to move here?"

"Yes."

Matt nods and smiles. "We have a few more people scheduled for interviews, so I will contact you with our decision soon."

He pauses for a few seconds, then continues with, "Are you going home today?"

"Yes, I'm leaving this evening. Is it okay if I use the phone to call a taxi to take me to Newton Center? I'm taking the train home from South Station."

"Someone might be able to give you a ride. Let me check with Yvette. I'll be right back."

A few minutes later, he returns and says, "Jason is leaving for the day. He said he can drop you off at Newton Center on the way home."

He shakes my hand again and I thank him for finding a ride.

Jason, one of the engineers, is as friendly as everyone else I met today. The ten-minute ride from the office to Newton Center flies.

When I return home at ten-thirty, Tom is sitting on the bed watching NY1, the city's twenty-four-hour news channel. Clips from Mayor Rudy Giuliani's press conference earlier that day dominate the TV screen. He holds a press conference every day, regardless of whether he has anything important or newsworthy to say.

Tom glances at me, then back to the TV. "How did it go?" he asks. The tone in his voice makes me wonder whether he really wants to know.

"It went well," I reply. "If they give me an offer, I will accept it."

Tom points the remote control at the TV and pushes the power button. He slides under the covers while the screen fades to black.

His silence speaks volumes. He isn't happy with my answer.

Job Offers

New York City and Washington DC, July-August 2001

Two weeks pass without any news from Matt. I wonder whether he found someone else for the job, but decide to wait another week before following up with him. He seemed sincere when he said he would contact me either way.

While I'm thinking about this, the phone rings. I answer.

"This is Shelly," a pleasant voice says. She shares the name of the company, a consulting firm in Washington, DC. "We received your résumé from Career Builder for our technical writer opening." Would you have a few minutes to talk about the position?"

I remember the name of the company. I applied for the job online the night I was in Newton.

"Sure," I say.

"We work with federal agencies. One of our biggest clients asked us to add a technical writer to our team to document a software product we're developing for them. You have the type of experience we need for this project. Are you still in the job market?"

"Yes."

"I see that you are living in New York. Are you interested in relocating?"

"Yes."

"We do not provide relocation expenses."

"I'm willing to relocate at my own expense."

"We would like to invite you to an interview. Would you have time to travel to our office this week? Our client is eager to fill this position."

We talk about options and set up an interview for the day after tomorrow.

Tom listens to my end of the conversation from the dining room table, where he's reading the *Staten Island Advance* newspaper. After I hang up, he lays the open newspaper on the table and asks, "Who was that?"

"It's someone from a company in Washington, DC. She asked me to come in for an interview on Thursday morning. I'm taking a train there tomorrow and spending the night. I'll be home on Thursday night."

Tom's face brightens, and he smiles at me. His eyes sparkle. "It would be cool if you can get a job there," he says.

Why is he excited about me working in Washington, DC, but he doesn't want me to work in Massachusetts? He should be happy if I get a job in either place, especially because he doesn't have any interest in keeping the pact we made when we moved to the Northeast. At least I'm trying.

We've traveled to Washington, DC twice since we moved to New York. Packing for both trips was nerve-racking because Tom believed someone was watching us and would try to follow us. But as soon as we boarded the Amtrak train at Penn Station, his fear of followers faded and didn't return throughout both trips. I couldn't understand why he became his old self again but didn't ponder on it because I was happy to have the real Tom back again.

Our first trip was in April last year, when we went to the annual cherry blossom festival. When we arrived, the flowers were at their peak. We walked hand-in-hand for miles enjoying the beauty of the trees and the monuments. We toured the Library of Congress and the Capitol Building. We visited as many Smithsonian museums as we could squeeze in. It was a special time, enjoying long walks and each other's company like we did so long ago.

Our next trip was on Independence Day to see the fireworks show at the National Mall. Watching fireworks is among our favorite activities during the holidays. When we lived in Seattle, we could watch the big shows from a viewpoint about a half-mile walk from our house. From there, we could see from the Queen Anne neighborhood, north of the Space Needle, as far south as Harbor Island, the industrial district between downtown and our neighborhood in West Seattle.

In Washington, DC, we arrived at the National Mall at noon

with plenty of water and some snacks and found a good viewing spot near the Washington Monument. The temperature was ninety-eight degrees and the humidity high. Although we wore light short-sleeved shirts and shorts, our bodies struggled with the heat because we were still adjusting to the climate in the Northeast. I worried that Tom's fair skin would burn. We continued slathering sunscreen all over his face, neck, arms, and legs while eagerly waiting for sunset and the show at dusk. My skin doesn't burn much because it's darker, but we applied some sunscreen on me just in case. Late that afternoon, Tom held our spot while I looked for a place to get sandwiches and cold sodas to go.

The sun finished its descent at eight-thirty, and the show started a half hour later. From our vantage point, the fireworks flying high and bursting behind the Washington Monument reminded me of a giant sparkler. I thought about another giant sparkler in Seattle, where the fireworks shoot off the Space Needle at midnight when the city greets a new year.

The show lasted a half hour. We left happy, satisfied, and grateful we could celebrate the anniversary of the United States declaring its independence from England at the nation's capital.

I didn't want either trip to end because I feared the real Tom would disappear again as soon as we returned to Staten Island, and that's exactly what happened.

The morning after my interview invitation, Tom rises before me and dresses. When I'm ready to leave, he hugs me, kisses me on the lips, and says, "Good luck." Why didn't he give me an affectionate sendoff when I went to Newton, but he is today? He said he didn't want me to get a job outside New York, but today this doesn't seem to be on his mind.

I spend the night at a Motel 6 in northeast DC. The next day, I call a taxi to give me a ride to the consulting firm at a tall granite building near downtown. I sign in with the receptionist in the lobby. A few minutes later, a woman with short curly light brown hair, dressed in a gray suit with a pencil skirt, white blouse, and black heels, welcomes me.

"I'm Shelly, the Human Resources Manager," she says while we shake hands. She escorts me to a large conference room with a wall of windows overlooking a panorama of the neighboring office buildings and a large oval walnut-stained table surrounded by black leather chairs in the middle of the space.

"Have a seat and make yourself comfortable," she says. "I'll check if my colleague is ready. We will be talking with you today."

She leaves and closes the door. A few minutes later, she returns with a tall man with short dark brown hair who's wearing a gray suit, gray tie, white shirt, and black loafers. He stops at the end of the table.

"This is Dave, our project manager for the work we're doing for the client," Shelly says.

He nods, smiles, and says, "Hello, nice to meet you," while extending his hand for a shake.

The interview lasts an hour and focuses on the project and my preferred process for working on large technical writing projects like theirs. Dave shares the name of the client and describes the software and its functionality. At the end of the interview, he says, "We really like your experience and would like to hire you. We need a decision immediately, because this job requires a low-level security clearance and it can take a few weeks before it's approved. We can start the paperwork while you're here to save some time, if you're interested."

I didn't expect to make a decision now. It seems like a great opportunity, but do I really want to do this?

You need to wait, Charlotte says. *It's too soon.*

Why didn't you tell this to me earlier?

Would you have listened to me?

I don't know. You know how much I need a job.

Sometimes you must wait. Everything will be okay.

How can everything be okay when I have too many bills to pay?

"I'm returning to New York tonight," I say to Shelly and Dave. "Will it be possible to finish the paperwork before I leave?"

"Definitely," Dave says. "We also need you to go to the FBI and get fingerprinted. If you do it there, the screening process will move faster. Our client has a tight deadline."

I want more time to think about this. If I had a choice, I'd accept the job in Newton, but I haven't heard from Matt. Will I hear from him? Now I have an offer, and this job is a good opportunity, too.

"Do you mind if I call my husband? I would like to talk to him before making a decision."

"Sure," Shelly says. She picks up the conference room phone from the center of the table and places it in front of me. "Dial nine plus the number," she says. "When you're done, open the door and we'll return."

Dave and Shelly leave. Dave closes the door behind them.

I dial our number. Tom doesn't answer.

"Hi, Tom," I say to the voicemail. "The company offered me a job, and I'm accepting it. I need to apply for a security clearance, so I'll fill out the paperwork before taking the train home tonight. I'll see you then."

Why didn't you listen to me? Charlotte asks as soon as I hang up.

I don't answer, yet the dread in my heart and the queasiness in my stomach are strong messages that my decision isn't the right one, but I must make the practical, sensible choice—accepting the offer presented to me. Waiting isn't an option. Besides, my nervousness about applying for a security clearance might be affecting how I'm feeling—although I haven't done anything that would show up negatively on a background check, unless the high balances on our credit cards affect the outcome.

I close my eyes and take a few deep breaths before opening the conference room door. Shelly and Dave arrive less than a minute later. They smile at me, but their muscles are tense when Shelly asks, "Well…what did you decide?"

"I'm accepting the position," I say.

Shelly and Dave's bodies relax, and they smile at me.

"Great!" Shelly says. "I will gather the paperwork and return in a few minutes."

After Shelly leaves, Dave shakes my hand again and says, "I'm looking forward to working with you."

I smile at him and nod. I'm afraid if I say, "I'm looking forward to working with you, too," my tone will be flat. Whatever would come out of my mouth would not match the enthusiasm they're looking for.

I arrive on Staten Island at ten o'clock, where Tom is sitting at the end of the dining room table waiting for me. When he sees me at the top of the stairs, he smiles.

"Did you get my voicemail?" I ask, sitting in a chair next to him.

"I did," he replies. "When do you start?"

"I don't know. I have to wait for the security clearance. It could take a few weeks. In the meantime, I need to look for an apartment."

Tom nods and smiles.

"Are you coming with me?" I ask. "You seem excited about this."

"I have to stay here and finish my classes."

"Finish your classes in what? You aren't majoring in anything."

"I have almost enough credits to get a certificate in business management."

This is the first time Tom mentioned a business management certificate. He probably thought it would make me upset, which it does.

"Why do you need a business management certificate when you already have a bachelor's degree in business?" I ask, trying to hold back my anger.

"Getting a certificate from NYU will help me get a job here."

"What you should have done, with all of the money we've spent, is get an MBA."

"I don't want to take the GMAT."

His response confirms why he didn't retake the first CFP exam. He's afraid of failing again. Taking the GMAT obviously scares him, too.

"There are schools where you don't have to take the GMAT, and they're just as good."

"They aren't NYU."

I'm too tired to win this battle tonight, but the time will come. He can't stay in school forever. We can't afford it, not even with my new job.

The next day, I start searching online for one-bedroom apartments in the DC metro area, schedule a few viewing appointments, and buy another train ticket. This time, I will spend a few extra days there to learn more about the area.

My last appointment scores the perfect place—a cozy one-bedroom in a safe, quiet neighborhood with ample natural light and air conditioning near a train station in Maryland for five hundred dollars a month. My commute is a five-minute bus ride to the train station, followed by a thirty-minute commute on the Metro to L'enfant Plaza and a five-minute walk to the client's office.

I sign the lease and start making plans to move. Then I follow-up with Shelly by email to let her know I've found an apartment, when I plan to move in, and to check on the progress of my security clearance. She doesn't respond. Maybe she hasn't heard any updates about the security clearance, so I will check in again next week.

A week later, Matt calls. "We've made a decision," he says. "We are impressed with your qualifications and would like to make an offer. Are you still interested?"

I'm interested but can't back out of my commitment in DC. Charlotte knew Matt would offer his job to me, but I didn't listen to her again.

"Unfortunately, I received another offer," I say. "A consulting firm hired me for a role in Washington, DC. I'm sorry to turn you down, but this offer is also a good opportunity and I couldn't pass it up."

I hear the disappointment in Matt's voice when he congratulates me and wishes me well.

The next day, I call Shelly again. Voicemail greets me after five rings. I leave another message but she doesn't call back. Why isn't she replying?

Another week passes. This time, my call goes directly to voicemail. I hang up and send an email.

I postpone packing, start searching for more openings online, and apply for a few. Four days later, the phone rings and the caller ID displays the name of the consulting firm.

"I'm sorry I haven't replied to your messages," Shelly says. "It has been crazy around here. Do you have a few minutes?"

"I do," I say.

Brace yourself, Charlotte says. *This isn't good news.*

I carry the phone to the dining table and sit.

"I hate to break this news to you, but our client decided that they do not want to add a technical writer to the team. Dave tried to convince them why it's important to have good technical documentation, but the client doesn't have enough money in the budget. Unfortunately, we don't have any more clients who need technical writing services, so we have to let you go."

I can't believe what I'm hearing, but now I understand why I felt uneasy during that interview. Charlotte was warning me. This consulting firm isn't the right place for me.

"I signed a lease in Maryland," I say to Shelly. "Now I have to break it, and that costs a lot of money."

"There are other jobs in the metro area," Shelly says.

That isn't the point. I was moving there for *this* job. I could have had the job in Newton. Now I don't have a job at all.

I reply with, "Thank you for the update." What I really want to say is, *Why didn't you tell me sooner? Why did you string me along? Why did you lie to me?* They never had a job for me. They were confident the client would add a technical writer to the contract, but the deal hadn't been sealed, and now I'm tossed aside like a bag of trash.

Next, I call the apartment management office in Maryland and explain the situation to the agent.

"We have a thirty-day money-back guarantee, and you're within that window," the agent says. "We can terminate the lease and give you a full refund for your deposit and first month's rent. We can take care of the details over the phone so you don't have to make another trip."

After we finish, I send an email to Matt about what happened and end with, "If you hear of any more technical writing openings in the Boston area, I would appreciate the leads."

Tom was at class when Shelly called, so I share the news with him when he returns home. I expect him to be angry, but he doesn't say anything. Maybe he's relieved because I'm not leaving New York after all. This city doesn't want to give me a job, but it doesn't want to let me go, either.

Matt replies two days later. "I am sorry to hear you lost your job," he writes. "We are still interviewing candidates. I will get back to you early next week."

When I interviewed in Newton, Matt said the company is looking for a candidate with the best fit for the company's culture. Almost two months have passed since my interview, and based on his brief message, they're still looking for someone with that perfect fit. They are serious about this.

I continue searching the job boards for openings in the Northeast and apply for a few more while wondering whether Matt will contact me again and what he will say. His reply to my email was on Thursday. Friday and the weekend pass. Monday, Tuesday, Wednesday…nothing from Matt. Thursday morning arrives, and I start to wonder whether I'll hear from him again.

The phone rings a few hours later.

"Hi, Cheryl. It's Matt again. I wanted to check in with you. As I mentioned last week, we were still interviewing candidates for the technical writing position. We finished the interviews this week, and after talking to everyone, we decided that we would like to extend a new offer to you. Are you still available?"

I couldn't contain my excitement. "Yes, I am!"

"We're increasing your salary, and our president approved a moving stipend. It's only two thousand dollars, but I hope it helps."

"It will. Thank you!"

Matt discloses my starting salary, which increased five thousand dollars a year over the original offer.

I accept the new salary.

"When would you like to start?" Matt asks.

"I can start on Monday," I say.

"Are you sure? Don't you need time to move?"

"My husband is staying here. He's a student at NYU. I will find a small place to stay in Massachusetts."

"Okay, if you're sure. If you want to take a couple of weeks to get settled here, we'll understand. We're happy to have you."

"I only need to bring a few things. I will see you on Monday."

When I tell Tom about accepting the job in Newton, he's quiet. We don't talk the rest of the weekend. When I leave to take the train to Boston, I kiss him on the cheek, but he doesn't kiss me back. He watches me descend the stairs from the living room in silence.

I make a reservation for three nights at the YMCA in the Charlestown neighborhood on the east side of Boston. The room assigned to me is like a hotel room, complete with a comfortable bed and private bathroom.

As soon as I settle in, I log onto the Wi-Fi with my laptop and start looking at the classified ads for small apartments. After scanning several ads, the sticker shock sinks in. Even studios near my new job start at fifteen hundred dollars a month, plus a deposit equal to the first and last month's rent. That price is low compared to the other ads I'm reading. I can't afford to pay this much money on rent in Massachusetts plus the rent on our apartment on Staten Island.

It's time for Tom to face reality. Whether he likes it or not, he's moving to Massachusetts.

A couple of days later during a one-on-one meeting with Matt, he asks how the apartment search is going.

"Not well," I say. "Everything is so expensive around here. Are there any affordable neighborhoods you can recommend?"

"Right now, prices are high because of the school rush," he says. "College students are returning. Usually the market calms down in

November."

I can't continue renting the room at the YMCA for two more months. Eighty-five dollars a night add up fast.

"Sounds like my best option is to find a room I can rent on a month-to-month basis and start looking for an apartment again in early November."

"That's what I recommend," Matt says. "If I hear of anything, I will let you know."

I scour the ads for rooms to rent near the T and schedule appointments to see them after work. Most are in questionable neighborhoods, not in good condition, or both. A week passes, then two, and now I'm wondering whether I will find a suitable temporary place until the apartment market cools off.

One day during the commute to the YMCA after work, I see an ad in the free *Metro* paper that looks promising:

MELROSE—Lovely rooms available in a house in a quiet neighborhood within walking distance of the Orange Line. Shared kitchen, living room, and bath. $750/month. All utilities covered. (781) 555-5555

I call as soon as I arrive at the YMCA, and a woman with a mild Boston accent answers.

"It's a beautiful house," she says. "I'm in a neighborhood surrounded by a forest. It's a ten-minute walk from the T, and you can rent month-to-month."

I schedule an appointment the next day after work. The scenic walk from the Orange Line passes a lake with maple trees lining its shoreline and continues into a housing development surrounded by the forest the landlord described. The street dead-ends at a cul-de-sac. All the houses are in excellent condition and the yards landscaped immaculately.

The landlord's house is near the end of the street: a rambler with white siding and sky blue trim, with two large picture windows at the right of the main entrance and on the north side. Trees across the street reflect in a smaller window left of the main entrance.

I climb the three steps to the landing and knock on the door. A woman with loose light brown curls wearing a blue jogging suit and matching slippers opens it. She smiles at me.

"You must be Cheryl," she says.

"I am. Are you Sylvia?"

"I am." She pulls the door wider and stands back. "Come on in."

As soon as I enter, I notice a narrow walkway through the living room formed by piles of boxes, topped with stacks of magazines and newspapers. We follow the walkway and stop at the entryway from the living room to the dining room. The dining room table is filled with neat stacks of magazines. When I turn around and look at the living room, most of it is filled with boxes and piles of newspapers, all neatly stacked. The only exposed space is a narrow path from the dining room to the couch and another short path from the couch to the TV, where the Channel 5 news anchors from Boston are talking but I can't hear them. Sylvia probably muted the TV before she answered the door.

Sylvia notices me scanning the piles and says, "I've been sorting this stuff. It will be gone soon."

She motions toward a hallway covered in low-pile, forest green carpet. "The rooms are this way."

On the way, we stop at the shared bathroom. It's immaculate with matching beige tiles on the floor and walls. The color of the toilet bowl, countertop, sink, and tub matches the tiles. A light blue shower curtain with a white liner hangs over the tub.

"Nice bathroom," I say.

"I have two rooms for rent," Sylvia says as we resume our walk. "You're the first person who answered the ad, so you have first choice."

Two closed walnut doors are at the end of the hallway. Sylvia opens the door on the left to a room that looks like it's from a furniture catalog. The bed is perfectly made with a cream-colored spread with a tiny pink flower print and forest green trim. Two pillows covered in shams matching the bedspread rest against a walnut headboard. The nightstand and rocking chair match the headboard. A closet extends the width of one wall. Low-pile, forest green carpet covers the floor.

"This is the smallest room," she says.

We walk into the other room, which is probably a master bedroom. The décor matches the other room.

"These rooms are beautiful," I say.

"Thank you," Sylvia says. "I'm an interior designer."

"Do you live here?" I ask.

"I'm using the basement. I remodeled it recently."

Maybe she's renting these rooms to recoup the cost of renovating her basement, but I don't ask. I don't need to know.

The lack of clutter in these rooms, compared to the living and dining rooms, puzzles me. Why would she have so much stuff piled up there and the other rooms could be showcases in a department store? Maybe she moved the stuff upstairs during the remodel and needs to sort through it, but that seems like a lot of work. Wouldn't it have been easier to do it while removing it from the basement instead of stacking it in the living room and dining room?

She said the stacks are only temporary. I can cope with it because I won't spend much time here. It's a comfortable, safe place where I can sleep. This will work until I can move into an apartment closer to the office.

"I'll take this room," I say.

Sylvia smiled. "Great! You can move in anytime. I don't need a deposit. You can write a check for the first month's rent tonight and move in tomorrow if you want."

"Sounds great."

We return to the sofa, and I write the check and hand it to her. She gives me a receipt, the login information for the Wi-Fi, and the house key.

"Feel free to use the kitchen whenever you want," she says.

"Thank you. I'll be back after work tomorrow," I say.

When I return the next evening, Sylvia isn't there. The TV is still on in the living room, muted. After I unpack my suitcase and backpack in the master bedroom, I turn on my laptop and connect to the Wi-Fi. I ate dinner at a pub near Haymarket, my connection point from the Green Line to the Orange Line, and will continue eating out for a couple of nights, then check out the kitchen before going grocery shopping this weekend.

Before I start working on my indexing project for a publisher in Indianapolis, I call Tom. I haven't told him about the new place yet.

When he answers, his voice is pleasant. "How was your day?" he asks.

"It went well," I say. "I'm working on an airflow controls guide for our laboratory research customers. We'll distribute it when we have booths at trade shows."

"Sounds interesting," he says. The tone of his voice sounds like he really means it.

"I have some news. I found a room to rent in a nice neighborhood and moved in tonight. I'm staying here until the rental market cools off. It's seven-fifty a month."

"How long will you stay there?"

"Probably two or three months. That's when prices should stabilize enough so I can find an affordable apartment close to work."

"Sounds like a good plan."

I wasn't expecting that response. Is Tom warming to the idea of living in Massachusetts?

I hesitate before asking, "How did your day go?" Maybe that question is benign enough so he doesn't believe I'm snooping.

"Good," he says. "It's a nice day here, so I went on a long walk."

"It's nice here, too. How's Tiger and TC?"

"Tiger is asleep on the bed, and TC is watching the birds from the top of the scratching post. Are you coming home this weekend?"

"Not this weekend. I need to finish an indexing project and go grocery shopping. I will see you next weekend. Speaking of that project, I need to go and work on it. Love you."

"Love you too," Tom says. I haven't heard him say those words for a long time. Why this shift today? Is my real husband back again?

When we hang up, I'm happy and relieved that we had a stress-free conversation. Has Tom decided that my decision to work here is a good one?

Three days pass, and every time I return to my room, I'm the only one in the house. I wonder what happened to Sylvia. I never hear her in the basement when I'm here. Is she staying somewhere else? The piles in the living room and dining room remain untouched. The TV is still on, muted, and I wonder if she keeps it on to make it look like someone is always at home.

Out of curiosity, I look closer at the stacks but don't touch anything. Box lids cracked open on top of some of the stacks reveal random items from cups to knick-knacks. There are also piles of newspapers tied in bundles. A thought briefly crosses my mind that Sylvia might be a hoarder. I've never met one, but I learned about hoarding during a psychology class in college.

On Saturday morning, I explore the kitchen. The color of the kitchen floor and counters match the bathroom, but the counters are packed full of boxes and stacks of magazines. The sink and stove are clear and clean, as is the kitchen floor.

Then I look through the cupboards to see how much space I have for groceries. They're packed with dishes, cups, and glasses.

There's no space to make room for anything—not even a toothpick.

My final stop is the refrigerator. When I open the door, a putrid odor greets me. I peek inside and see rotten vegetables and fruit, a chunk of cheese covered in a thick layer of mold, and a pint of milk with a sell-by date of two years ago. There's no way I'm trying to clean up this mess. I'll buy non-perishable healthy snacks to eat in my room after work. In the morning, I can pick up something for breakfast on the way to the office and grab lunch in the café in the office building downstairs or in the neighborhood.

This is only temporary. After enduring Tom's lock and chain around the refrigerator for months, I can survive in a hoarder's house until I can rent an apartment. I'm trading one form of abnormal for another until I can find a way to have a normal life again.

The September 11 Attacks
Massachusetts and New York, September-November 2001

Today is September 11, 2001, and I'm standing at the bus stop at six-thirty in the morning, waiting for my ride to the office and looking forward to my day. Yesterday started my fourth week at the company in Newton, and although I'm spending most of the week two hundred fifty miles away from Tom, I'm enjoying the extra time alone. I miss him but not what he has become, and the longer I'm away from him, I wonder whether my hopes of returning to the normal, happy life we shared in Seattle are simply a dream. Sometimes I ask Charlotte about this, but she never shares her insights.

This job is perfect for me. Because I work in the marketing department, my projects cover the gamut and I love the variety. I'm mostly editing and writing marketing materials so far, but Matt says when the upgraded system is closer to release, I will start updating the technical documentation.

I've never worked in the airflow controls industry, so I'm learning a lot. My love of learning is what attracted me to studying journalism in college and steered my career toward technical writing.

Matt is a kind, genuine person, who respects everyone as individuals regardless of their job titles. He treats his employees fairly and spends time getting to know us on a personal level. During a meeting with him in his office about a week after I started, he invited me to dinner at his house with his wife and family.

"Please bring Tom if you can," he said. "We would love to meet him."

I politely declined. I didn't feel comfortable introducing Tom to Matt, out of fear that Tom would be suspicious—either because he would think I'm plotting a conspiracy against him with my new boss and wife, or he would be ambushed at dinner. Even if I felt comfortable bringing Tom, he still wouldn't want to go, and it would feel awkward if I went alone.

When we both worked full-time, Tom never wanted to mix business and personal activities. The only time he broke this rule was when my supervisor from my first technical writing job invited us to The Metropolitan, a fancy restaurant in downtown Seattle, for Christmas dinner with his wife, the other coworkers from our department, and their spouses. We enjoyed ourselves, but Tom never wanted to repeat the experience. He never explained why, and I didn't ask. I believe this comes from his sales training, where he didn't want to show favoritism to some people over others in a professional setting.

While I wait for the bus, I try to forget about Tom's behavior. The weather this morning is perfect: sunny and in the low sixties, with a gentle breeze tickling the maple leaves. They'll change colors soon, and I imagine what they'll look like. This will be my first fall season in New England, and I'm looking forward to it. I've heard stories about how beautiful the fall colors are here—so beautiful that people travel here from all over the world to admire them.

It's a peaceful morning, and I want it to last forever. I want Tom's paranoia to stop so we can share peaceful mornings, afternoons, and evenings together forever.

An hour after the bus drops me off at the office, I go to the graphic designer's desk to talk about drawing some pictures for a marketing booklet I'm updating. Patty doesn't hear me walk up behind her because she's searching for something online. The site she wants to read won't display on her screen. She types the web address into her browser again, and the same message displays: "404 – Page not found." She sighs and shakes her head, and her straight short blonde hair waves with the movement.

"What's going on?" I ask.

"My boyfriend just called," she says while staring at the screen, tapping keys and pressing buttons on the mouse. "He said two planes just hit the World Trade Center. I'm trying to find some information about it."

"What?"

Patty looks at me with her greenish-blue eyes, her creamy face solemn. "It's true…no joke. He's at home, watching the news. Two passenger jets flew into the World Trade Center and exploded. The towers are on fire."

She resumes searching for websites with updates about the crashes while I watch over her shoulder and slowly process the news. My mind struggles to accept this news is true.

None of the sites Patty tries to launch respond because of the heavy traffic.

Then the phone rings at my desk. Tom is on the line.

"I'm okay," he says as soon as I pick up. No *hi, how are you?* Just *I'm okay.*

Of course he should be okay, I think. *He should be at home at our apartment on Staten Island!*

"Where are you?" I ask, expecting no reply from him.

"I'm at Battery Park," he says. "Two planes hit the World Trade Center. The top of the towers are on fire. The police have barricades set up and won't allow us to go anywhere."

I'm surprised he revealed his location. Is he distracted from what's going on there?

"We just heard about it here," I say. "We're trying to find more information online, but the sites keep crashing from the heavy traffic."

"We can see the smoke from here," Tom says. Battery Park is one-half mile south of the World Trade Center.

I can't hear any background noise on Tom's end of the line. It's quiet…eerily quiet. If he's in Manhattan, where are all the usual sirens, honking horns, and people rushing and yelling when there's an emergency? I wonder whether he's really there, but why would he say he's there if he isn't? He might believe someone tapped into our call and he doesn't want them to know where he really is.

"I took the ferry to Manhattan and stopped at the barber shop next door to the ferry terminal to get a haircut," he says. "When I left, the towers were on fire, and someone said that two planes struck the buildings. The police told us to go to Battery Park and wait."

He pauses and the strange silence returns. Then he says, "I was on my way to a workshop in one of the towers and decided to get a haircut at the last minute."

This is the most information Tom has shared on his whereabouts in weeks. He doesn't seem worried about anyone spying on him today, so I conclude he's being honest with me.

"That haircut probably saved your life," I say. If he went straight to his workshop, he would have been inside one of the buildings when the planes struck. That thought frightens me.

The strange silence lingers. Maybe it's so quiet because the roads are closed and all the emergency crews are at the World Trade Center, but from Tom's location, I should at least hear faint sounds of sirens from fire trucks and ambulances in the background.

"Is the ferry running?" I ask. "Can you go home?"

"It's still running, but they're talking about shutting it down," Tom says.

"Please take the next one home."

"Okay."

"And call me when you're home."

"Bye," he says and hangs up.

Hopefully Tom will call me when he's home. I never know what he will do or when his paranoia will flare up. If he decides someone is following him or I'm interfering, he won't contact me. And if I call, he won't answer the phone. But what if he can't come home? With the chaos unfolding at the World Trade Center, the police might stop anyone from leaving and entering Manhattan.

The phone on my desk rings again. This time, it's Matt.

"Hi, Cheryl. I'm just checking on how you're doing. "Have you heard from Tom?"

"Yes, he just called," I say. "He's in Manhattan at Battery Park. He stopped at a barber shop next door to the ferry terminal to get a haircut on his way to the World Trade Center. That's when the planes hit."

"I'm glad he didn't make it there and he's okay. I've been thinking about him."

"Thank you, Matt. I appreciate it."

Matt's comments touch me. No one else I've worked for would have taken the time to call and ask about our well-being at a terrible time like this. His gesture makes me more grateful to have a manager like him.

While we talk, I hear people rushing in the background and muffled announcements over a public address system.

"Where are you?" I ask.

"I'm at Logan. I was booked on a flight to New York this

morning, but it was canceled."

"I'm glad you're okay."

"So am I." He pauses, then continues with, "I need to make a few more calls. I'll be back in the office this afternoon. We'll catch up then."

After our conversation ends, my thoughts shift to Tom again. Where is he? Is he really on his way home? I start searching the web for any news about the plane strikes, but the sites continue crashing.

I return to Patty's desk. "Did you find anything?"

"Not online," she says. "My boyfriend called again and said two more jets crashed—one into the Pentagon and another in a field in Pennsylvania. The authorities believe terrorists hijacked the planes."

"Wow, this is hard to believe, even though it's really happening."

"Yeah, it's scary."

Here we are in a small office building in a quiet neighborhood ten miles west of Boston, where we now feel unsafe and disoriented in a world that's suddenly out of control. The bits of news that manage to penetrate our bubble are like the beginning of a horror movie. What else will happen today, tomorrow, or days or weeks from now? No one knows, which adds to the cloud of fear that envelops us. Everyone is hunkered in their cubicles and offices, deep in their thoughts, trying to contact family, and desperately searching online for more developments. All meetings today have been canceled.

At noon, I take a break in the kitchen. Jesse, one of our two IT people, sets up a TV at one end of the dining area and tunes it to WHDH, Channel 7 in Boston, for updates on the attacks. A few minutes after I sit at a table, a video clip shows both towers collapsing, steel and stone buckling, sinking, and crumbling into a giant dust cloud rising from the ground.

Panic rises inside me. My mind freezes while my body stiffens, then weakens into putty. If I weren't sitting, I'd fall on the floor.

I'm thankful that Tom didn't show up for his workshop in the towers, but I have not heard from him since nine-thirty this morning. Where is he? Is he all right?

I return to my desk and call Tom's cell number. "All circuits are busy," a recorded voice says. "Please try again later."

That's when I remember that some of the cell towers routing phone traffic were on top of the World Trade Center. The lines still working are jammed from people checking on their loved ones. I try calling every ten to fifteen minutes but continue getting the "circuits are busy" message.

I log into my personal email in case Tom sent a message there. Nothing from him, but I see messages from my former coworkers in New York City. Our former administrative assistant started the thread and so far, twenty of the thirty people she contacted sent replies. None made it to Manhattan today. Some are on vacation, others started their commute into the city but the trains shut down before they could arrive, and two people called in sick. One person writes that a former colleague from another job works near the World Trade Center. His colleague was at the office when the planes hit and saw several people jump from the towers when they were trapped and discovered there was no other way out. I try to imagine how this person feels after watching these victims fall to their deaths but can't. Nothing could prepare anyone for coping with such horror.

I think back on the monthly fire drills when I worked in Lower Manhattan. Every time we reported to our assigned stations, the firefighters who led the drills told us if there was a real fire, we couldn't use the elevators. We must take the stairs. But in our building, the doors to the stairwells were locked from the inside. That meant that if we tried to take the stairs from one floor to another, we would be trapped in the stairwell. There was no other way out.

One day during a drill, one of my coworkers asked, "Will the doors to the stairwells be unlocked if there is a fire?"

The firefighter couldn't answer his question.

I wonder if this is why so many people in the World Trade Center couldn't escape through the stairwells today. Since the doors were locked in the twelve-story building where I worked, they're probably locked in the other office buildings in Manhattan for security reasons. A measure designed as protection from intruders created a death trap.

While I read these messages, more former coworkers reply and say they're safe and unharmed. I reply that I'm now working outside Boston and am safe at the office. I'm grateful and relieved my former coworkers weren't harmed today. Fate steered them away from danger.

At two o'clock, Tom calls again. "I took the last ferry from Manhattan," he says. "It left at one-thirty. They're not saying when it will run again."

"I'm glad you're home. Please be careful."

That night after work, I listen to NPR on my alarm clock radio. I hope to hear new information about what happened and whether the emergency crews found any more survivors. I return every night, desperate for sound bites of good news or updates on what caused this tragedy, but the same information repeats with different spins and analyses about the destruction in New York City, the Pentagon, and the crash in a field near Shanksville, Pennsylvania. I continue listening until my body insists it's time for bed.

Somehow I manage to sleep well after silencing the radio, most likely from mental exhaustion caused by this tragedy and the ongoing unpredictability of my life—Tom's roller-coaster behavior, my juggling act to keep our bills under control, and the upcoming battle to force him to move to Massachusetts. The only stable part of my life is my job, although I'm a new employee. This company has low turnover. I haven't met anyone yet who has worked there less than five years. Tom still isn't happy I moved to Massachusetts, but I need to do what's best to help us survive financially and for my career. I'm grateful for having this job after turning it down the first time.

But something must give. My patience stretches longer than most people, but eventually the band will break. What will happen then, I don't know. I've dedicated almost four years of my life supporting Tom in a career change that's going nowhere. I've grabbed the reins of our marriage and am holding on, but I don't know how to steer the horse.

Tom's reactions to the September eleventh aftermath are unusual. When the police shuts down Staten Island in response to tips about suspicious characters or activities, he's excited about the news and calls me to share it. He acts like a child having fun at a carnival. If I were there, I would have been scared and felt trapped. Why would someone react this way to such a destructive, senseless, horrifying event that destroyed thousands of people's lives?

I recall our trip to Manhattan a week after the crashes, during the first weekend ferry service resumed from Staten Island to Lower Manhattan. Most of Lower Manhattan was off-limits. The public could walk only in designated areas, roped-off walkways set up by the police that reminded me of the experiments from my Psychology 201 class, where I trained a white rat named Burrito to find his way through a maze for a treat—except here, there weren't any treats. Lower Manhattan was covered in a thick layer of ash and dirt, where water trucks roamed twenty-four hours a day, spraying the streets to subdue the dust clouds. The smoky air smelled like the remnants of a giant electrical fire, stung our eyes, and made us cough. When the wind blew in our direction, we could smell the smoke on Staten Island.

We walked as close as we could to the site of the towers, now called Ground Zero. The walkways gave us a view of the site, about two blocks away through the skyscraper tunnels. The rubble was up to six stories high in spots—piles of mangled steel, stone, broken glass, and dirt. Like the others who stood there and stared at the destruction, we were numb. Some people snapped pictures, while others managed to mutter, "Oh, my God," or "I can't believe this."

We stood there in silence for almost an hour, staring at the scene before returning to the ferry terminal. We didn't talk during our walk or even during the thirty-five-minute ride to Staten Island. We sat in silence throughout the short taxi ride from the ferry terminal to our apartment. And we didn't talk much the rest of the day, and when we did, we said nothing about the towers.

On Staten Island, we're constantly reminded of what happened, because we can see the smoke from the fires from our living room and kitchen windows. At the Catholic church across the street, the funerals are non-stop during daylight hours. As soon as a half dozen pallbearers carry a casket outside and load it into a hearse, another funeral starts. Barges cross the harbor every hour, escorted by bright orange NYPD rafts, carrying rubble from Ground Zero to the Fresh Kills Landfill. That's where workers sift through the debris to find evidence and body parts. Watching these scenes when I'm here on the weekends is mind-numbing.

After Tom's unusual behavior wears off a month later, his obsessions about the invisible people snooping on him and trying to contaminate him return stronger than ever. Now, he calls me at the office at least three times a week, starting the conversation with, "Someone broke into the apartment again today." Then he would add that either someone took something or moved things around.

"What's missing?" or "What did they move?" I ask, depending on which version of the report Tom delivers. He never answers either question.

After a week of these calls, he adds a request: "I want you to call the management office and tell them that someone broke in."

There are three problems with this: First, I'm not there, so if I call, the caller ID at the management office will display my number from an area code outside New York City. Second, if there really was a break-in, Tom should call the police and file a report. The police probably won't do anything because Tom has no evidence of a break-in. Third, I can't fill in any details if anyone wants a report, because I never saw what happened.

Hasn't Tom thought about this? No, he can't in his irrational mind. And now he wants to push me deeper into this unbelievable tale.

The first time he asks me to do this, I ask, "Have you called the police? If someone broke in, you need to file a report."

He doesn't reply, so then I ask, "Did you call the management office?"

I hear a few seconds of silence on the line before he says, "They won't believe me."

"If they won't believe you, then why would they believe me? How do you know they won't believe you?"

"I called and they won't do anything. It's because they're involved."

"When did you call? And how do you know they broke in? The only time they would come in is to fix something, and we'd have to give them permission to enter."

"I want you to call them."

I wonder how many times he called the office already, or whether he called them at all. I doubt he called them, because he usually delegates the phone calls to me.

To diffuse the situation, I say, "Okay." After Tom hangs up, I return to work and push our conversation from my mind.

An hour later, he calls again to say no one responded, to which I reply, "There's nothing they can do."

"You helped them break in!" Tom shouts.

"I can hear you. You don't have to yell at me. And, no, I didn't help anyone break in. They weren't there. No one was. If anyone was there, you could tell me what was missing or moved."

"You know who did it. You told them when I'd be out today."

"How can I know where you're going, when I'm working in an

office two hundred fifty miles away? You never tell me your plans. How do you think I feel when you blame me for things I'm not doing? Why would you believe I'd do something to hurt you? The person being hurt here is me."

"I have to go," he says and hangs up.

Tom stops asking me to make these calls a month later. I don't know if it's because he figured out I wasn't doing it or whatever prompted him to ask was replaced with another obsession. I never ask. I don't want to know, and he probably wouldn't tell me. I'm tired of fighting these battles. When will the real Tom return?

The Hit and Run

Massachusetts and Staten Island, November 2001-February 2002

Matt was right about the rental market relaxing in November. Early that month, I find a one-bedroom apartment for thirteen hundred dollars a month on the bottom floor of a five-story brownstone built in the 1920s on Commonwealth Avenue, two blocks from Boston College in Brighton. The locals' nickname for the street is "Comm Ave."

The commute on the T, with a connection to a bus, is a half hour each way. If I drive, it's ten minutes. I don't drive very often because parking is hard to find in the neighborhood without a permit, and I can't get a permit because our car doesn't have a Massachusetts plate. Tom wants to keep the car on Staten Island. Sometimes he drives here on the weekends, or I will take the train to New York and we'll drive back to Brighton together.

During one of those trips, I bring Tiger and TC. Tiger's glucose levels have been stable since I started my new job, but he still needs regular blood tests to monitor his condition. I found a vet who specializes in cats less than a mile away, which has worked out well.

Tom doesn't comment on the apartment, and the longest he usually stays is three days. Although the apartment has a few quirks, it's a comfortable place to live. The living room and bedroom have hardwood floors, which are an advantage when the dust whips up from the Green Line trolley passing by on Comm Ave every fifteen minutes to a half hour from five in the morning until midnight. They're easy to clean with a dust mop, but as soon as the dust settles from another passing trolley, the floor is dirty again.

The kitchen is double the size of our kitchen on Staten Island, and its layout is efficient. Linoleum covers the floors of the kitchen and bathroom. Each room is equipped with old-fashioned, accordion-shaped cast-iron steam heaters, which heats the apartment too well at times. When the system cranks up on cold nights, the temperature reaches ninety degrees, so I have to open a window or two to cool off. Tenants can't adjust the heaters.

Since I've moved in here, I've started a subtle campaign to convince Tom to move to Massachusetts. He's interested in Civil War history, so I'm trying to expand his interests into the American Revolution. The more he discovers, the more he will want to know, and what better way to learn than to live where history happened? He became interested in other periods of history during trips to research information for my travel articles when we lived in Seattle. The American Revolution is another point on the timeline with different stories.

Although I'm interested in history in general, my favorite topics to explore are in Northwest history from the mid-1800s through the 1920s. I admire the people who overcame challenges that seemed impossible to survive in rugged, isolated, breathtakingly beautiful country. Maybe what I've learned from their resiliency during my research can help me with my struggles with Tom. Maybe it is already, but I haven't thought about it until now.

Since I've moved to Massachusetts, I've visited the sites along the Freedom Trail in Boston and strolled parts of the famous Battle Road from Lexington to Concord. Immersing myself in these places brings the stories I read in history classes to life.

So, when Tom comes to Brighton on the weekends, I plan trips to these sites to share my experiences with him. After we walk the Battle Road a few times, we gravitate toward his favorite section, a one-mile stretch starting at the Hartwell Tavern. Sometimes the tavern is open for tours, hosted by volunteers dressed in period clothing. Behind the tavern, Minutemen give musket demonstrations. Seeing living history up close sparks Tom's curiosity, and soon he's researching places we can explore when he's here.

The paranoia doesn't follow Tom to Massachusetts. We're free from the intruders while we enjoy walks on the Battle Road, the Freedom Trail, and in Brighton. It's like we're dating again or in the early years of our marriage—walking hand-in-hand, soaking in the scenery, and treasuring our time together, often without words.

Could the absence of Tom's paranoia when he's here be related to being in a new place? I noticed the same pattern after he moved to Staten Island. Or is it because he's in a more relaxed atmosphere? Maybe being apart during the week makes him want to spend quality time with me in the few precious hours we have on the weekends.

Although Tom visits some weekends, I'm traveling back and forth the most by train. I hire a catsitter to check on Tiger and TC while I'm gone. Commuting five hundred miles round-trip most weekends gets tiring. I dread the trips to Staten Island because I never know how bad Tom's moods will be until I arrive.

A month and a half after my move to Brighton, Matt schedules a private meeting with me in his office.

"I have some news to share with you," he says. "I am leaving the company in two weeks to start a new business. I have dreamed of doing this for a long time, and now I have the opportunity to move forward."

This is a surprise and it's hard to know what to say, other than "Congratulations, Matt. I'm sure you will be successful."

"Thank you. I will miss everyone here, but we will probably cross paths when my business gets off the ground. I am still working in the industry."

"What will you be doing?"

"My business will provide commissioning services. With the latest changes in the industry, it's a growing niche."

"It seems like a good market, based on what I've read and learned since I started working here."

Matt nods. "I want to assure you that you'll have excellent support after I leave. Todd is stepping into my role."

I've worked on some small projects with Todd already. He's a kind, patient person who seems to want everyone he works with to be successful. Although I will miss Matt, I look forward to reporting to Todd.

"Yes, he will be a great marketing director," I say. "This will be a good career move for him."

Two weeks later, Tom calls me at the office within minutes after I arrive.

"Someone hit our car this morning," he says.

"What did you say?" I ask. Is this a new delusion? The people who are following him are now slamming into our car?

"I said, *someone hit our car this morning.*"

He's telling the truth, Charlotte says.

I don't want to hear this. I paid off the car loan six months ago. We have a 1996 Honda Accord and take good care of it. It should last many more years. This is not a good time to buy another car.

The apartment complex on Staten Island doesn't have parking for its residents, so we park our cars on the street. I've never felt comfortable about this because drivers often speed along the streets surrounding the buildings. The speed limit is thirty-five miles an hour but often they're traveling fifty, sixty miles or more.

"Did you see what happened?" I ask.

"A black Jeep was speeding down Saint Mark's Place. It slipped on a patch of ice and slammed into the car. It pushed the car on the sidewalk. The grill fell off the front of the Jeep."

"Did the driver stop?"

"No. After hitting the car, the driver sped off and left the grill behind."

"Did you get the license plate number?"

"I couldn't see it from here. All I know is the car is from New Jersey."

"Did you call the insurance company?"

"Not yet, but I will this morning. I took pictures and video of the damage."

When we hang up, I'm drained. I'm struggling with the bills and now this. Hopefully the damage can be repaired, but Tom's description doesn't sound promising.

Then it dawns on me that today is our thirteenth wedding anniversary. *Happy anniversary*, I think. *What a way to celebrate.*

I'm nervous about Tom handling the claim with the insurance company, but I must rely on him. He tends to procrastinate, even when he isn't paranoid. I can't take time off work unless I use paid vacation time, which I don't want to do. I can't afford to take time off without pay, and it's too difficult to get it approved without explaining the situation to Todd. I don't want Todd to know what's going on. Maybe giving Tom this task will distract him from thinking about the people he believes are after him.

It's hard to concentrate on editing the new marketing brochure Todd drafted when my mind wants to focus on the car. If it's a total loss, the insurance company will give us a payout, but it will not be enough to buy another car. The money from our investments and savings is draining fast. It will probably be hard to get another car loan with our escalating credit card debt. My schedule is full, so I can't accept new side projects. Why did this happen now?

Tom calls after lunch. "The claims adjuster left a few minutes ago," he says. "He says the car will probably be a total loss. He'll know more tomorrow. They towed the car to the Honda dealership, where they'll take a closer look at the damage."

"This isn't good news," I say. "We can't afford to buy another car."

"They will give us a check for the car's value," Tom says.

"But how much will that be if the car is totaled? It won't be enough to buy a car—even a good used one."

"We'll manage."

"How? I can't squeeze in any more freelance projects. My salary barely covers our bills. You need to find a job."

I've run out of ways to perform miracles. Unless a truck dumps a load of money on my doorstep, we'll have to manage without a car until we can scrape up enough for a down payment or Tom finds a job.

"We'll manage," Tom says again. "I'll keep you updated. Happy anniversary."

He remembered. He always remembered until we both settled in New York, but then we stopped celebrating. Tonight, I will treat myself to a steak dinner and dessert at the Ground Round near my apartment in Brighton and spend the rest of the evening editing a psychology workbook for a publisher in Boston. I'll stretch out on the futon, lean my back against the wall, and edit the manuscript on my lap.

Tiger and TC will jump on the futon when the mood strikes and either curl up in a corner or lie against my legs—on opposite sides of me, of course, because Tiger doesn't like to cuddle with TC. I'm happy my furry friends will be there to keep me company but am sad that Tom and I will not celebrate our wedding anniversary together again.

The next morning, Tom calls me at the office. "The claims adjuster said the car is a total loss," he says. "The insurance company will evaluate the car's worth and give us a check for the value."

"Could they give an estimate?" I ask.

"No. They won't commit to a number. The adjuster said they'll call me in a few days."

The insurance company settles for eight thousand dollars—more than I expected. When Tom calls with this news, he says, "They left a voicemail. I'm waiting a few days to call back."

"Why?" I ask. "They're ready to issue the check. Call them so we can get the check and start looking for another car." At least we'll have a nice down payment, and we can qualify for a loan to cover the rest—that is, if the lenders don't balk at our credit card balances.

"If I wait, they'll increase the settlement."

"What are you talking about? This isn't a sales negotiation. They won't change their minds. Waiting delays us from getting the check. Please call them so we can wrap this up."

"I will call them," Tom says, but he doesn't say when he'll do it.

Two weeks pass. During that time, I ask Tom several times about following up, but his response is, "I haven't had a chance yet."

"Why not?" I ask. "You can call when you're not in class. You're not taking classes all day, every day."

"How do you know where I am?" he asks. "I knew you were interfering!"

"That's ridiculous! If you don't follow up, I will. This has gone on too long."

"I will call them."

"When?"

"I said I would call them!"

"I will give you one more day. If you don't call them by then, I will."

Tom calls the insurance company the next day to accept the offer. He deposits the check as soon as it arrives in the mail.

The funds from the settlement are spent quickly after the check clears the bank—not on another car, but to cover expenses for the Staten Island apartment and the credit card charges for Tom's classes.

When we get another car, I lease a 2002 Honda CR-V from a dealer in Brighton. I don't want to lease because we're planning to keep the car after the three-year term, but several battles with Tom wears me down. I fill out the application at the dealership without Tom, who refuses to go with me for reasons unknown.

When the accountant handling the paperwork notices Tom hasn't been employed for five years, she asks if I want to include his name on the lease.

"I thought both of our names had to be listed because we're married," I say.

"It isn't necessary. You can lease the car in your own name."

We complete the application without Tom's name on it, I sign it, and the lease is approved. When I tell Tom later, he's furious. My explanation that the application probably wouldn't have been approved if he were included because he wasn't working only accelerated his anger.

My frustration continues to grow about the bottomless money pit. The investment in Tom's education isn't one anymore. He no longer has goals for his career change, and he isn't looking for a job. And, from what little I know, he's taking classes that aren't stretching his skills and knowledge. I can't get any information unless I spot his notes from classes on the table or on the office desk that he forgot to put away before I return to Staten Island on the weekends. No longer do I see textbooks from his classes when I'm there, which means he's either hiding them from me or he isn't attending classes and finishing his assignments. If I confront him, he won't tell me.

I wait for advice from Charlotte, but she's silent. Or she's not ready to reveal it. Or she wants me to figure this out without her help. She's teaching me a lesson because I didn't heed her advice about moving to the Northeast three years ago.

Cheryl Landes

My Revelation

Brighton, Massachusetts, November 2002

Tonight, I sit at the desk in the bedroom of my apartment. Tiger and TC are curled in matching tortoiseshell tabby balls, sleeping on opposite corners of the futon behind me. Outside every five to ten minutes, the Green Line trolley squeaks and rattles on the track in the middle of Comm Ave on the way to either Boston College or downtown Boston. The antique cast-iron steam heaters inside the apartment gurgle when they switch on to ease the chill.

I'm still moonlighting as an indexer and editor, but since the dot-com bust two years ago, editing work is in higher demand. My project tonight is editing a Psychology 101-level workbook that accompanies a textbook about mental illness. Each chapter starts with a summary of a different mental health condition and its symptoms, followed by a case study of a patient. I finish editing the first three chapters and start reading the next one about a topic I experienced first-hand during high school with Bubby, my second stepfather, who was diagnosed with schizophrenia.

"Schizophrenia is a brain disorder that affects a person's view of the world," the summary begins. "People suffering from schizophrenia have an altered perception of reality. Often they have a significant loss of contact with reality. They might see or hear things that don't exist, speak in strange or confusing ways, and believe others are trying to harm them or they're constantly watched. This blurred line between the real and imaginary makes it difficult to carry out the activities of daily life. Often in response, people who have schizophrenia withdraw from the outside world or act out in confusion and fear."

Pay attention to this, Charlotte says.

The Best I Can Do

My mind is focused on editing, so why did she chime in? She should know I'm paying attention to the text.

I ignore her and continue.

"The common symptoms of schizophrenia are delusions, hallucinations, disorganized speech, unpredictable behavior, and so-called 'negative symptoms' like lack of emotional expression, lack of interest or enthusiasm, an apparent lack of interest in the world, and speech difficulties and abnormalities."

Some of these symptoms remind me of Bubby. He didn't care for anyone, except for himself. He had extreme mood swings when he didn't like something or things didn't go his way, and that's when he became violent. When he believed something happened, he blamed Mom, my sister, and me. His outbursts often included verbal lashings, beatings, or both. Mom, my sister, and I lived in constant fear because we never knew what would trigger his bad moods or how violent he would get.

Charlotte returns, saying, *You're on the right track, but you're missing something.*

What are you talking about? I want her to go away so I can meet my deadline, but there's a familiar feeling about this—something not related to my stepdad.

You'll meet your deadline, Charlotte says, *but you need to pay attention to this chapter. Step out of editing mode and read it carefully.*

Now I'm on the defensive. *When I'm in editing mode, I am reading carefully. Why do you say I'm not?*

You can't ignore this. It's important!

I sigh. She's too persistent tonight to leave me alone until I do what she wants, so I shift into reading mode with the next paragraph.

"Schizophrenia can appear suddenly, without warning, in some people, but for most, it develops slowly with subtle warning signs and a gradual decline in functioning long before the first severe episode. Many friends and relatives of people suffering from schizophrenia report knowing early on that something was wrong, but they didn't know what it was."

While I'm reading this paragraph, I'm still thinking about Bubby's behavior, but these words don't match my experiences with him. He was diagnosed long before Mom met and married him. So, why am I recognizing the patterns here?

Keep reading, Charlotte says. *This is not about your stepfather.*

What are you talking about? I don't know anyone else who has schizophrenia.

Yes, you do. Keep reading.

I shake my head and continue.

"John is thirty years old. Six months ago, he was promoted to a manager of a construction company. Soon he began to change by becoming increasingly paranoid and acting out in unusual ways. He became convinced that his boss, the owner of the construction company, was watching him through surveillance bugs planted in the office phones. As John continued to change, he began to believe his coworkers were also 'in on the conspiracy.' Then he started hearing voices telling him to find the bugs and destroy them. When he responded by smashing the phones and screaming that he wasn't going to put up with the 'illegal spying' any more, the frightened owner called the police, and John was hospitalized."

I stop reading and stare at the page with a new, distressing awareness: John is Tom!

In my struggle to find answers during the past seven years, I've overlooked the truth clearly in front of me: Tom has lost touch with reality. Two years before he was laid off from his job, he began fearing that people were following him. After his layoff, he gave up on his career change when the job search became tough and morphed into a professional student to escape. The more he tries to escape, the more his fears manifest into a larger conspiracy, where the followers bug our home and send someone to watch him by driving around our neighborhood. He believes I share his daily schedule with other people, although he keeps his activities secret. And Tiger's need for insulin shots to treat his diabetes triggered Tom's belief that someone is contaminating him with a clear substance he can't smell.

How did I miss this? I minored in psychology in college, and I didn't recognize Tom's symptoms of paranoid schizophrenia! Because his symptoms grew over time, I couldn't identify them. We're like frogs in a cold pot of water on the stove who don't know we're being boiled alive until it's too late. This is why I couldn't spot the pattern, the warnings that he's slipping deeper into mental illness.

That water is bubbling in our lives, and if I can't cool it down, the pot will boil over. Has it boiled over already? I don't know. My mind is in panic mode.

Our support system, friends and family, is three thousand miles away, and they don't know what's going on. How can I tell them? Who will believe me? I can't believe this, so why should they?

I stare at the study guide while my heart beats faster and ask myself, *What am I going to do?*

The Swans

Massachusetts and New York, Spring 2003

I choose to do nothing. Well, not really *nothing*. I think about options. My top priority is for Tom to move to Massachusetts. If I start talking to him about how serious his paranoia is and how much he needs counseling now, it probably will stop him from moving here. The only way to start easing my financial burden is to end the lease on the apartment on Staten Island.

Although I know what must be done, I'm afraid to talk to Tom about counseling. How will he react? When his paranoia is in control, he often gets angry. The real Tom is a patient, kind person, but his fear from the people following him constantly, listening to his conversations, watching him, or contaminating him makes him defensive. That's when he starts blaming me for being involved. If he's agitated during his delusions, he yells at me, which I don't understand. If he's concerned about someone interfering, wouldn't the yelling attract them to him? They can hear everything he says.

Tom has never been violent; it's not part of his nature. I don't believe he could be now, but at the same time, how do I really know? He isn't the same person I knew before paranoia invaded his life.

While we were dating, I talked to Tom about my experiences with Bubby—how violent he was and the verbal abuse and physical beatings I endured. I ended with, "If any man tries to lay a hand on me again, I will walk away and never come back." I don't know why I said that. I never thought Tom would hit me or treat me badly in other ways.

Tom listened to me quietly and gently held my hands. "No one should treat another person that way," he said. "I'm so sorry you had to go through this." Then he wrapped his arms around me and held me gently for a long time.

Does he remember this conversation now? How much has his paranoia clouded his memories? Will the time come when he forgets I am his wife, his loving partner and best friend? I don't know, and this scares me, too.

Tom knows I want him to move to Massachusetts. I've talked to him about it many times since I started working here. At first, I tried to appeal to his interest in American history. During walks on the Battle Road in Lexington and Concord and the Freedom Trail in Boston, I've slipped the topic into conversations with variations of, "When we're both settled here, we can check out some more historic places. We've barely scratched the surface."

Tom reacts to my comments with either silence or changing the subject to any topic not related to New England, but he hasn't said, "I don't want to talk about it anymore," which makes me hopeful he'll come around. At the same time, I'm feeling my strategy isn't strong enough to win him over. He knows I'm trying to sell something to him that he doesn't want to buy.

Now, I'm playing a card I didn't want to use but probably will be more effective. It's a pitch focusing on another reason he'd like to live here: "You can continue studying at the Harvard Extension School."

He listens but doesn't react, but I can tell he's thinking about it from the curiosity he can't hide in his eyes. I've planted the seed. Now I need to continue nurturing the desire so it sprouts into action.

Last fall, Todd approved funding for me to attend a graduate-level certificate program in educational technologies at the Harvard Extension School, and I'm halfway through it. I didn't know Harvard had an extension school until I found this new program during a web search for courses in instructional design for online learning. My coursework is helping the company develop online courses for our sales representatives and field technicians, which, when our program is fully developed, will substantially reduce travel costs for onsite training. It's also a great skill to add to my résumé, and that's another reason I proposed it to Todd as one of my performance goals. Online training is a new field, and the demand for experienced instructional designers is growing fast.

When I started looking for a new apartment closer to work after the company moved from Newton to Acton late last year, I wanted a one-bedroom in a place where I could easily upgrade to a two-bedroom when we give notice on the apartment on Staten Island. In January, I found the perfect arrangement in Waltham. The complex has one-, two-, and three-bedroom units. It's also in a convenient location—a fifteen-minute commute against the rush-hour traffic flow on Route 2. When I talked to the leasing agent, she said I could upgrade, if needed, before my lease renewal next year with no penalties.

I moved here in March. My one-bedroom is on the ground level of a three-story brick building, overlooking a forest. A creek flows at the edge of the property and connects to a reservoir about a quarter mile away. There's a trail along the stream to the reservoir where I walk after work most days. I look forward to this quiet time to enjoy the outdoors and escape my stressful life, even if it's only for an hour.

The setting is perfect for the cats, too. They have a picture window in the living room where they can watch the birds, squirrels, and any other creatures that pass by.

A week after moving in, I spot a large nest on the bank of the creek, protected by some bushes. It appears to have been here for a long time, but some fresh twigs and leaves are woven into it. I've never seen a nest so large; the closest was a bald eagle's nest at Discovery Park in Seattle. Tom and I hiked the trails in the park often, especially in the spring, when eaglets hatched to a pair of adults who returned every year. This nest was near the top of a bald tree that overlooked the park and Puget Sound—the perfect place for the adults to scout for prey to nourish their young. We spent hours watching the family, sharing a pair of binoculars Tom received during one of the food company's sales campaigns. We loved watching wildlife together, so I'm hoping my discovery at the creek encourages Tom to revive his interest in nature.

When Tom comes to Waltham for a long weekend, I intentionally don't tell him about the nest. He'll probably believe I'm trying to coerce him into a trap for his imaginary adversaries, but at the same time, I hope he explores the creek on his own. Getting outside in nature might help him forget about the stress he's under from the chaos in his mind.

On Monday when I return home from work, he greets me with a kiss on the cheek and says, "Did you know there's a nest on the bank of the creek?"

He went for a walk today! I'm elated.

"I've seen the nest, but it's empty," I reply. "It looks like something is adding fresh twigs and leaves to it—maybe getting ready to use it."

"There are three eggs in the nest, and I saw a pair of swans swimming nearby," he said with excitement in his voice.

"Let's go for another walk and take a look," I say.

He didn't hesitate to join me. We both need this beautiful distraction.

Sure enough, three large eggs are in the middle of the nest. A swan swims in circles a few feet away, keeping an eye on the eggs. Tom and I stand at a safe distance, which allows us to watch but not scare the swan.

We stay for a half hour, immersed in this small world. While we stand there, Tom reaches for my hand and holds it gently. It's peaceful like the days when we watched the eagles in Seattle, sat at viewpoints waiting for brilliant sunsets, admired panoramas at the end of trails, and listened to the gulls and waves at the beach. I don't want this day to end because Tom is back. Is nature rescuing him?

Soon, Tom wants to spend more time in Waltham to see the swans. For his next trip a week later, he's here for an entire week, and each trip afterward grows longer.

When I return home from work every day he's here, he has new reports about the swans—variations of, "They're sitting on the eggs. It looks like they take turns keeping the eggs warm."

Based on his reports, I can tell he's spending a lot of time outside watching them from a safe distance. The wonder and magic of new lives soon to be hatching into the world bring him calm and happiness. The people in his mind have disappeared. He doesn't talk about them anymore. The swans have replaced them.

Every night after work, we take another walk along the trail after work and stop to check on the swans. Then we walk to the end of the trail and watch the sunset over the reservoir. As the sun slides below the horizon, the golden rays reflect on the water and sparkle like tiny stars on the ripples in the current. The water transforms into a kaleidoscope of red, pink, lavender, purple, and navy blue as the sky above matches the colors in brighter hues.

Our romance rekindles. We walk hand in hand along the trail and watch nature with our arms wrapped around each other. I'm treasuring every moment with my real husband.

One late afternoon when I return home from work, he says, "Something happened to one of the eggs. It's cracked and has a hole on one side. The swans are still sitting on the other two eggs."

We check the nest again from our safe distance. The hole in the egg is big enough for a small animal to burrow through, likely to enjoy the yolk as a meal. I mention to this to Tom after we return to the apartment so our voices don't disturb the swans.

"That's probably what happened," he says.

The swans leave the empty egg on one side of the nest while they continue taking turns keeping the other two eggs warm.

Two weeks later, the cygnets hatch—two powder gray puffballs with a head, beak, and webbed feet that are hard to see under their fuzzy feathers. Soon their parents have them in the water, swimming around the nest. As they grow, their fuzz transforms into snowy white feathers.

Tom continues to keep watch over them while I'm at work, and we check on them every day after I'm home. At the same time, the flame of our relationship reignites to the bliss we knew in the Pacific Northwest. Life is good, except for struggling with the bills, but now I'm hopeful that Tom has recovered from his paranoia and will pursue his dreams again. This is the break we desperately need.

The cygnets grow quickly. As the weeks pass, they're swimming longer distances with their parents by their sides. They glide effortlessly, gracefully across the water, just like their parents.

One night, three months later, Tom and I take our usual walk. We hold hands while strolling along the creek and searching for the swans, but they're gone.

"Could they be in the reservoir?" I ask. "The youngsters are probably strong enough to swim there now."

We walk to the end of the trail. In the middle of the reservoir, the changing colors in the water highlight the silhouettes of the four swans. They swim farther away from us, heading toward the setting sun. Deep down, I know we'll never see them again.

Good-bye. I wish you well. Thank you, parents, for allowing us to watch your babies hatch and mature into beautiful beings. Thank you for bringing my husband back to me. Hopefully the gentle breeze delivers my thoughts to them.

We stand at the end of the trail, quietly watching the reservoir until the stars twinkle. We turn around and walk back to the apartment holding hands, immersed in our own thoughts. I miss the swans already, and judging by the downcast look on Tom's face, he does, too.

The next day, Tom packs to return to Staten Island, and I drop him off at the Alewife T station in Cambridge to connect to the Amtrak line from South Station. During the drive, he asks, "Next weekend, will you come to New York?"

"I'll be there late Friday night at the usual time," I reply, looking forward to spending more quality time with him.

When we arrive at the passenger drop-off area, he kisses me and says, "I love you."

"I love you, too."

I watch him enter the station and follow the hallway to the turnstiles until I can't see him anymore.

The loneliness quickly sinks in during my short drive back to Waltham. It feels cold and fractured, like the old slate sidewalks in the Saint George neighborhood where our Staten Island apartment is located. Uneasiness creeps in, too. Something doesn't seem right. Tom's recovery during the weeks the swans hatched and nurtured their young is a miracle, but suddenly I'm worried about what will happen when he returns to Staten Island. Will the intruders find him again? If they do, can Tom fend them off? Is Charlotte warning me that a change is coming?

On Friday night after work, I drive the five hours from Acton to Staten Island, along the usual asphalt trails through Connecticut and White Plains, along I-80 and the New Jersey Turnpike, and across the Goethals Bridge. David Sanborn, Dave Koz, and Brian Culbertson serenade me with smooth jazz instrumentals from the CD player while I anticipate another relaxing weekend with Tom, strolling along the Promenade down the hill from our apartment and taking the ferry to Manhattan for a longer walk in Central Park. I also think about the swans that brought him back to me and wonder where they are now and how they're doing.

Tom is awake when I arrive, and he greets me with a hug and kiss. He seems like his old self. But other things haven't changed, like the chain wrapped around the refrigerator, now secured with a combination lock instead of a padlock. A shoestring is tied on the office door to deter anyone from opening it.

If the people left Tom's mind like I thought they did, why would he still have these barriers?

Tom needs help, Charlotte says. *He needs counseling. The swans were a temporary distraction.*

I don't want to believe her, but she's right. That's why I felt uneasy after he left. The weeks we spent together watching the swans raise their young made him forget about the people following him. Tom loves animals, this was a new experience for him, so while he focused on this beautiful event, his fears faded. When the swans swam away and he returned to Staten Island, the people returned and won't let go. Will they ever let go? Can Tom ever be strong enough to let them go?

I keep my thoughts to myself. I'm disappointed and sad, but nothing I say to Tom will change this. Now I feel lonelier than the day Tom left Waltham.

We don't go anywhere this weekend, except to buy takeout at the tiny Chinese café a block away. Tom doesn't talk much. I can tell from his mood that he's distracted and distraught. I pity him but don't have the strength to talk to him. I pity myself for losing my real husband again.

When I get ready to leave on Sunday afternoon and say goodbye to Tom, he doesn't hug and kiss me. Instead, he says, "I want your keys to the apartment and the gate."

I can't believe what I'm hearing. "Why?"

"Because I don't want you in the apartment anymore when I'm not here."

"How can I do that when I'm working two hundred fifty miles away? This is my apartment, too."

"I don't want you telling them what I'm doing."

What a change in a week. His lack of trust in me is deeper than ever, and I still can't understand what I did to cause this. The farther I drive from Staten Island, the lonelier I feel.

TC is waiting at the door when I arrive in Waltham. I pick him up, using one of my palms as a foundation for his back feet, and he rests his front paws on my shoulder. He softly rubs my check and chin, purring louder with every stroke. I wrap my free arm around him and hold him close for comfort until he's ready to break free, then sit on the couch. After I'm comfortable, TC and Tiger jump on the couch, on opposite sides of me. Tiger kneads my thigh gently, and TC places his front paws on my other thigh and rests his head on his paws.

I stroke both of them, accepting the comfort they give to me while thinking about the dreary trip this weekend. I've lost Tom again, probably forever this time.

The week passes slowly, and I go through the motions of commuting to work, marking off items on my to-do list, driving home, and repeating everything the next day. TC and Tiger sense something is wrong in their catlike ways. They stay close when I'm at home, keeping watch over me as if they think I'm about to shatter into a zillion pieces. Maybe I am, but I'm too stubborn to crumble. I can't give up.

TC jumps on my lap, asking for hugs, while Tiger watches. At night, they sleep on opposite sides of me until dawn. Sometimes when I wake up, I can't move because their weight stretched the covers tightly over me.

Tom calls me at the office on Friday, just before lunch. "Are you coming down this weekend?" he asks.

I'm surprised he asks. "I'm not planning on it," I say.

"I want you to come."

"I didn't think you wanted me there anymore after you took the keys away from me."

"Call me when you're here. I'll let you in."

Before I can reply, he hangs up.

Usually when I drive to Staten Island for the weekend, I pack a bag before going to work so I don't have to backtrack twenty-four miles. I don't want to do it today, either, but I want to know why Tom wants me to come. He won't tell me if I call him back.

Leaving at four o'clock places me in rush-hour traffic, when lines of cars crawl through the toll booths on I-90, the Mass Pike. Then the struggle continues in Hartford, followed by Waterbury at the exit to the mall, which is always the worst. Often I'm stopped in traffic there. By the time I reach southwestern Connecticut, the roads are clear until I'm on the New Jersey Turnpike.

Tonight, the drive is worse. Heavy rain begins pouring north of Hartford, accompanied by thunder and lightning ripping across the sky. Visibility is terrible. I stop at a diner for some comfort food, a garden salad and roast beef dinner.

While waiting for my order, I call Tom. After six rings, the call forwards to voicemail.

"Tom, I'm in Vernon, north of Hartford. A storm is blowing through, and visibility is almost zero. I'm eating dinner at Denny's to wait it out, so I'll be late. Call me when you get this message."

Forty-five minutes later, the rain slows to a shower. Tom hasn't called back. I pay the check and continue the drive.

It's ten-thirty when I arrive in Saint George. Luckily, I find a parking spot in front of the apartment across the street. I look up at the windows to our apartment, where the lights are off and the curtains drawn. I call Tom, no answer.

"Tom, I'm parked outside, across from the apartment," I say to the voicemail.

He doesn't call back. No lights shine in the apartment windows. I don't see him outside, either.

He's here, Charlotte says.

I wait ten minutes and call again. The call goes to voicemail.

"Tom, I'm here. I called ten minutes ago. Please let me in."

I don't want to ask the guard to let me in because he'll charge a fee for not having my key, which will cause a ruckus with Tom if his paranoia is flaring up. It probably is because he's not responding to my calls.

I call again and get the voicemail. "Tom, I'm giving you five more minutes. If you don't come down to let me in, I'm driving back to Waltham."

Five minutes pass. No response, no lights in the apartment.

Go home, Charlotte says. *You've waited long enough. He's not coming.*

Why didn't you tell me sooner? I could be in bed by now, getting a good night's sleep! You know I didn't want to come here this weekend.

When I arrive at home at three-thirty in the morning, I call again. I don't care if I wake him. That's the least punishment he deserves from refusing to let me in after a long drive.

No answer. I leave a voicemail.

"Tom, I'm in Waltham. You didn't answer the phone when I arrived. I called three times and left messages. Why didn't you let me in?"

A few hours later, Tom calls while I'm sitting on the couch, nursing a headache and sipping a cup of coffee with Tiger curled on my lap. I'm astonished I don't have a migraine after my erratic sleep this morning. Lack of sleep can trigger my migraines, too.

"Where are you?" he asks.
"I'm at home," I reply. "Where were you last night?"
"I was here."
"Why didn't you let me in when I called?"
Silence.
"Are you there?" I ask.
"I'm here," Tom replies.
"Why didn't you let me in when I called?"
Still no reply.
"Why aren't you answering my question? If you were at home, why didn't you let me in?"
"I was here," Tom repeats.
"If I drive there again on the weekend and you don't let me in, I'm contacting security. I am not driving five hours only to turn around and come back. After what happened last night, I'm seriously thinking about not driving to Staten Island anymore on the weekends. You can come here."
"I don't want you asking security to let you in," Tom says. "They're not coming into this apartment."
"They wouldn't enter the apartment. They'd only let me in."
"You're not contacting security!"
"Okay, then, I'm not driving there anymore on the weekends. How do I know you won't let me in again?"
"I have to go. I'll call you later."

You made the right decision, Charlotte says. *You need to set some boundaries with him. Staying in Massachusetts on the weekends is a good start.*

"How many boundaries can I set with him until it's too much?" I reply. "If I set too many, will he feel trapped because of his paranoia? If he does, how will he react?"

Tiger looks up at me as if he's asking, "Are you talking to me?"

"I was thinking out loud," I say, rubbing his back and staring into his big green eyes. "But now that you're looking at me, do you have any suggestions?"

He squeezes his eyes, and I feel the vibration from his purring.

"Thank you," I say. "I need all the comfort I can get."

A Reunion with Friends
Seattle, June 2003

Although I understand what's going on with Tom now, I'm still determined not to tell anyone about his mental illness. No one would believe me. They don't see this side of Tom because he doesn't openly show his paranoia around other people.

If Tom's family found out about this, his mother's depression would worsen. When her children are with her or call her, they never talk about anything that could make her sad. One time when she and I were alone during a visit to Coos Bay, she mentioned that she takes antidepressants.

I can't tell Mom, either. She's a compulsive worrier, to the point where she loses sleep when she's focused on bad news that affects her family. So, whenever I write to her, I say everything is going well at work and with Tom's studies. I don't call her because she's on the road a lot with her partner, a long-haul truck driver. Sometimes she calls me when they have a break between loads. If Tom is with me when she calls, I don't answer because I'm afraid he'll get mad if I talk to her about what we're doing.

After I moved to the Northeast, I intentionally did not take any trips to Seattle. I knew if I went there, I would never return, but this changes when I receive an email from the American Society for Indexing (ASI) that its annual indexing conference is scheduled in Vancouver, British Columbia, in June. I ask Todd if the company will pay for the conference and if I can take a few vacation days in Seattle. Because I'm indexing our product manuals, he approves the expense.

I've limited contact with my friends since leaving the Northwest, primarily because I don't know what to write or talk about. I don't want to tell them about Tom's unpredictable behavior and his unsuccessful career change. When we're in contact, our conversations are short because I use email. Talking by phone is too risky because it's easier for them to ask questions, and they'd expect answers. With email, I can control the conversations.

Of all my friends, I miss Lily and Betty the most. As soon as I make travel reservations, I email my schedule to them and ask if we can meet for lunch. They reply the next day, and we set a date and time after the conference. I'm excited that the timing works out. Finally, I can see them in person again and chat like we did before I left Seattle. I can enjoy a nice conversation without talking about Tom. That's because I'm not saying anything about his mental illness. If anyone asks about him, I'll stick with the high-level basics.

We meet at Cutters near Pike Place Market. On the way there, I arrive early to spend some time walking through the market. I stop to rub the pig's nose at the entrance in hopes the legend is true—the action will bring me good luck. I need a lot of it. I take a few more steps inside and stop in front of the Pike Place Fish Market to watch the fishmongers toss salmon from the bins across the counter to wrap for the customers. Sometimes the pink flesh of the salmon shows under the silver skin.

Tom and I loved to stop at this "Flying Fish Place," as we called it, and watch the fishmongers when we lived here. We laughed at their jokes and antics from our view in the crowd of spectators, mostly tourists snapping pictures. A pit forms in my stomach, and I wish the old Tom were here now, laughing with me. But today, I'm smiling at the fishmongers, not laughing. I'm happy to be here but sad, too. Everywhere I look, my beautiful memories of a world that slipped away too soon linger with the fishy smells in the market.

I follow the pathway in the north wing through the market, filled with smaller fish counters and tables with local honey and jam, fresh produce and flowers, and photographs and handmade crafts. Some of our favorite vendors are still here, which rekindle more memories of blissful times browsing the market on Saturday or Sunday mornings years ago and fuel my longing to return to Seattle permanently.

When I emerge from the north entrance facing Cutters a block away, I see two women standing outside the restaurant and recognize them immediately. Betty is slightly shorter than me, wearing her trademark khaki slacks and jacket with a white button-down blouse. The gentle breeze rustles the loose curls in her short light brown hair. Lily's shoulder-length straight dark brown hair, parted in the middle of her head, stays in place from her shelter just inside the alcove. She's wearing a dark blue windbreaker, black slacks, and a blouse with tiny teal flowers on a white background.

"There she is!" Lily points at me when she sees me waiting for the light to change across the street. The three of us wave at each other.

After I cross the street, we hug and squeal like teenage girls, prompting a few stares and glares from passersby. We don't care; we're overjoyed to see each other for the first time in more than three years.

The host seats us at a table with a view of the green space between the restaurant and the market. The sun is out, and people are lying on the grass reading books or leaning on the concrete fence on the west side admiring the view of Elliott Bay and the Olympic Mountains. Others walk along the sidewalk and disappear into the market. The glass skyscrapers along Second and Third Avenues rise in the background.

"It's so good to see you again! It has been too long," I say.

"We've missed you," Betty says.

"Yes," Lily says, "and I've missed our long lunches."

The server stops at our table to take our drink order. When she leaves, we read the menu, and an item catches my eye.

"They still have the green pea salad," I say. "Now I know what I'm getting." Green pea salad and grilled coho salmon. Tom loves this salad, too. When we occasionally treated ourselves to lunch here, we always ordered one apiece. I push the memory aside.

After we order, I ask, "What's been going on? Catch me up."

Lily and Betty look at each other.

"I'll start," Lily says. "Larry and I are remodeling the house. We added a sunroom next to the kitchen. It has a lovely view of the forest and creek at the edge of our yard.

"Larry is still working as a technician at the phone company. He celebrated his fifth anniversary there in November. And, speaking of anniversaries, we just celebrated our twenty-fifth wedding anniversary!"

I wonder if Tom and I will make it to our twenty-fifth anniversary. Our fourteenth anniversary was in January, but we didn't celebrate this year.

"Congratulations!" Betty and I say simultaneously.

"How's Brandon doing?" I ask. Brandon is Lily's son, an only child.

"He's doing well," Lily says. "He started a job at Boeing in January. His engineering degree is paying off already. He graduated from college in December."

"He was always a fantastic networker," I say.

"Yes. He met a recruiter from Boeing during a job fair on campus. The recruiter was impressed with him and offered him a job less than a week after they met. I'm so proud of him."

"Congratulations to Brandon!" I say.

"He has a girlfriend, too," Lily says. "They met during their sophomore year in college and have been dating ever since."

"Any wedding plans yet?" Betty asks.

"Not yet," Lily says. "I think they want to wait until they've worked a little longer."

Lily's words remind me of Tom again. We met in college and waited to marry until we both had full-time jobs. It was too stressful to go to school full-time, work several part-time jobs with different schedules, and nurture a marriage at the same time. I graduated two years before Tom and worked for the State of Oregon in Salem until Tom graduated and started his sales job in Seattle. We married six months after Tom moved to Seattle. There was a time when it seemed like this happened only yesterday, but not anymore. My real husband exists only in my memories.

I don't want to think about this now. I'm here to enjoy precious time with Betty and Lily. Who knows when I can see them again?

"Lily, how's your job going?" I ask.

"I was promoted again in April, my second in the three years I've been there," Lily says. "I loved instructional design, but when the opportunity came to be a project manager, I took it. The company paid for my training and the PMP certification."

"That is huge! I've heard that exam is tough to pass," I say.

"It is but worth the effort."

Our food arrives. While we eat, we watch the view outside. Dark clouds gather, followed by a brief shower. Some people run for cover; others flip their jacket hoods over their heads or open umbrellas and continue strolling or reading as if nothing happened.

Betty chuckles. "Well, now we know who the tourists are," she says.

Lily and I laugh. It feels good to laugh again.

"What's happening with you?" I ask Betty between mouthfuls. The pea salad and salmon are as delicious as I remember. Memories of Tom eating here with me creep in again, but I quickly push them away.

"I decided to semi-retire," Betty says. "I just finished a short part-time contract, writing a policy and procedures guide for a small company. Now, I'm decluttering our house. Rex is retiring from his federal job in five years, when he's eligible to draw his pension. When he retires, I will, too."

"Do you have any big plans for retirement?" I ask.

"We're planning some long bike trips." Betty and Rex started cycling shortly after she, Lily, and I met. They never had children.

Retirement isn't in my future anymore. If we hadn't depleted most of our investments and savings, Tom and I could have comfortably retired at fifty-five. Before Tom's layoff, we talked about traveling during our senior years. Tom wanted to visit Vienna during the Christmas holidays, I wanted to explore Switzerland, and we both wanted to go on a safari in Africa. We wanted to return to England and spend more time there; our fifth anniversary trip whetted our appetites. But Tom's failed career change and deteriorating mental health shattered these dreams. By the time we reach retirement age, will I recognize Tom anymore? I barely recognize him now. Why did mental illness target him? Why is it destroying our lives?

"Tell us about Massachusetts," Betty says. "What's it like living there?"

Stick to the basics, I remind myself. *Tom's mental illness isn't darkening our conversation like the clouds we just saw outside.*

"It's much more relaxed than New York City," I say, "and we have four real seasons. The stories about the fall colors are true. They're the most vibrant I've ever seen. So far, the winters aren't as cold and summers aren't as hot as New York. Maybe it's because New York has so much asphalt.

"I love my job. I'm the only writer at an airflow controls company. My title is technical writer, but I also help with their marketing materials and instructional design. It's great experience, and the people there are wonderful to work with. There's almost no turnover—only one person has left since I started there to start his own company. My position is a new one. Before they hired me, they'd bring in a temp when they needed help with the writing."

"How's Tom's career change going?" Betty asks.

I don't want to answer but can't avoid it. *Stick to the basics. Be brief.*

I opt for "Okay" in the most upbeat tone I can manage.

Immediately, I regret my word choice. I should know better. Betty isn't the type of person who gives up easily, especially when she believes something is wrong.

"What's he doing now?" she asks while Lily watches us. Lily will speak up, too, when she decides the time is right.

"He's in school, working on some certifications."

"Does he have a job?"

"Not yet."

Betty shakes her head. "I don't understand why he doesn't have a job yet. He's been out there for four years. He should have his CFP certification by now."

"He should be working," Lily says, looking at me, then at Betty and back at me. "He can study and work at the same time."

"He had several interviews," I say, "but no offers."

"How long ago?" Betty asks. She's determined to hear the whole story, even if she has to pull it out of me piece by piece. I don't want to talk about this. I want to forget about this and enjoy myself for a day. Only one day. Is that asking for too much?

Stick to the facts. Don't talk about his mental illness. It hasn't been diagnosed yet.

"About two years ago," I reply. "He had several interviews with finance companies and no offers. Then he started looking for another job in sales. He had one interview with a competitor but no offer."

Betty shakes her head again, then leans toward me. "That's too long. Hiring managers don't like that." After our contracts ended, Betty worked in human resources briefly at one company and recruited at an employment agency, so she's familiar with what hiring managers look for in job candidates.

"No, they don't," Lily says. "Hiring managers expect that someone Tom's age will work and go to school at the same time when they're changing careers."

"I think there's more to this story than you're telling us," Betty says. "I know that's harsh, but I'm concerned. Something is wrong."

"I agree," Lily says. "You can tell us. We will listen. That's what friends do. We're here to support each other."

I study my hands folded in my lap while thinking, *I would rather run away instead of continuing this conversation*, but there's no way out. They're waiting for an answer. I live in a bizarre world every day but still don't believe what's happening. How will anyone else? Of all the people I know, Lily and Betty are the most likely to understand what I'm going through. One thing's for certain—they won't stop asking until I tell them the truth. I take a deep breath and hope they don't notice, but they will. They're tuned into every detail, which is why they're successful in their chosen career paths.

"Tom failed the first CFP exam before we left Seattle, and he never tried to retake it. I think he's afraid he will fail it again. He interviewed for several job openings in finance in New York before I moved out there. He had twelve interviews at the last company that called him, which isn't unusual at the finance companies, but after that, he never heard from anyone again. By the time I arrived, he'd stopped looking for a job. He became a professional student. He tried to find another sales position about a year later but gave up after one interview. He's still in New York."

Finally sharing this with my trusted friends is a relief. The concerned expressions on their faces indicate they believe me, which makes me relax a little, but I'm still nervous about where this conversation will lead.

"This isn't good," Betty says. "You can't continue supporting him there when you're working full-time in Massachusetts."

"I'm trying to convince him to move to Massachusetts," I say. "He doesn't want to come. I don't know why. He won't tell me."

"He needs to tell you," Lily says.

"He won't," I say and quickly look away, hoping they don't see my watery eyes. Do I really want to tell them this? I don't know if I can without shedding tears.

Lily notices. "Are you okay?" she asks.

I wipe my eyes, shift my gaze to her, and nod.

"Why won't he?" Betty asks.

I look at my lap, still struggling with an answer. I'm hanging on by wadding my cloth napkin and gripping it for comfort. When I'm able to regain my composure, I say, "It's because he doesn't trust me."

"Why would he not trust you?" Lily asks. "You'd never do anything to betray him."

"He believes I'm interfering in his life. He says people are following him and contaminating him. He says I'm telling these people where he is and what he's doing and helping them with the contamination by using an odorless, colorless substance. The obsession with contamination started after Tiger was diagnosed with diabetes and needed insulin shots."

Betty and Lily stare at me with shocked looks on their faces.

"I don' know what Tom is doing because he won't tell me, and I've never done anything to cause him to lose his trust in me. Sometimes I ask why he doesn't trust me, but he never answers. He looks at me with a blank expression on his face or ignores my question and continues talking about his delusions."

"You need to talk to your doctor about this," Betty says.

Lily nods. "Yes, you do."

"What can she do?" I ask. "I don't understand how my primary care physician can give me advice on this. She doesn't have a background in mental health."

"You need to talk to her," Betty says. "This is serious. She will know what to do. You can't go on like this any longer because you don't know what will happen. It will only get worse."

"Please talk to her," Lily says.

"Okay," I say. I'm not convinced she can do anything, but I won't know until I see her.

"And please keep in touch," Lily says. "We want to know how you are."

"I will. Thank you for listening. I thought no one would believe me if I talked about this, so I've kept it inside. That's why I haven't stayed in touch very well since I left Seattle."

"You're not doing that anymore," Betty says. "If we don't hear from you, I will be calling you."

I smile. "I know you will."

After I return to the hotel in our old West Seattle neighborhood, I sit on the bed and sob. I don't want to leave Seattle tomorrow. I want to stay here and forget about Tom's paranoia. I wish I could call Tom, tell him we're moving home, and he'd return the next day and our old life here could start again. We could live happily ever after in this place we love—or at least I hope Tom still loves it as much as when he wanted to live here after he graduated from college. He refuses to talk about Seattle anymore.

    I regret we left Seattle. Would we have lost so much if we'd stayed? Will we ever regain what we've lost? Maybe my doctor can answer my questions. This is the only reason I can find for boarding my flight to Boston in the morning. Now, I'm counting on her to help me wake up from this never-ending nightmare.

Counseling

Massachusetts, June 2003

The next morning after clearing security at Sea-Tac and finding my gate for the flight to Boston, I call my doctor's office and schedule an appointment. It's in two days.

When I arrive in Waltham, I call Betty to tell her I'm home.

"How was your flight?" she asks.

"Boring, which is great," I say. "I like the new non-stop route Alaska Airlines has from Seattle to Boston. Usually when I fly cross-country, I have to connect somewhere."

"Have you thought more about talking to your doctor?"

"Yes. I scheduled an appointment on Thursday morning before my flight left Sea-Tac, but I still don't know what to tell her."

"Tell her what you told us at lunch."

"I'm afraid she'll think I'm crazy."

"She won't. You can do this."

Betty's right, Charlotte says. *You can do this.*

The morning of my appointment, I'm still struggling over what to say. My mind tries to organize the words during my ride on the T from Cambridge to Boston: *My husband is mentally ill.* But how do I know this? I came to this conclusion from editing a Psychology 101 workbook. Tom hasn't had counseling, so he doesn't have a diagnosis. Could he even get a diagnosis if he went? He won't go to a medical doctor anymore, so convincing him to get counseling isn't likely.

What if my doctor doesn't believe me? I'll be talking to her about Tom's bizarre behavior, which could be fodder for a fiction novel. Lily and Betty claim she will believe me. They were deeply concerned after I opened up about Tom's fears of people following him constantly and contaminating him, and about him not trusting me anymore.

If my doctor doesn't believe me, it will be an tough conversation—as if it isn't tough enough already. My words might convince her that *I* need counseling, not Tom.

I tend to keep my problems to myself. I don't want anyone feeling sorry for me because most people don't want to hear about my troubles or anyone else's. They have their own. My grandparents taught me that it's best to conquer life's problems without relying on others to help. Despite what I learned from them, they were always there to support and protect me until their deaths some thirty years ago, but even now, I often sense they're watching over me. Sometimes it seems Charlotte's advice is coming from them. Could that be possible, an inner voice communicating with spirits? If it is, why do I often resist her? I listened to my grandparents when they were alive.

The medical assistant leads me into an exam room less than five minutes after I arrive. I sit on the hard bed still struggling for words to tell the doctor. At this point, I'll have to speak and hope for the best. I've never felt comfortable with improv.

My doctor, a petite woman with straight, shoulder-length light brown hair, walks in five minutes later. She smiles at me and says, "Hello."

She sits in front of the computer and reads the screen. "According to your chart, you're not due for a follow-up for six months," she says. "How can I help you today?"

"I'm not sure," I say. "I was talking to two of my closest friends a few days ago about something and they suggested that I schedule an appointment to talk to you about it. I don't know if there's anything that can be done about it."

"I will do my best," she says. "What is it?"

"It's my husband. He has become paranoid, and it has been getting worse during the past year. He believes people are following him constantly. A few months ago, he also started claiming that someone is contaminating him."

My doctor watches me with a concerned look on her face.

"His behavior has changed his life completely," I continue. "He has lost interest in everything. It's affecting my life, too, and I don't know what to do about it. I feel like I don't have a life anymore."

"What is your husband's name?" she asks.

"Tom Landes."

My doctor turns to the computer, taps a few keys, and scrolls with the mouse. While she's reading, she says, "He scheduled an appointment with me a month ago. He canceled the day before his appointment and didn't reschedule."

"I wasn't aware of this," I say. "I'm surprised he scheduled an appointment. He hasn't seen a doctor since he was laid off from his job six years ago. I didn't know about the appointment because he doesn't tell me what he's doing anymore. He says I'm communicating his whereabouts with the people he believes are following him."

She shifts her gaze toward me, and I stare into her warm hazel eyes. "I know this sounds strange," I say. "I'm living this, and I can't believe it, either."

"I believe you," she says. "I know it was hard for you to come here today and talk to me about this. What you shared with me isn't good. Your husband needs counseling, and I urge you to talk to him. But I also recommend that you see a counselor. I can give you a referral. It's required by your insurance."

"I don't understand why I should see a counselor when Tom needs help."

"Talking to a counselor will help you, too. Ideally, you can convince Tom to go with you, but even if you go alone, it will make a difference in your mental and physical health. You need to take care of yourself."

I've never thought about counseling benefiting my health. It wouldn't hurt to try it. I could always stop if it doesn't work, but I'm still skeptical until Charlotte breaks in with, *Keep an open mind. She knows what she's doing.*

"I will try it," I say to the doctor.

"Great! There's a counselor I highly recommend near your office. I will send a referral to her, and someone will call you to set up your first appointment. I want you to schedule a follow-up with me in a month. If anything changes before then, please call me."

After returning home, I call Betty. "She believed me," I say, "but she referred me to a counselor. I don't know how that will help, but I agreed to try it."

"I'm glad you did," Betty says, "It will help. A counselor can guide you when you need advice. She can give you comfort and hope."

"I can understand the guiding part, but how can a counselor give me comfort and hope? I spend an hour talking to her and then come home to the same stress and uncertainty. I have to mentally prepare myself every time I go to Staten Island or Tom comes here because I never know what type of mood he'll be in. It hurts so much when he blames me for interfering in his life. What happened to our marriage being a partnership, where we support each other? The first nine years of our marriage, it was perfect. Now it's lopsided. I'm trying to keep everything together, but it feels like everything is falling apart. It's like I'm taking care of a four-year-old child in a forty-eight-year-old body."

"It's daunting," Betty says, "but a counselor can comfort you by reassuring you that you're doing the best you can. This isn't your fault. Whatever caused Tom to change was affected by something he's going through—not anything you've done. I believe his layoff triggered this. He doesn't know how to handle it, and he escaped into his classes. His paranoia is probably his way of rationalizing his career change not going the way he wanted. He's blaming someone else instead of taking responsibility and moving forward."

She pauses. "I hope this didn't come across as trivial. It is serious."

"Maybe this is his way of coping, rationalizing, whatever…but if it is, it has taken over our lives. He's constantly in fear, and I'm the only person he communicates with—except for his brother in Coos Bay occasionally by phone—so he lashes out at me."

"That's another reason he needs to see a counselor. A counselor can help him sort out his feelings and help him to return to a healthy life. Men take job losses harder than women. They identify with their roles more than women. To them, their job is their life."

"I think you're right. I've been through two layoffs and bounced back. It took about three months both times, but I didn't give up, either."

"Have you talked to Tom yet about seeing a counselor?"

"Not yet. My doctor advised me to talk to him about it today, but it isn't the right time."

"Why are you waiting? His condition will only get worse, and it might put you in danger."

"I have to convince him to move to Massachusetts first. I can't continue covering expenses on two apartments. I'm afraid if I talk to him about counseling now, he won't leave Staten Island. Sometimes he seems to like the idea of coming here, but he hasn't committed. We're barely hanging on financially, and I don't know how much longer we can continue surviving on only my income. Most of the money from our savings and investments is gone."

"What are the terms of your lease on Staten Island?"

"We renew every twelve months. Our current lease expires August thirty-first. We'll get the renewal notice on July first."

"That's two weeks away."

"That's when I'm telling Tom that we're not renewing."

"You need to stand firm when you tell him. He'll probably balk."

"Probably, but he has no choice. If he refuses, I'll open a bank account here in my name only and switch the direct deposits of my paychecks. He'll have to figure out another way to pay the rent."

"Wait a minute—does this mean you have joint bank accounts?"

"Doesn't every married couple?"

"Oh, dear, you should have separate accounts. Rex and I have had separate accounts since we married. We agreed to be responsible for certain bills and split the payment for the mortgage. What will you do if everything falls apart?"

"I don't know—take it one step at a time like I've always done. I'm overwhelmed. As soon as I win one battle, there's another one to fight. Often, I don't know which battle to fight first."

"Your counselor can help you with that, too. Please tell her what we talked about today. She needs to hear this."

"I will. Maybe I'm reluctant to see her because I'm so overwhelmed. I've been going through this for so long alone that it doesn't seem possible to get help from anyone."

"You can and you will. And remember, I'm always here. Call me anytime."

Two hours after I arrive at work the next morning, the receptionist at the counselor's office calls. "Our next opening is today at three o'clock," she says. "Usually we don't have an opening for a new patient so soon, but someone rescheduled. Can you make it then?"

Today? Am I really ready for this now?

Go, Charlotte says. *The timing is perfect!*

"Yes," I reply to the receptionist. "I will see you then."

I hope you know what you're doing, I say to Charlotte.

You're doing the right thing, she says. *Thank you for listening to me!*

The counselor's office is on the bottom floor at the back of an office building on Route 2A, with a forest surrounding it in a horseshoe shape. Walking through the back door makes me feel edgy, like I'm sneaking around, doing something suspicious. In a way, I am because I haven't told Tom what I'm doing. Whether I will, I don't know. I don't even know if I'll return after this appointment.

Maybe her office is strategically located here so her patients don't worry about anyone recognizing them in this small town. They can park in a secluded lot and enter and leave her sanctuary privately. So can I.

When I walk through the door, only the receptionist is there. The waiting room is a small inviting area framed by white walls, with a powder gray carpet, matching love seat and four chairs with overstuffed cushions, and an empty white oak coffee table in front of the love seat. I associate gray with depression, but the sunlight from the window casts a comforting glow over the scene. Maybe the intention is to create a neutral setting for the patients, and gray and white are the best colors to achieve this.

After checking in, I barely sink into one of the chairs before the counselor opens the door of her office, steps in front of it, and looks at me. She's dressed in business casual: a white blouse with gray slacks that match the décor. The brightest colors I notice are her brown hair, cut into a bob at jaw level and parted on the left side, and a necklace with alternating light blue and clear glass beads.

"Hello. You must be Cheryl," she says in a friendly, calm voice. "Come in."

I pass in front of her, and she closes the door. Her office décor matches the waiting room, except there's a white oak desk in front of another picture window, a charcoal leather chair behind the desk, and two gray chairs with thick cushions in front of the desk. Ponytail palm trees in cream-colored pots flank the desk. A floor-to-ceiling bookshelf matching her desk reaches across the wall behind the chairs in front of her desk, filled with psychology, medical, and health and wellness books. There's no couch like the therapists' offices in the movies.

"Have a seat," she says, motioning to the chairs in front of her desk.

I sit in the chair closest to the door and stare out the window while she settles in her chair. Vibrant green maples and oaks dominate the view. Watching the gentle breeze brushing the leaves makes me relax a bit, but I'm still nervous about talking to this stranger behind the desk.

She leans forward, looks into my eyes, and asks, "How can I help you today?" Her blue eyes match the beads in her necklace and appear genuinely concerned for me, but her question seems strange to me. Why, as a counselor, would she ask me how she can help? I suppose it's better than asking, *How are you today*, because she already knows something is going on; otherwise, why would I be here?

"My medical doctor referred me," I say. "She thought talking to you would help me with a problem I'm having with my husband."

The counselor leans back in her chair but her eyes stay fixed on mine. "What's your husband's name?"

"Tom."

"Okay, thank you. So, please tell me what's going on."

"I don't know where to start. I'm new at this."

"It's okay. Take your time."

I pause, studying the ponytail palm tree in the pot in front of me, hoping it will give me some clues on where to begin, but there aren't any. I suppose this conversation is the same as talking to my doctor—I need to start somewhere and see where it leads. Will this counselor believe me like my doctor did?

"My husband is extremely paranoid. He believes people are following him all the time and listening to his conversations."

The counselor is frozen in the same position, watching me but not showing any emotions. Is this what she's supposed to do? I don't know how to respond to this.

"When did you start noticing this?" she asks.

"It came and went starting the last two years of his job," I reply. "Then, when he was laid off, it got worse. Now it's out of control."

"How long ago was this?"

"It started eight years ago. He was under a lot of stress in his job then."

"What type of work did he do?"

"He was a sales rep for a *Fortune 500* food company. He was one of their top performers."

The counselor picks up a pen and begins writing on a white

legal pad on her desk. When she's finished, she looks at me again, expressionless, and asks, "Can you describe his behavior? When he's paranoid, what does he do?"

How do I even begin to answer these questions?

Start from the beginning, Charlotte says.

"At first, he briefly talked about someone following him on his sales routes. He couldn't describe who it was, but he referred to the person as a man. His accounts gradually became more frequent and vivid."

I stop, unsure whether I should continue. Not seeing or hearing any reactions from the counselor unnerves me.

She watches me for a few seconds, then says, "Please continue."

"He stopped talking about these people after his layoff. He decided to change careers from sales to finance, which he studied in college. I supported his decision, and he started taking courses to prepare for the tests for the Certified Financial Planner certification. He took the first test but didn't pass."

I pause, expecting her to respond, but she only sits in her chair and watches me.

"As he continued studying to retake the exam, he'd say that when I was at work, he saw someone in an old gold Chevy passing our house at the same time every day. He believed the driver in the car was watching our house. He couldn't describe the driver, except he said it was a man. When I asked why someone would do this, he wouldn't answer. He'd continue with his story, but aside from the color and model of the car and the driver being a man, it was always vague."

I look down at my hands folded in my lap. "It was scary."

The counselor leans back in her chair again. "Why did you feel scared?"

"I couldn't understand it. He was convinced this was happening, but I couldn't see what he saw. I didn't understand why anyone would want to follow him. The more he talked about this, he added that someone bugged our house. Why would anyone be interested in snooping on him, on us, constantly? I concluded that they aren't. No one cares what we're doing. I tried to tell this to Tom, but then he started blaming me for being involved. He stopped trusting me. I've never done anything to cause him to lose his trust in me."

I look up at the counselor again. "Why would I betray the trust of someone I love? I've asked that question to him many times, but he won't answer it."

"Why do you think he doesn't answer?" the counselor asks.

"I believe he knows, deep down, he can trust me, but his mind is clouded with whatever convinces him those people are interfering. If he really doesn't trust me, then why does he talk to me about what he believes these people are doing? My attempts to rationalize this don't make the situation any easier.

"It hurts when he blames me." I choke on those words and quickly look at my lap to stop any tears that try to escape. Somehow I manage to stay in control.

"It's okay to cry if you need to," the counselor says.

"I'm okay," I reply, but I'm not okay. Navigating this counseling experience is tough.

"Did Tom retake the exam?" the counselor asks.

"No. I think he was afraid he would fail it again. Every time a new test was scheduled, he never went."

"What happened to his career change?"

"When this started, we lived in Seattle. To break in, he needed to move to New York City. He went there four years ago, on the promise that he would continue studying for the CFP and pass it. I had signed a one-year contract at Microsoft a few months before he left, so I stayed behind to finish the term. He started looking for entry-level jobs in finance and received some interviews. One looked promising, but after twelve interviews, the company never contacted him again. He gave up and turned into a lifelong student, and he still hasn't tried to retake the CFP exam. He's still living in our apartment on Staten Island, taking classes at New York University, but we're giving notice when we receive the lease renewal next month."

We're definitely not renewing the lease in Staten Island in July. Where did that come from? Maybe talking about this makes me feel more confident about winning the battle I'm expecting over this. Maybe counseling will help me.

"Is he working on a degree?"

"All I know is he finished a certificate in business. I don't know what classes he's taking now. He won't tell me what he's doing because of his lack of trust. This is frustrating for me because I'm trying to support living in two locations on my income and it's not enough."

Now the counselor is writing more notes than watching me.

When she finishes, she asks, "When did you start your job in Massachusetts?"

"August 2001."

"Have you talked to him about getting a job to help you?"

"Countless times. He always has excuses. Either he wants to look for a certain type of job in finance or he blames his inability to get a job on the people he believes are following him. I've begged him to get a job in anything to help cover the rent and utilities. He can't be choosy anymore because he hasn't worked since he was laid off from his sales job in December 1997."

"That must be frustrating for you," the counselor says.

"It is," I say. It's far beyond frustrating now.

"I've stopped talking to him about finding a job because there are so many other things I'm trying to juggle," I continue. "His deteriorating mental state makes everything more challenging, but 'challenging' isn't the best word to describe this. It's overwhelming."

The counselor takes more notes, then says, "We have only a few minutes left today. Based on what I've heard, we have a lot to work through. I would like to schedule sessions twice a month, if that's okay with you. Your insurance will cover them, minus your co-pay."

My co-pays are fifty dollars per session. It's another bill to add to my budget, the budget that's a moving target every month. Whether counseling will be worth the money, I'm still not sure, but today was only the first session. She spent most of the time gathering information from me, which she needs to move forward. It's similar to my research for technical writing projects. If I don't take the time to do this, how do I know what to write about?

"That's fine with me," I say.

"Great. Stop by the front desk, and Samantha will set up your next appointment."

During my drive home, I feel better, despite struggling to get my bearings on the counseling process. It feels good to talk to someone who listens, even though I'm paying her to listen. Whether she will or can give me any advice looms as a question in the back of my mind. If I follow this new journey long enough, maybe it's possible.

It is possible, Charlotte says. *Give her a chance. She will help you find your way.*

I call Betty an hour after returning home.

"How did it go?" she asks.

"Okay, I suppose," I reply. "It felt more like an information-gathering session instead of counseling, but we need to get acquainted so she knows how she can help. She wants to see me twice a month. My insurance will cover the cost, except for a fifty-dollar co-pay."

"Aside from that, how do you feel?"

"A little better, maybe. I'm still trying to process my first hour with her. It's hard to read her—what she's thinking. She isn't emotional; she's like a researcher observing subjects." I think back to the experiments in my psychology class, when I trained Burrito, my rat, to navigate a maze for a treat at the end. He was a quick learner. "When she responds, she asks me questions."

"Like she's guiding you without giving the answers?"

"It seems that way." If only my life were that simple...

Tiger's Grief

Waltham, Massachusetts, July 2003

Today is moving day. It's a short one this time. I've upgraded my lease in Waltham from a one-bedroom to two-bedroom apartment in preparation for Tom's move here. The new apartment, a two-story brick townhouse, is directly above my old one. The building is on a tiny hill and the back of my old apartment is partially underground, so the entrance to the new apartment is around the corner on the opposite side. The living room, kitchen with a dining area, and a half bath are on the bottom floor; two bedrooms and a full bath are upstairs. We'll convert the small bedroom into an office.

While I carry my belongings to the new apartment, Tiger and TC are tucked away in their carriers in a corner of the living room in the old apartment so their curiosity doesn't catapult them into an adventure outside. I don't want to chase them down, or worse yet, they get stuck in a tree.

When I'm finished, I carry them to the new apartment and release them in the living room. After emerging from his cat carrier, TC stretches in a downward dog yoga pose, followed by circling the perimeters of the living room and half bath, sniffing every inch, and disappearing into the kitchen.

I expect Tiger to repeat TC's routine. Instead, he hunches inside his carrier and stares through the open door.

"C'mon, Tiger," I say. "Check out our new home."

He won't budge.

I reach in and gently place my hands on both sides behind his front legs, then ease him out of the carrier. When I let go, he sits on the floor in the middle of the living room, stares at a spot above the window, and meows. He cries, howls, then wails, like a mother grieving over her dead child. I've never heard sounds like these from a cat.

Then Charlotte breaks in with *something bad will happen soon.*

Cheryl Landes

Deaths in the Family
Massachusetts, August-December 2003

Less than a week after the apartment manager on Staten Island sends the lease renewal, Tom drops off his thirty-day written notice at the office. He doesn't complain about the move. He only talks about the move when we're making plans to shuttle the contents of the apartment from New York to Massachusetts.

As soon as we finish moving and unpacking, I learn why Tom changed his mind: My conversations with him about the Harvard Extension School worked. He applies for a business certificate program there and is accepted. He's eligible for financial aid because he registered for two classes per semester, the minimum requirement to qualify. The student loans will cover his tuition, books, and basic living expenses. I'm not happy about owing more money but don't share my opinion with Tom. Maybe he will make some connections who can refer him to job openings.

Every day for the past two weeks, Don has called with news about Tess. Tom talks to him, so I hear only one end of the conversation. Every time Tom hangs up, he says, "Don said he doesn't think Mom will last much longer. She's worse today." Tom never shows any emotion when he talks about this.

Based on some of Tom's replies to the conversations with Don, I'm under the impression Don is trying to persuade Tom to visit Tess again before she dies. We haven't returned to the Oregon Coast since we moved to the Northeast, and Tom never talks about the possibility.

After moving to New York, we bought postcards to send to their parents, who are in separate nursing homes, twice a week. The postcards were a highlight for the residents where Tess stayed. Every time the mail was delivered and she received a postcard, anyone who was able to walk to her room wanted her to read it to them. It was sweet but sad at the same time to think that they probably never received any mail from their families or had any visitors, either.

We continued sending the postcards from Staten Island until I moved to Massachusetts, but Tom hasn't talked about it since then. Because he hasn't sent any cards to them after moving to Massachusetts, I wonder if he stopped after I moved here two years ago.

I ask Tom if he plans to go to Coos Bay. "You should see Tess before something happens."

"No," he says.

"She would like to see you one more time. If you don't go, you will regret it after she's gone."

"I said good-bye to them before I left Seattle." He spent two weeks in Coos Bay before he moved to New York. Before he went, he only said, "I want to spend some time with Mom and Dad before I leave"—never that this was the last time he planned to go there. He was close to his parents, especially Tess. I think about the Psychology 101 workbook describing the symptoms of paranoid schizophrenia, where people who suffer from this condition lose interest in the world. Has Tom lost interest in his family? Often it feels like he's losing interest in me.

A week after this conversation with Tom, the dire news comes. "Don said she probably has less than twenty-four hours left," Tom says as soon as I arrive at home after work that day.

We've expected this day to come for years, but it doesn't make matters easier when the time draws near. Tess has had many health problems that started long before Tom and I met, but she always managed to pull through. Now, at eighty-nine, her body is tired, and it's ready to rest. I try to say a prayer for her—as if I know what praying means anymore. I've prayed for a lot of things since we've moved to the Northeast, but none of my requests are granted. Maybe the higher powers have abandoned us, too. I hope when it's time for Tess to go, at least Don will be with her and she leaves peacefully. I know he will; he visits her three or four times a week and calls her when he can't. Everyone who knows her will remember her fondly, and her spirit will always be in our hearts.

I wish Tom would change his mind about going to Coos Bay to

be with her. He still has time, but it's fading fast.

Tom and I don't talk the rest of the evening. Tess' impending death must be agonizing for him, but he isn't showing it. I retreat to a freelance project in our home office upstairs, and he stays downstairs and watches prime-time crime shows on TV.

The next morning before I leave for the office, I gently place my hand on Tom's shoulder while he lies on the bed with his back facing me and say, "If Don calls you, please call me at the office. I'm taking my paid bereavement time. I get three days off." I'm still hoping he changes his mind about traveling to Oregon.

"Okay," Tom says, before he rolls over and pulls the covers over his head.

This is the first time anyone close to Tom has passed away during his lifetime. Over the years, I've lost great aunts and uncles, my great-grandmother, my grandparents, an uncle (Mom's oldest brother) and his wife, and my sister. In high school, two boys in my class died two weeks apart: one in a motorcycle accident and one by suicide. They were both sixteen.

Waiting for someone to die never gets easier. With Tess, I have mixed feelings. I will miss her, but I don't want her to suffer any longer.

Todd arrives at work a half hour later. After he settles in, I stop at his office and tell him about my mother-in-law. "Take the time you need," he says. "If you want to leave early, that's okay, too."

"I'll wait," I say.

Two hours later, at ten o'clock, Tom calls my office phone. "Don just called," he says. "She's gone."

"I'll see you soon," I say.

On the way home, I wonder how Tom is handling this. When he called, he talked as if it's simply another day.

He's still acting this way when I arrive. I find him wandering around the living room, organizing notes from his classes and recycling papers he no longer needs.

"How's Don?" I ask while visualizing him sitting in his law office, calling Sam, Ron, other family members, and friends with the news. He'll keep himself busy with making arrangements for the funeral and other details related to Tess' death.

"He's okay," Tom says without looking at me. His avoidance of eye contact and continued sorting are clear messages he wants to be left alone, so I go upstairs to write a paper for my class at the Harvard Extension School. In two semesters, I will graduate from the certificate program in educational technologies.

The next two days are the same: Tom tinkers in the living room, and I work in the home office. I want to talk to him, but when I try, he changes the subject.

Since Tom has moved here, I've stopped talking to Betty on the phone because he would accuse me of sharing too much information with her and add her to the list of conspirators. Now I send emails to Betty and Lily once every week or two to let them know I'm okay and for updates on what's happening in their lives.

Don still calls every day. I can hear Tom's end of the conversation from the home office because it's directly above the living room. In every conversation, Don asks Tom to come to the funeral, but Tom says, "No."

A week after Tess' funeral, Tom surprises me with an announcement when I return home from work. "I have an interview tomorrow afternoon," he says.

My heart soars. Finally, he's looking for a job again!

"That's great!" I reply. "What are you interviewing for?"

"I applied for a volunteer position."

"What will you be doing?"

"I can't tell you."

If he's afraid someone is listening, why did he tell me this much? I'm disappointed he isn't interviewing for a paying job, but I'm hopeful the volunteer experience—whatever it is—will help him find work soon.

"I need the car tomorrow to drive to the interview," he says.

"I need it to commute to work," I say. "What time is the interview? Depending on when it is, I can take a longer lunch break and drive you there, or I can leave work early."

"I can't tell you."

"You already said it's tomorrow afternoon. I need the car. The only way I can commute to work is by car. There's no easy way to take public transportation from here to the office."

"I can drive you to work and pick you up."

This is not a good idea, Charlotte says.

I ignore her. He needs to get some recent experience so he has a better chance of finding a job.

"All right," I say. "We need to leave here at seven a.m. I get off work at four."

You're making a mistake!

How can I be making a mistake? He needs this experience.

He shouldn't drive in his condition.

It's too late now to change my mind. It would start another battle, a battle I don't have the energy to fight.

The next morning on the way to the office, Tom drives carefully, which reassures me that Charlotte's warning is a false alarm.

When we arrive, I kiss him on the cheek and say, "Good luck with the interview."

He smiles and drives off.

At the end of my shift, he's waiting in the parking lot.

"How did the interview go?" I ask after sitting in the front passenger seat and fastening the seatbelt.

"Great!" Tom replies. "They offered me the position."

"That's fantastic! What will you be doing?" I didn't expect an answer, but he seems excited about talking about his accomplishment.

"Data analysis for a non-profit near downtown Waltham. I'm working there three mornings a week."

"Which organization?"

We're approaching a two-lane rotary on Route 2 by the penitentiary in Concord with five different roads feeding into it like giant spokes on a wagon wheel. Suddenly, Tom's mood changes.

"Why are you asking?" he asks, his face filled with fear. "You know where it is. They told you."

"Who told me?"

Tom pulls into the rotary from the Route 2 spoke. He doesn't see the car that exited Route 2A a few yards away and is now less than ten feet from us. The driver hits the brakes just in time to miss us, which triggers a series of honking horns from her and the other angry drivers already inside the rotary. Tom doesn't notice.

"What are you doing?" I yell at Tom. "That car almost hit us!"

Tom looks straight ahead and drives as if nothing happened. He's lost in the fog of his delusion, and my words aren't penetrating it. We're sitting only two feet apart, but there's no way I can reach him without grabbing him or the steering wheel, which would make matters worse.

The Best I Can Do

We ride in silence the rest of the way to Waltham. I'm on edge, wondering whether we'll make it. The thought of Tom having an accident never entered my mind before we approached the rotary. This is why Charlotte warned me.

Thankfully, we arrive home safely. When Tom parks in our spot, my muscles relax and I take a deep breath. He doesn't notice.

Inside the apartment, he drops the keys on the coffee table, and I grab them as soon as they land. Tom notices.

"I need the keys," he says.

"No, you don't," I say. "You're not driving the car anymore. You can walk or take a taxi. Waltham Center is only two miles from here."

"I can drive you to work and pick you up."

"No. If that driver hadn't been paying attention at the rotary tonight, you would have caused an accident—a bad accident. You're not driving the car anymore."

"You're doing this because your name is on the lease."

"No. I'm doing it for your safety—and mine."

Tom huffs and stomps upstairs. The bathroom door slams.

I sit on the couch, lean back, and close my eyes. TC jumps on the couch, crawls on my lap, and props his front paws on my chest. He rubs his head on my chin, purring louder with every stroke. I hug him while he continues rubbing.

Good! You've set another boundary, Charlotte says. *You need to set more of them.*

How many do I need? If I set too many, how will he react? I ask a second time. She didn't answer when I asked the first time.

You'll know when the time comes, she replies.

Why can't you tell me now?

This is all you need to know for now. Take one step at a time.

She makes it sound so easy. Can't she see how hard this is?

TC stops rubbing and lays his head on my chest. I rub his head, between his ears, with my chin. He squeezes his eyes in approval, and the volume of his purring rises. The sound and his warmth lull me to sleep.

During lunch the next day, I stop at the UPS Store in Acton to check our mail. I dread seeing the pile of bills in the box every time I come here. Back in the car, I open each envelope to check the balances. None have changed much, except for the cable bill.

The statement shows a balance of three hundred dollars, up from the usual fifty dollars a month for our basic service. The statement is much longer, too—four pages instead of two.

I start reading the statement but soon stop, shocked from the seeing the long list of charges for movies from the adult channel, which were purchased on weekdays in the middle of the afternoon. Obviously I'm not watching these, and Tom has never expressed interest in X-rated movies. Would he be watching these now? If he is, why? Or is there a mistake on our bill?

I call the cable company as soon as I return to the office. "The charges are from your location," the customer services representative says. "Is anyone at home at this time of the day?"

"Yes, my husband is," I say, "but he hasn't done this before."

"Well, the orders were definitely placed from your account," she says.

Why would Tom do this? Is his paranoia now fueling some strange sexual fantasy? I can't think of any other reason. Whatever it is, this can't continue.

"Is there a way I can remove the pay-per-view channels from my account?" I ask.

"We have a child lock. It blocks access to those channels."

"What do I do to set it up?"

"If you want it, ask me, and I can set it up for you now. It will take effect immediately."

Tom's name isn't on the cable bill and the rest of the utilities for the apartment. When I moved from Brighton to Waltham, I didn't add his name when I transferred the accounts. He's not a leaseholder on the apartment, either; I listed him as a tenant. The leasing agent didn't add him as a leaseholder for the same reason as the car dealership—no employment history since 1997. So, if I block access to the adult channel, Tom can't call the cable company to reverse it.

"Please do it," I say.

"Just a moment while I set it up." I hear the customer service representative tap keys at the end of the line. About thirty seconds later, she returns and says, "It's activated. If anyone tries to access the pay-per-view channels from your TV, they'll be blocked."

"Thank you. Now I need to make payment arrangements for this bill. I can't cover the entire balance this month."

"Sure. Give me a few more seconds to look at your account."

She splits the payments over three months, which will help me cover the rest of the bills, but it will be tight.

When I come home from work, Tom doesn't greet me. His first question from his vantage point on the couch is, "What happened to the cable service?"

I stand at the end of the couch, facing him. "What do you mean, 'what happened to the cable service?'"

"All the pay-per-view channels are blocked."

There it is: He was watching the adult channel! He confessed without knowing it.

"I called the cable company today and blocked them."

Tom's face turns red when he yells, "Why did you do that?"

"Take a guess on how much the cable bill is this month."

Tom glares at me.

"It's three hundred dollars because of a long list of charges from the adult movie channel. Why are you watching X-rated movies?"

Tom picks up his textbooks from the couch. "It's none of your business." He stomps upstairs.

"It is my business!" I yell. "I'm paying the bills!"

He slams the door of the home office and slides the chair from under the desk. Then, silence.

I go to the kitchen to refill Tiger and TC's food and water dishes. They hear the familiar sounds of dinner being served and rush in from different directions. While they're munching, I make a small salad and a turkey and provolone sandwich. Tom can fix something for himself, if he decides the food in the refrigerator isn't contaminated, because I'm not going anywhere tonight. If not, he can wait or walk somewhere to buy his own dinner. He could use the exercise because he has been gaining a lot of weight. So have I because we're eating too much fast food.

After Tom moved to Waltham, I set two more rules: We both have keys to the apartment, and he isn't barricading the refrigerator. He didn't say anything when I announced these boundaries, but he refuses to eat here unless we buy takeout. He believes McDonald's and Panera Bread, which are next door to each other in the shopping center a quarter mile away, are the only places that sell food free of contaminants. Occasionally he will buy something at Star Market, a grocery store in the same shopping center, but most of the time, he prefers McDonald's.

While I sit at the table eating, Charlotte returns with, *You did the right thing today. Now it's time to talk to him about counseling. You can't delay this any longer.*

I'm still meeting with the counselor twice a month, usually during my lunch breaks. Whenever we can't schedule an appointment midday, I'll skip lunch and leave work an hour early.

Every session, she asks about whether I've talked to Tom about counseling, and I reply with, "The time isn't right yet."

Then she asks, "When will the time be right?" But she never directly tells me what to do. She only asks questions and lets me draw my own conclusions, but her wording of the questions steers me in a specific direction. I know I need to talk to him, but I'm stalling because I'm scared of his reaction. He has transformed into a spoiled child who pushes the limits, and now that I'm setting more boundaries, his behavior is getting worse.

Charlotte breaks in again. *You can't focus on his behavior. You need to take care of yourself, like you're doing now by eating a healthy meal.*

Okay, I say. *I'll talk to him after work tomorrow.*

The next day, I don't talk to him because of another distraction—a call from Don at the office with more news from Coos Bay.

"Dad's health is declining fast," he says. "The doctors say he won't last much longer."

"Oh, Don, I'm so sorry," I say. "He has lived a long, productive life, but this doesn't make things any easier." Al turned ninety-six earlier this year.

I'm surprised Don called me directly with family news, but maybe it's because he wanted me to hear what's happening without a messenger in between. Maybe he senses that Tom isn't telling me everything.

"Have you told Tom yet?" I ask.

"Yes, just before I called you," Don replies. "He didn't say much after I told him."

"He hasn't talked about Tess at all since you called after the funeral."

Don sighs. "He must be taking her death harder than I expected."

"I wish he would talk to me about it, but I can't force him."

"Hopefully he will change his mind. He needs to talk to someone."

When I come home after work, Tom is agitated. He's looking for something in a stack of papers next to a textbook on the coffee table. He shuffles the papers several times, spreads them across the table, followed by wandering around the living room, rearranging papers on the desk across from the couch, and pulling books from the bookshelves and flipping through the pages. He mumbles words I can't hear or understand.

"What are you looking for?" I ask while standing in front of the living room door, watching him.

Tom ignores me. His back faces me while he continues searching the bookshelves. He returns to the coffee table and shuffles the papers again.

"Tom, what's going on?" I ask.

He stops shuffling and looks up at me.

"Where did you put my homework?"

"I haven't touched anything, Are you sure it isn't on the coffee table? Maybe it's upstairs in the office. Did you look there?"

"It's not in this apartment! What did you do with it?"

"Nothing. Why would I do anything with your homework?"

Tom resumes shuffling the papers on the coffee table while I watch.

"Tell me what it looks like, and I'll help you find it," I say.

"No. I'll do it myself."

"You'll find it if you calm down," I say on the way to the kitchen to feed the cats.

When I'm finished, he's still searching and muttering. I retreat upstairs to the home office to finish an assignment for my class. The conversation about counseling will have to wait. I can't talk to him while he's angry.

The next day, Tom seems to be in a better mood when I come home after work. *You must talk to him now*, Charlotte says. *It's time to get this out in the open.*

I sit on the couch, facing Tom on the other end. "I'd like to talk to you about something," I say.

He looks at me with no expression on his face. "What about?" he asks.

"I'm concerned about how paranoid you feel, about the people who are following you and trying to contaminate you. It scares me when you talk about your fears and how stressed you are about them. It hurts that you don't trust me anymore because you believe I'm helping these people do bad things to you."

Tom sits still and stares at me with no expression.

"This is affecting our marriage," I continue. "We don't enjoy being with each other anymore. I've noticed you've lost interest in the things you like to do and the things we enjoy doing together. I believe talking to a counselor will help sort things out."

Tom's face turns red. "I'm not seeing a counselor!"

"Tom, this isn't getting any better without counseling. This has been getting worse for a long time and it accelerated after Tess died. Her death hit me hard, too, but I think it has affected you much more than me. It has also made your paranoia worse. You don't notice it, but I do, and it scares me."

"There's nothing to worry about. I don't need to see a counselor!"

"I can go with you. I think it would help both of us if we go together."

"We don't need marriage counseling!"

"This isn't about marriage counseling. It's about talking to someone about these people who are trying to hurt you and figuring out how to make them go away. This isn't natural. You're constantly in fear, and they aren't leaving. They shouldn't be here."

I didn't want to say, "This isn't normal," although it really isn't normal. But, after all these years, the abnormal has become normal. What *is* really normal anymore?

"I don't have a problem," Tom says. "You do."

Did I just hear him say that? How can he believe I have a problem? Is this why he's blaming me for the "interference" in his life? He isn't able to admit it's in his mind, so shifting the blame to me is how he copes.

"How do I have a problem?" I ask. "Tell me why you think I have a problem."

Tom stands and glares at me while the shades of red deepen on his face. "I'm not going to counseling. This conversation is over!" He climbs the stairs and slams the door to our home office.

I stay on the couch, prop my elbows on my lap, and bury my head in cupped hands while shaking my head. How can I get through to him? Will I lose him forever?

"Meow," TC repeats in a musical tone from the kitchen. He runs into the living room, singing all the way, then jumps on the couch, props his front paws on my shoulder, and rubs my cheek. I pick him up and hold him close, which raises the volume of his purr. He lets me hug him for a long time while he rubs my cheeks and chin.

"You're so sweet, my little buddy," I whisper to him so Tom can't hear me. I don't want Tom to interrupt this comforting kitty moment.

TC stops rubbing and lays his head on my shoulder. I've never met a cat who enjoys hugs as much as he does, this scrappy alley cat who adopted us from sleeping in the birdbath in our backyard in Seattle after his former humans moved away and abandoned him. Here he is now, consoling me in his catlike way while getting the attention he loves.

"TC, what am I going to do? Why won't Tom listen to me? How can I get him to listen?" I feel the vibration of TC's little motor against my chest.

It's time to talk to Don about this, Charlotte says. *He needs to know what's going on.*

What can Don do? I ask. He's three thousand miles away. How can he help his brother from so far away?

You need to tell him.

The next day, I take my lunch break at the Acton Arboretum, my favorite walking spot near the office. Even on a cold winter day like today, my stroll through the dormant gardens and along the woodland trail is a relaxing, refreshing diversion. It's a nice place for contemplation. Today, I'm thinking about when to talk to Tom again about counseling and when to talk to Don about Tom.

After last night's conversation with Tom, I don't know if I will ever be able to convince him to get counseling. I didn't tell him about my counselor because I'm afraid it will discourage him. He'd get angry about me sharing information with her. Because he doesn't trust anyone, could he confide in a counselor if he agrees to see one? He probably can't.

Last night, I thought we could have a productive conversation by focusing on my observations and how these make me feel. I thought this approach would work because it wouldn't make Tom defensive, but my observations and feelings didn't reach him. Does this mean he has stopped loving me? Can he care for me anymore?

When should I talk to Don? I think about the struggles he's facing now with Tess' death and Al and Nancy's worsening health. Nancy was diagnosed with cancer earlier this year, and it's now at Stage 4. My news will add to his stress, but someone else in the family needs to be aware of this and Don is the best person to talk to.

I need to take some vacation time before the end of the year; otherwise, I'll lose it. It's early December, so I'll ask for some time off around the holidays to have a longer break. I can call Don one morning while Tom is at the non-profit, shortly after Don arrives at his office for the day.

Todd approves my vacation request from Monday, December 22, through Friday, January 2. Combined with the paid holidays and the weekends, I'll have two weeks off.

Two days before my vacation, Don calls again with news that Al died. Tom reacts the same as when Tess passed. After Tom tells me that Al will be cremated and there will be a small memorial service after Christmas, we never talk about his parents' deaths again.

At eleven o'clock Eastern time on Monday morning, I call Don's office.

"I heard the news," I say, "and I'm calling to express my condolences. What a tough year it has been!"

"No kidding," Don says after thanking me.

"How's Nancy?"

"She's better. Last week, she had to go to the emergency room for another blood transfusion. Her white blood cell count drops lower than normal from the chemo treatments. She's sensitive to even the lowest dose."

"That's terrible. She's in my thoughts and prayers."

"I appreciate it."

"Is she at home now?"

"Yes. I've hired a private nurse to take care of her while I'm at the office."

Don and Nancy have been married for seventeen years. Both married later in life, and this is their first and only marriage. They love each other deeper than when they were dating. When Don is working, he always stops at home and checks on Nancy during his lunch hour to make sure she has everything she needs—even though she's under a nurse's care.

There was a time when Tom and I were like this—doting over each other through the good and bad. I miss those days.

"I need to talk to you about something," I say. "It's something you should be aware of."

"What is it?"

"It's about Tom. He has changed a lot since you last saw him. The changes aren't good."

"He seems fine when we talk on the phone."

"He has extreme paranoia. He's constantly afraid someone is following him, and lately, he believes the people who are following him are contaminating him. It has been getting worse since Tess died. I've tried to talk to him about counseling, but he refuses to go."

Don clears his throat. "Well, I'm sure that whatever it is is just a passing phase."

Great...he doesn't believe me. Now what do I do?

"I have a conference call in a few minutes," Don says. "Thank you for calling."

After Don ends the call, I listen to the dial tone for a few seconds before hanging up, dazed at his reaction. If anything happens, I can't contact him. No one else in the Landes family will want me to contact them, either. I've never felt so isolated in my life.

Cheryl Landes

The Breaking Point

Massachusetts, January 2004

When I return home after work today, Tom sits on the couch reading a textbook for one of his classes at the Harvard Extension School. When he hears me open the door, he looks up and smiles.

"Hi! How was your day?" he asks in a pleasant voice.

His question takes me aback. I haven't heard a greeting like this from him for so long that I've forgotten how to respond. Every time I come home now, I brace myself and try to anticipate what I'll encounter when I walk through the door. It changes every day, but often there's an element of blame from Tom about something he believes I've done that day.

But with Tom's mood being different today, more like his old self, I decide to follow along.

"It went well," I reply. "We finished last-minute details on the presentations for the national sales meeting. Everyone is flying there tomorrow."

Tom nods.

"Thank you for asking," I say. Maybe if I give him some positive reinforcement, he'll be more cordial every day when I come home from work.

I stop short of asking him about his day, which was my natural reaction long ago when he started these conversations. How will he react? Will he accuse me of snooping on him again? Often, a simple question like this one triggers a long lecture about the people interfering in his life and his assumptions that I'm involved.

Maybe tonight is different. Maybe I can have a real conversation with him, so I choose to continue.

"How was your day?" I ask.

"It went well," he says. "I've been studying most of the day." He places a bookmark in the textbook and closes it. "Let's go to Panera for dinner tonight."

Tom still doesn't want me to cook, but that hasn't stopped me from buying food to stock in the refrigerator and freezer. I make my own breakfast before work, but when I come home, Tom wants to eat out. I'm glad he chose Panera Bread tonight because I'm tired of eating at McDonald's.

At Panera Bread, Tom orders a cup of mushroom soup and a turkey sandwich, and I order my favorite soup, tomato basil, with a half turkey sandwich. We sit in a booth and eat in silence. Although Tom seems pleasant enough, I'm uneasy. Something feels off tonight.

When we return home, Tom sits on the couch and resumes studying, and I go upstairs to finish an assignment for the final class in my certificate program. After I catch up, I go to bed.

A half hour later, Tom climbs into bed and initiates sex. Soon after he penetrates me, he says, "I want you to say, 'Fuck me'."

He's never made a request like this, and it baffles me. From our first time together, intimacy has been a loving, sweet time of sharing a special private bond. Why would he ask me to do this when he knows it's uncomfortable for me? He knows I never use the "f-word."

I don't respond.

"I want you to say, 'Fuck me'," he says again. "Fuck me."

My mind grapples with his repeated request. Where is this coming from? Is this what he was hearing when he watched the movies on the adult channel? The cable bill didn't list the names of the movies, only where the movies were purchased. Even if I saw the titles, I wouldn't recognize them. I don't have any interest in watching X-rated movies.

"I want you to say, 'Fuck me'!" he demands, followed by a hard thrust that catches me off guard. I groan from the impact.

"Fuck me!" he continues saying in tandem with each thrust. The force is so hard, it feels like he's trying to drive a poker through the length of my body.

Each thrust is pushing me closer to the head of the bed. Soon my skull bangs the wall in response to each plunge. I manage to push the pillow under my head between the wall and the top of my head to buffer the blows, then try to brace the rest of my body from moving any closer to the head of the bed. It's impossible to stop the movement because of Tom's strength and his weight. I'm trapped, and my body trembles from fear.

The horror continues for another five minutes, until he ejaculates. He dismounts, pulls on his shorts, and goes downstairs. I curl on my left side in a fetal position and quietly cry myself to sleep. Tom has violated the only part of our marriage that was still intact. I feel drained, defeated, and dirty. This is the only time I've felt this way when we've had sex.

The next morning, I awake in the same position when the sun starts to rise through the bedroom window. TC is sleeping on top of the cat tree next to the window, and Tiger is curled in a ball at the base. I'm struggling to believe it's daylight already. I must have slept for six hours, but it feels like I didn't sleep at all. My neck and shoulder muscles are sore, and my eyes feel dry and scratchy, like someone poured a bucket of sand into each one. My cheeks are moist from leftover tears, and my eyelashes are matted with salt granules from tears that dried overnight.

I feel the top of my head for any bumps from hitting the wall last night. No bumps, no tender areas that might be bruised, and no headache. It's a miracle I'm not injured physically. Apparently I effectively cushioned the impact in time with the pillow.

I sit up and look at the other side of the bed. Tom isn't there. He probably slept on the couch all night, and he's probably mad because I wouldn't give in to his demands, but I don't care. There's no excuse for his behavior.

Taking a shower soothes my eyes and slightly improves my energy, but the water doesn't wash away my sadness and pain from Tom's cruelty. He didn't make love to me last night; it was rape. Why would anyone who's supposed to care for his partner treat her this way?

Why am I allowing this to happen? Why do I believe that if I keep trying, I can make everything better? Tom doesn't want to admit there are problems between us. In his mental state, he probably can't understand how serious this is, but I can't use this as an excuse to justify his behavior. What happened last night is a clear signal that I'm no longer safe in this relationship.

I stand in front of the mirror and look at my face while brushing my teeth. My eyes are red, and dark circles swell like tiny cups under my lower eyelashes. My mind flashes back to my teenage years, when Bubby beat me for no reason and said I was stupid and worthless and would never amount to anything. Then I realize I've replaced one type of abuse with another. Why am I continuing to allow Tom to treat me this way? He refuses to get counseling. Why do I keep hoping he will change his mind? He doesn't trust anyone. Until he can admit he needs help and trust others enough to get help, he can't take that step. Why doesn't he see that this is tearing our lives apart? We're both living in misery, but he won't admit it.

This must stop.

What should I do? I ask Charlotte. I know the answer, but I want her to guide me.

I return to the bedroom to finish getting ready for work. As soon as I'm dressed, Tom rushes upstairs, wearing a short-sleeved gray sweatshirt and khaki pants from yesterday, and stands in the doorway of the bedroom. His eyes are wild and his face is red.

TC and Tiger sense the tension. They dash between Tom's feet into the hallway and down the stairs. Their warning makes my heart pound faster.

Tom glares at me and yells, "Why did you tell them what I did yesterday?"

"What are you talking about?" I ask, trying to calm my shaking body.

"They know where I am. You told them!"

"Tom, I don't know who these people are, and I don't know what you did yesterday—other than you were here. I was at work all day, working."

"You're interfering with my life! Why are you doing this?"

Don't answer, Charlotte says. *It's time to go.*

"I have to leave now, or I'll be late for work." I'm afraid to say that when I leave, I'm not coming back.

Tom's face turns deep red and his eyes widen. "You're not going anywhere until you answer me!"

He's completely blocking the door to the bedroom, my only way out.

It's time to go, Charlotte repeats. *You need to go now!*

I pull my suitcase from the closet, open it on the bed, and start packing.

"What are you doing?" Tom yells.

"I'm leaving. I can't take this anymore," I say while filling the suitcase with clothes.

Tom stands in the doorway watching me with a stunned look on his face.

I zip the suitcase and look at his red face. The wildness in his eyes has been replaced with a confused look.

How will I get past him? What will he do if I try?

Go! Charlotte says.

I grab the suitcase handle, pull the suitcase off the bed, and walk toward Tom while my heart pounds and my body trembles. He moves aside and watches me pass in front of him, through the doorway, to the end of the hallway, and into the home office, where I grab my laptop. He follows me down the stairs, through the kitchen, and into the living room, where he stops at the front door while I walk outside and climb into the SUV. When I'm backing out of the parking spot in front of the apartment, he's watching through the living room window with a stunned look on his face.

During my fifteen-minute drive to the office, the tears flow freely while I fight to stop them. I need to compose myself before walking into the office. Usually I can control my emotions, but not today.

My marriage is dying—well, at this point, it's dead. I thought ours would be different. I thought we would always be together. On our wedding day, I believed the cliché of living "happily ever after." I didn't have any reason to *not* believe it. During our four years of dating, we survived the challenges of finishing our degrees at the University of Oregon through full-time course loads, working multiple jobs, and barely making it financially. Then in front of a justice of the peace and thirty relatives and friends in a ceremony at the historic Deepwood House in Salem, Oregon, we promised we would cherish and take care of each other for the rest of our lives. Now I'm breaking that promise, but Tom broke it first when he stopped trusting me.

This time, if Tom asks me to return, I can't. I don't know if he'll try, but I must be strong and unwavering if he does. When I left Tom while we both lived on Staten Island, I promised myself if this happened again, I'm moving forward on my own. I've gone beyond what's possible to keep our marriage together without Tom's help. He doesn't understand—or maybe in his state now, he can't understand—how much this is affecting our lives at every level. And now, it isn't safe for me to live with him anymore. No longer do I know what he's capable of doing, and I don't want to find out.

When I arrive at the office, I sit in the car and calm myself by focusing on the tallest snowbank at the edge of the parking lot and taking deep breaths. When the tears stop, I wipe my eyes with a tissue and take a few more deep breaths before leaving my sanctuary. I enter the building through the back door to the kitchen and retreat to the women's restroom to freshen up. My face watches me in the mirror with eyes red and swollen, purple circles underneath. Washing my face doesn't lighten the color much, but the warm water against my skin feels good.

I don't want anyone in the office to see me like this. I'll hide in my cubicle and focus on updating a product manual. If anyone invites me to meetings today, I'll excuse myself with, "I have a deadline," and suggest a new time for next week. When I left the office yesterday, my calendar was clear.

My plan doesn't work well, except for no meetings and hiding in my cubicle. It's Friday, and with the entire marketing department out for the sales meeting except me and the administrative assistant, others taking long weekends or vacations, and everyone else taking advantage of the quiet time to catch up on their projects, it's quiet in our office cocoons. But in mine, it's hard to concentrate on technical prose with the events from last night and this morning stuck in my head. Sometimes tears surface again while I fight them back, and I can't keep the dam plugged much longer.

My cell phone rings, startling me in the heavy silence. Don is on the line from his office in Coos Bay. I never expected him to call me again after our last conversation.

"Hi, Cheryl," he says. "I'm calling to check on you. Tom called a few minutes ago and said you left."

I take a deep breath. I never thought Tom would call Don about this; after all, wouldn't he have to tell Don about what led up to this? Don would ask questions, but Tom could avoid answering them.

"Remember our phone conversation before Christmas?" I ask.

"Yes."

"That's why."

"Oh. I'm sorry. I didn't know it was that bad."

"It has been for a long time. I can't take it anymore. Tom needs counseling, but he refuses to go."

Don believed you during that call, Charlotte says, *but he didn't want to accept what you said. He's struggling to believe this could happen to his youngest brother.* Her words comfort me, and now I'm hearing the concern in Don's voice, which reassures me.

"Have you talked to him about it?" Don asks.

"Yes, but he gets mad and says he doesn't have a problem. I do."

"How long has this been going on?"

"It started before we left Seattle. It got worse after he was laid off. He was fine for the first three months after he moved to New York, but then it returned, worse than before. Now it's constant."

"I had no idea. When I talk to him on the phone, he sounds okay."

"He hides his behavior from everyone, except me."

"Maybe this explains why he wouldn't come to Mom's funeral. I offered to pay for your airfare, but he wouldn't accept it."

I didn't know about Don's offer. Maybe he thought Tom didn't want to tell him we couldn't afford to fly there on short notice. Maybe he thought it was the only way he could convince Tom to go.

"Thank you for offering," I say. "I wasn't aware of this, and I appreciate your generosity. I tried to talk Tom into going, but he didn't want to. He said that he said good-bye to Tess and Al during his last trip to Coos Bay. Then he refused to talk about it anymore."

"What are your plans now?"

"I haven't thought that far ahead yet. For now, I will find a place to stay and sort things out. I hope this convinces him that he needs help, but with everything else that has happened, I'm not sure it will. I'm trying to stay as positive as possible. There's always hope."

Hope. There's that word again. Where did it come from? I'm not feeling hopeful today. Why did I say this to Don?

You aren't feeling it today, but you are hopeful and positive, Charlotte says. *You're strong. You're a fighter. You can do this.*

"I hope it works out," Don says. "Let's keep in touch."

After we hang up, I look at the clock on my computer screen. It's twelve-thirty. I'm not hungry, so I try to resume updating the manual, but my thoughts can't focus on the upgraded gateway system. I feel the lump in my throat build again, followed by the tears that want to escape.

I stare at the screen, where the words in the manual blur through my watery eyes. I wipe them with a tissue, but tears spill over my eyelids. As hard as I try, I can't stop the flood.

Take a break, Charlotte says. *Get something to eat. You need to take care of yourself.*

I decide to take the rest of the day off, then save the manual, back it up on the network, and shut down the computer. The updates can wait until Monday. Before leaving the office, I search Google for the Motel 6 closest to the office and find two of almost equal distance, one north of here and one west. I'll pick one later and check in tonight for a few days.

Cheryl Landes

Stepping Forward, Sliding Backward
Massachusetts, January-March 2004

It's quiet at Applebee's in Westford when I arrive for a late lunch. The server seats me in a booth next to a window with a view of the parking lot and the woods in the background, where the naked branches of the trees reach skyward. Their collective vulnerable pose resonates with me today in my fragile state as I continue struggling to hold back the tears through reading the menu, ordering a burger and fries, and eating. A few escape, and I absorb them with the black cloth napkin covering my lap.

After lunch, I check into the Motel 6 in Tewksbury, the closest to Applebee's. Through intermittent streams of tears, I search craigslist for rooms to rent near the office. One ad looks promising in Acton. I write the phone number in my spiral notebook to call tomorrow, when hopefully I can compose myself long enough to talk to another person.

Ernie, the landlord, agrees to meet me at ten o'clock the next morning and gives me directions. The room is in a large two-story lemon cheesecake colored house built in the 1700s New England style, less than ten minutes from the office in a quiet neighborhood of equally large houses in matching architecture with yards surrounded by forests of tall maples, oaks, and pines.

The asphalt driveway runs parallel to the east side of the house, then curves downhill behind it to the left. I drive around the corner, park in a spot in front of the back door, and knock on the door. A man with a slight slouch in his shoulders, wearing a red and white plaid flannel shirt and khakis held up with red suspenders, opens the door. His white hair reveals little baldness, but the wrinkles in his face and hands show his age.

"Are you Ernie?" I ask. "I'm Cheryl. I called about the room for rent."

"Yes, come in," he says in a booming, crackling voice that reminds me of a professor lecturing in front of hundreds of students in an auditorium without a microphone.

We enter through a large kitchen and turn to the right, where there's a doorway to an office. On the way, Ernie pulls a chair from the dining table. He places it in front of a large walnut desk in his office and says, "Have a seat."

He sits behind the desk in a walnut swivel chair with green cushions tied to the back and seat. At the left of his desk are floor-to-ceiling bookshelves filled with law books. A window with a view of the forest is behind him.

"The room is upstairs on the top floor," he says. "It has a private bath. You'd share the kitchen with the rest of the tenants."

I nod. I didn't expect to have my own bathroom.

"I must inform you that most of the tenants are men," he says. "The only woman who lives here is the daughter of the tenant across the hall from the empty room."

"I don't mind," I reply. I'm looking for a safe place where I can sleep, and I don't plan on interacting with anyone else here if he allows me to rent the room. I will be nice to them if I see them in passing, but I'm not going out of my way to be sociable. I have too much to handle on this new path forward.

"I'd like to see the room," I say.

I follow him up a steep stairway, which ends at a hallway. On the left, another hallway runs the width of the house, and I see two doors on each side. Ernie unlocks the door on the right, which opens into a room with a couch facing another doorway into a bedroom furnished with a double bed, nightstand, and desk. A full bathroom is through another doorway off the room with the couch.

This is a small apartment, not a room—the perfect place for me to start over.

Ernie stands inside the entryway with his arms crossed and watches me while I look around.

"I'll take it," I say.

"All right," he says, "but first, I need you to fill out an application and complete a background check."

"That's okay," I say. "I can do it now if you'd like."

We return to his office, and he hands the paperwork to me. I don't know if he'll accept my application, but I won't know unless I try. I'm not telling Ernie about Tom; it's none of his business. All he needs to know is I have a good, stable job, and an excellent rental history. He didn't mention checking my credit. It isn't very good anymore. I don't know if he can reject my application over an unhealthy credit score.

When I hand the completed application to him, he says, "I'll call you with my decision next week."

The rest of the weekend passes quickly, except when I think about Tom and how our world has turned upside down. It's especially tough on these cloudy January nights under the hidden moon, in a hotel room a few yards from the railroad tracks. I didn't notice the tracks after checking into the hotel until one-thirty the next morning, when I heard a train pass with its wheels squeaking on the steel rails. A row of trees behind the building shields the tracks from view, but when I look out the window while the train is here, it's clear where it is from the lights streaming among the trunks. I wonder what the cars carry and where the train is going, then think about where I'm heading and what will happen to Tom. We're on separate paths now, and finding a small place of my own is my second step. The first was leaving Waltham.

Tom hasn't called since I left. After hearing from Don on Friday morning, I expected Tom to call me later that day. Maybe Tom assumes I will call him first because I'm the one who left. I'm not ready. I don't know when I'll be ready.

On Tuesday morning, Ernie calls my cell phone while I'm at my desk rewriting a sales bulletin. "I accepted your application. You're welcome to move in anytime."

I want to jump around in my cubicle to celebrate. Instead, I say, "Thank you. I'll be there tomorrow after work." It's too late to cancel my hotel room tonight.

My cell phone rings again an hour later. Tom's name displays on the screen, and I hold my breath, debating whether I should answer.

It's okay to talk to him, Charlotte says.

But what will I say?

You'll know what to do.

I pick up on the fifth ring.

"How are you?" Tom asks. "I've been thinking about you."

"I'm fine," I say in my most pleasant voice. "You sound well today."

"Are you going to class tonight?" he asks.

We have classes at the Harvard Extension School on Tuesday and Thursday nights—different subjects, same time.

"I'm planning on it."

"Can you give me a ride?"

Now that I'm gone, he doesn't have easy access to transportation and it's too far to walk to Alewife to catch the T to Harvard Square. The cost of taking a taxi back and forth adds up. I didn't think about this when I left, but is it my responsibility? Guilt creeps inside for stranding him.

"I'll pick you up at five o'clock in front of the apartment," I say.

"I'll see you then," he says.

After I hang up, my mind is a mangled mess of guilt and regret. Did I make a mistake? I didn't, so why am I thinking this way? It's too late to turn back, but I can be supportive.

It's okay to be supportive, but you must remain strong, Charlotte says. *You can't go back to him.*

She's right. She's always right.

Tom is waiting outside the apartment door with his backpack slung over his left shoulder when I arrive. I watch him walk to the passenger side of the car, climb in, and shut the door. He glances at me with an uncertain look while fastening his seatbelt. I don't say anything. I can't think of any words to say. During the fifteen-minute drive to the Alewife parking garage, the only sounds we hear are the passing cars and the hum of the engine of my Honda CR-V.

A parking spot is available on the second level near the entrance to the main stairway to the subway platform. I pull in and turn off the engine. Its sound is replaced with the echoes of cars climbing and descending the ramps, and driving around each level of the garage to find a place to park.

Tom breaks the silence with, "Let's talk for a minute. We have time."

I look at him but don't reply.

"When are you coming home?" he asks.

"I'm not," I reply. He needs to know.

His eyes widen. "Why?"

"I can't continue living like we are. Remember in New York when I left, you said things would get better? They didn't. They're worse."

Tom's blank face stares at me.

"Do you remember that conversation we had in the Au Bon Pain?" I ask. "It was when we met on the third night after I left. You came to Manhattan, called me at work that afternoon, and asked if we could talk there."

His confused look tells me he doesn't remember.

"We don't have a life anymore," I continue. "You believe I'm trying to harm you when I'm not. We can't enjoy our lives together because of your constant fear. You're not the same person I married."

"I don't know what you're talking about," he says.

He really doesn't understand how his behavior is affecting your lives, Charlotte says.

I can't explain it to him, I say to her. *I'll never be able to explain it to him, will I?*

That's up to him.

"We should leave now," I say to Tom.

We walk to the subway platform, board the train to Harvard Square, sit side by side on the plastic seats, and read the ads on the walls of the subway car while I think about our brief conversation in the garage. Will Tom remember what I said? Will he think about it and ask for help from a counselor? Does he understand what's happening to us?

The train stops at the Harvard Square station. We climb the stairs, exit the station, and cross Mass Ave. to campus. Tom says, "I'll meet you at the entrance to the station after class."

I nod and we part quietly while cars drive by and students chat with each other on their way to classes, the Coop, or to grab a bite for dinner.

Class is a blur. I'm present but not listening to the lecture. This entire evening is like an awkward dream. My mind moves back and forth like I'm watching a tennis game, except the ball is flying back and forth from guilt for severing the bond between Tom and me and my need to move forward. Being together for so long complicates breaking the physical and mental connections.

After class, Tom is waiting at the designated location. When he sees me, he doesn't say hello. We walk side by side in silence to the turnstiles and continue when we emerge on the other side. During the train ride, we read the ads again.

The silence continues throughout the drive back to the apartment in Waltham. When Tom gets out of the car, he doesn't say "goodnight." I don't, either. He walks into the apartment and shuts the door. No lights come on inside.

I back out of the parking spot and drive to my apartment in Acton. My mind is too numb to think. When I arrive, I change and go straight to bed.

This routine continues. There's no conversation, unless Tom is agitated from a delusion. He talks vaguely about interference from someone while he studied or about someone trying to contaminate him. He says someone is monitoring him from the apartment below. I listen but never respond, which makes him angry and prompts him to say variations of, "You're involved" or "You're contaminating me."

I'm tired of talking about this. Anything I say to him won't make any difference.

Something else I didn't think about when I left Tom was the cats. They're with him. This makes me feel guilty again because I've been their primary caregiver, and I promised I would never abandon them. Now, I've broken that promise.

Tiger hasn't needed insulin shots for a few months, but he still needs blood tests twice a month to check his glucose levels. So, now I pick him up for his appointments at the cat clinic in Brighton every other Saturday morning. Tom never objects.

At Tiger's first appointment after I left Tom, I decide to talk to the vet about the situation. I don't know why this seems important, but the thought won't stop nagging at me.

I ask the vet to add a note in Tiger and TC's records to contact me if Tom brings them there for any treatments. The vet says he will.

The stress is making me forgetful. I'm diligent about keeping my calendar and task reminders updated in Microsoft Outlook at the office, but sometimes something escapes my attention when I'm not in front of the computer.

Last week, I scheduled an eight o'clock meeting with Russ, who recently became the Vice President of Marketing, and three of the product managers to talk about a new project. On the way to the office the morning of the meeting, I stop at Starbucks to pick up a latte and lemon poppyseed scone. It's my only chance today for any meal that resembles breakfast.

While standing in line, someone behind me taps my shoulder. It's Russ, looking at me with a smile on his face rivaling the Cheshire Cat's in *Alice in Wonderland*, which deepens the dimples in his cheeks. His brown eyes sparkle as if he's ready to tell a joke.

"Aren't you supposed to be somewhere else right now?" he asks.

I feel my face flush. *Oh, no, it's my meeting! How did I forget it? But, wait a minute...*

"Aren't you supposed to be there, too?" I ask Russ while trying to recover from my embarrassment.

"I'm on my way," he replies through his smile. "But first, coffee to go!"

I've never been late for a meeting I've scheduled and feel horrible about my absent-mindedness. When I arrive at the office ten minutes later, I reschedule the meeting with an apology inserted above the agenda. The product managers accept the updated invitation with no comments as does Russ, who arrives in the office ten minutes after me.

Two weeks later, Todd schedules a meeting for my annual performance evaluation. I've always received high marks on my performance evaluations, and during this one, the trend continues almost to the end, when Todd says, "I've noticed you're making more mistakes lately."

I think about my rescheduled meeting. Todd wasn't one of the attendees. Did Russ or one of the product managers tell him?

I don't ask, but Todd mentions some errors in my writing. All my work is reviewed and approved by the subject matter experts before it's published. Did they review my drafts or just skim them? How did I miss these mistakes?

"This is not reflective of the outstanding work you have done for us for the past three years," Todd says. "If you need to talk to me about anything, I'm here."

I'm not ready to tell him how my life has turned upside down and don't know if I ever will be. No one at the office knows what I'm going through because I don't want to be the juicy topic of the grapevine. It's a small company, one hundred ten employees, so word spreads fast.

"I'm sorry," I say. I want to add that *it will never happen again*, but in my current state, can I be so sure? Instead, I continue with, "Thank you for bringing this to my attention."

For the next week, the results of the performance evaluation haunt me. I spend extra time checking and double-checking every document I write to ensure they're error-free. I agonize over whether I should talk to Todd about Tom. Todd has never done anything to make me distrust him.

My reluctance comes from an experience early in my career, when I was a file clerk for a government office. Five months after I started working there, my left hand and wrist were injured. The doctor said I had a repetitive motion injury from filing papers forty hours a week and qualified for workers' compensation. After I applied and was approved, my manager constantly tried to find evidence that I faked my injury. She didn't stop until I accepted a promotion to an executive secretary in another department.

Four days later, I'm still on the fence about talking to Todd, but this is about to change. It starts when I check voicemail for the landline at the apartment in Waltham. I still check messages there, without Tom's knowledge, in case someone calls for me. The only message today is from the cat clinic, left yesterday afternoon.

"Hi, Tom," the vet says. "I have the results from Tiger and TC's tests. All the tests were negative. I didn't notice anything to be concerned about during their exams, either. They're in boarding until you return from your trip. You said you thought you'd be back in five days. Please call my office to confirm when you'll pick them up."

Why didn't the vet call me when Tom dropped off the cats? Obviously he didn't add the note to Tiger and TC's records.

I go to Todd's office, say something came up that I need to take care of, and I'll be back as soon as I can.

"Take your time," he says. "I hope everything will be okay."

After arriving at the cat clinic, I stop at the front desk, a white crescent-shaped counter in the middle of the waiting room where the receptionist, a woman with brown hair in a bob cut who's probably in her late thirties or early forties, sits behind a large monitor. She's wearing a pink sweater, and her gold-rimmed glasses rest mid-nose while she taps the keyboard. She greets me with, "Hello. May I help you?"

"I need to speak with the vet."

"Do you have an appointment?" she asks.

"No, but it's important. My two cats are his patients."

"He's with a patient," she replies. "Is there anything I can help you with?"

"Maybe. I received a voicemail this morning that my husband dropped our two cats here for exams and a series of tests. In the message, the vet said they're in boarding for five days. They should not be here. I asked the vet to call me if my husband brings the cats here for treatment. I take care of their appointments. My husband has a mental health condition. He's extremely paranoid and cannot think clearly because of his delusions."

"What is your name?"

"Cheryl Landes. The cats' names are Tiger and TC. My husband's name is Tom. The last time Tiger had an appointment for a blood test to check his glucose levels, I asked the vet to put a note in Tiger and TC's files about this."

"Please have a seat while I talk to him. It will be a few minutes before he finishes with his patient."

Ten minutes later, the receptionist calls me to the front desk. "He still isn't available. Would you like to wait?"

I believe the vet is avoiding me. He knows he made a mistake. I should have asked the receptionist to add the note to Tiger and TC's files but didn't think about it at the time.

"No," I say. "I'll take the cats with me."

When I signed the lease for the apartment in Acton, I didn't ask the landlord whether he allowed pets. He didn't say anything, so I assumed it would be okay. Tiger and TC need me to care for them. I can't leave them with Tom anymore.

The receptionist tallies the charges. "The balance is six hundred dollars," she says.

"Six hundred dollars!" I shout without caring who hears me. "For what?"

She shows me the itemized bill, which includes a comprehensive exam for both cats, a long list of tests, and thirty-five dollars a day for boarding each cat. They've been here for two days.

"TC had his annual check-up in December," I say, struggling to withhold my anger. "He's in excellent health, so he didn't need another exam so soon. Tiger is diabetic. I have his next appointment for a blood test set up for next week. I scheduled it after our last appointment. The vet knows I bring Tiger here twice a month for these tests. None of this lab work Tom requested was necessary, and the vet knows this, too. I can't afford to pay this bill."

"We need payment in full before you can take the cats," the receptionist says.

"I can't pay in full today! I didn't authorize this treatment. The vet should have contacted me for permission before treating them and allowing them to board here. If I had known, I would have refused treatment and picked them up."

"I'm sorry, but you can't take the cats home until the bill is paid in full."

"I don't have enough money to pay in full today, but I can make payments."

"We don't have payment plans, but we have a grant program from a generous donor to help people in tough financial situations. The maximum grant is four hundred dollars. Can you pay two hundred dollars today?"

I can't afford two hundred dollars, either, but the cats need a safe place to stay. There's barely enough room on one credit card.

"Yes."

She hands a form to me. "Fill this out for the grant. When you're finished, we'll finalize the payment."

My body shakes while I fill out the form. It's hard to hold my hand steady to write. What was on Tom's mind when he brought the cats here? He was too obsessed with his delusions to think about how he would pay this bill. What would he have done when the receptionist gave him the balance and said it's due up front? By the time he returns, the bill would be a few hundred dollars higher. Probably the outcome would be a call from the receptionist, asking me to pay.

Tom seems to believe we have an open checkbook or I can work harder to make more money. He doesn't understand there's a finite number of hours in the day. I'm exhausted from working full-time, moonlighting when I can get extra projects—which are harder to find with the publishers downsizing—and my overwhelming stress. He doesn't care. It's all about him and the invisible followers.

After paying the bill, I load the cats into the car and drive to Waltham to pick up their food and supplies. While I'm there, I go upstairs and look for Tom's suitcase, which he stores in the bedroom closet. It's gone, as is several of his favorite shirts and pants that hang on the rod in the closet.

When I arrive in Acton, I leave the cats in the car until until I finish setting up their food and water dishes and litter box in my apartment. By doing this, I can assure them that this is their home now, hopefully for a long time. They've faced a lot of disruption since we moved to the Northeast. I want them to know they can rely on me to take care of them like I did before leaving Tom.

After releasing the cats from their carriers, I call Tom while they explore the apartment. No answer. I hang up without leaving a message. He'll be surprised when he returns in three days and discovers the cats are gone, but I don't care. He should know where they are if he can think rationally.

Three days pass, then four, and Tom hasn't called. I wait another day and drive to Waltham to check the apartment. No one is there, and nothing has changed since I picked up the cats from the vet.

When I return to Acton, I call Don at his office in Coos Bay.

"Have you heard from Tom?" I ask.

"Not recently," he says. "Why?"

"The vet left a voicemail last week about the cats. Two days before the vet called, Tom dropped the cats off for boarding for five days. I haven't heard from him. I checked the apartment this afternoon, and he's not there. I think he might have gone to New York."

"Why would he go there?"

"I don't know. It's just a hunch."

"Did he talk about going anywhere before he left?"

"No. I didn't know he was gone until the vet left the message. After I received the message, I picked up the cats. They're staying with me now."

"This isn't like Tom."

"Tom has changed a lot since the last time you saw him. He looks like the same person, but his personality is completely different because of his paranoia."

"I'm sorry. I wish there was something I could do."

"If I don't hear from him tonight, I'm filing a missing person report in the morning. I'll call you when I find out anything."

With everything I've gone through with Tom, why should I worry about him going somewhere and not returning when he said he would? In his mental state, I don't know what he's thinking. Maybe he didn't know where he was going and randomly chose a place. It's possible if he feels threatened by his followers and he's trying to escape their grip. But if he isn't aware of his surroundings, he could run into trouble—especially if he's in New York.

I believe he's in New York because it's a city of contrasts. It's the place to go if someone wants to be seen, but it's also the place to go if someone wants to get lost. Tom falls into the latter category. He could fade into the background and become anonymous, which would be his way of protecting himself from his tormentors.

Tom doesn't have any friends in the Northeast. The only two people he's in contact with are Don and me.

No news comes overnight, so the next morning, I leave Acton early to check the apartment in Waltham. Nothing has changed.

My next stop is the police station. The woman sitting behind the counter is reading some papers on her desk when I walk up. She barely looks at me when she asks in a monotone, "May I help you?"

"I'd like to fill out a missing person report," I say.

"How long has the person been missing?" she asks.

"Eight days," I say. "It's my husband. He has an undiagnosed mental illness. I'm afraid something happened to him."

She asks some basic questions and takes a few notes on a small pad next to her phone. When I mention we're separated and tell her about the voicemail from the vet, she looks at me above her gold-rimmed glasses and asks, "So, you don't really know he's gone, do you?"

"Yes, I do. His suitcase is missing, along with his favorite clothes in the closet. I checked again this morning, and they're still gone. The vet is the last person who saw him before he left. He has not called me or his brother in Oregon. We're the only two people he keeps in contact with."

"Usually in cases like these, they'll return in a few days," the woman says.

"How do you know?" I ask. "This isn't like my husband. When he says he will be back at a certain day or time, he's never late. He has been gone for eight days. The vet said in the voicemail that my husband told him he'd be back in five days when he dropped off the cats. He hasn't returned."

"Have you talked to the vet?"

"No. When I went to the cat clinic, he wouldn't talk to me. It's because he treated the cats without my authorization, and he didn't want me to confront him about it."

"I don't think you have anything to worry about," she says. "If you don't hear from him in a couple of days, contact us again."

"But he's already been missing for more than twenty-four hours, so technically, he's a missing person. Can I file the report, please?" I don't understand what she doesn't understand about this situation. Is she brushing me off because I said Tom suffers from a mental illness?

"I'll take care of it," she replies. "Have a nice day."

Will she? I don't believe her, but what else can I do but leave? She's tired of dealing with me.

On the way to the office, I think about whether I should call Don again. I don't have any news for him yet, so I decide to wait until I do. This new unpredictable behavior from Tom worries and scares me. Scenarios of terrible things that could happen to him whirl in my mind throughout the day, along with my guilt for leaving him, but I can't break my promise to myself. Charlotte continues to remind me that *you can't go back. You must remain strong. You can do this.*

After work, I'm exhausted and hungry. I stop at an Asian restaurant in Maynard, order a Happy Family entrée and bowl of hot and sour soup, eat the soup and part of the entrée, and ask the server for a box to take the rest home. There's enough for lunch tomorrow.

Tiger and TC are asleep on opposite corners of the bed when I arrive. TC looks up at me and yawns when I hang up my coat in the closet, then promptly returns to his nap. I rub between his ears, which triggers a soft purr but no movement. Tiger is planted deep into kitty dreamland.

"I'm joining you two. It has been a long day."

Two days later, Tom calls mid-afternoon while I'm at the office. "I went to the vet today to pick up the cats. He said you have them."

"That's right, and they're staying with me. Why did you order all those tests? TC is fine and Tiger has another blood test scheduled next week."

"They were contaminated. So was I."

"All the tests were negative."

Silence.

"Where were you?"

After a long pause, he asks, "When are you bringing the cats back?"

"As I said, I'm not. They're staying with me. I'm not leaving them with you when I don't know where you'll be from one day to the next. They need someone who will take care of them, not dump them at the vet, disappear for more than a week, and run up a six-hundred-dollar bill. Then I'm stuck with paying the bill."

"I would have taken care of it."

"With what? You're not working!"

I hear a click at the end of the line, followed by a dial tone.

After I calm down from this conversation, I call the non-emergency number at the precinct to report Tom's return. The woman who answers listens but doesn't put me on hold to search for the report. When I finish, she says, "Well, now, he's back, isn't he?"

I hang up. Just as I expected, no one filed a report. The person I talked to never intended to file one, probably because I disclosed Tom's mental illness. What would happen if someone disappeared and was in serious trouble? Probably nothing. What a messed-up system we have.

Now I wonder what Tom will do next. His new level of unpredictability might force me to drop everything to resolve more crises. Anything could happen now.

Tell Todd, Charlotte says. *You can trust him.*

I schedule a meeting for the next morning with the subject line, "Follow-up from my performance evaluation." Todd accepts the invitation within five minutes after I click the Send button.

After I close the door to his office and sit in a chair in front of his desk, he looks at me curiously and asks, "What's up?"

"I'm going through something you should be aware of," I say. "I didn't know how much it was affecting my work."

A lump forms in my throat, and I shift my gaze from Todd to my lap to compose myself. Instead, I start falling apart.

"I'm sorry," I say as tears start flowing down my cheeks. "I'm usually not like this."

"That's okay. Take your time," Todd says. He pulls a tissue from a box on his desk and hands it to me. I wipe my wet eyes and cheeks.

"It's my husband. We're separated. He has been extremely paranoid for a long time, and it reached the point where I couldn't live with him anymore. I've begged him to go to counseling, but he refuses. I even offered to go with him."

"I'm so sorry," Todd says. "I want you to know that I will not share this with anyone else. If you need to take any time off, just let me know."

The river of tears slow to a trickle. "Thank you. I don't need to take time off now, but I might have to leave during office hours to take care of some things. If I do, I will make up the time." I don't want to use all my paid leave or fall behind in my work.

"Do whatever you need. I'm here to support you."

I wish I had everything under control. It feels like I'm in an earthquake that refuses to stop shaking my world.

"My wife is a psychiatrist," Todd says. "If it's okay with you, I can ask her if she can recommend any organizations that can help."

"I'd appreciate it. It's impossible to find information." I've been searching and coming up empty. My counselor hasn't referred me to any organizations and I haven't thought about asking her. Maybe the topic hasn't come up because she doesn't believe I need to contact them.

"I will talk to her tonight," Todd says. "If you need anything else, please let me know."

I'm relieved after talking to him but fearful of what might happen next.

It's okay, Charlotte says. *He will support you. You can trust him.*

The next morning, he stops at my cubicle a few minutes after he arrives at the office.

"Do you have a minute?" he asks.

"Yes," I reply.

"Let's talk in my office," he says.

I follow him. He closes the door, sits behind his desk, and pulls a large Post-It note from a side pocket of his brown leather briefcase.

"My wife recommended these organizations," he says as he hands the note to me. "Hopefully they can provide some help. If not, let me know, and I will talk to her again."

Four organizations are listed on the note with phone numbers.

"I will call them," I say. "Please thank your wife for me."

Todd nods and smiles. "My offer still stands. If you need anything at all, please let me know."

The meeting hall, a wing at the back of the Unitarian church in Bedford, seems humongous with only twelve people sitting in a circle, waiting for our first session to start. We're here for the twelve-week Family to Family class hosted by the Middlesex affiliate of the National Alliance on Mental Illness (NAMI). Through a series of phone calls originating from those four phone numbers Todd's wife gave to me, someone referred me to NAMI. Claire, the volunteer I talked to there, recommended this class.

"It's for caregivers of people with mental health conditions," she said, "and it's taught by trained instructors who have family members coping with mental illness. Every week, we have class for an hour and a half. Then we take a short break and have a support group for an hour. We talk about what we've been facing for the past week."

As our conversation continued, she convinced me that the class could help me. "We cover information you can't find anywhere else."

Now that I'm here, I question myself. Tom and I are no longer together, so am I really a caregiver anymore? How can this class help me?

As I look around the circle, the other students appear tense while we quietly wait for the first session to start. Some stare out a window to avoid eye contact with anyone. Others sit with fingers laced in their laps, twirling their thumbs and watching them with feigned interest.

I wonder if they're thinking what I'm thinking: *Why am I here?* We wait, hoping that whatever we committed to will deliver solutions for our loved ones and ourselves.

Like me, they've probably searched for days, weeks, months, or longer to find information or resources to help their loved ones and themselves, and probably hit the same roadblocks I have. I've heard so many excuses from organizations advertising they're here to support us on why they can't or won't—that is, when they answer their phones. Many of my calls head straight to voicemail, where I'm greeted with, "Please do not leave a message because we do not have enough staff to return calls."

When someone answers who doesn't treat my call like a hot potato or says I need to call a different number, they ask me the same two questions:

"Is your income less than ten thousand dollars a year?"

"Do you have children?"

I don't fall into either category, so their response is always the same: "We can't help you."

After hearing this for the umpteenth time, I ask, "Who can survive on ten thousand dollars a year in Massachusetts? You can't even rent an apartment for that amount."

"Oh, you'd be surprised," was the unhelpful response. The woman at the end of the line didn't elaborate, and I wonder if anyone who qualifies gets any help, either. Probably there are excuses for not providing assistance to them, too.

Why do these organizations exist, other than to collect donations? Where does the money go? I probably don't want to know. One thing's for sure: When I can afford to donate money again, they won't be on my list.

The two instructors enter the meeting hall five minutes before class is scheduled to start. They're two heavy-set women. Their graying hair and wrinkles make me assume they're over fifty, but the stress from coping with their loved ones' challenges probably accelerated the aging process. One woman wears a loose-fitting, short-sleeved, button-down blouse with red flowers and black vines on a white background and black slacks. The other woman wears a pastel green smock and navy blue pants.

They sit in the only two chairs available in the circle, say "hello," introduce themselves, and share brief backgrounds on their experiences. Both women have adult children with different conditions that started when they were young. The woman wearing the flowered blouse says her daughter was diagnosed with anxiety and obsessive compulsive disorder (OCD). The other woman says her son struggles with schizophrenia but currently, he's stable.

These ladies don't call themselves "instructors." "We're facilitators," the woman wearing the flowered blouse says. "We're here to help you learn more about mental illness, the symptoms and conditions, treatments, self-care, our rights as caregivers, how to communicate with your loved ones, and how to advocate for them. The information we will share with you has been developed by experts in the field. Our goal is to equip you with the tools you need to help you and your loved ones navigate your personal journeys. We want you to know that you are not alone. So often, that's how we feel as caregivers, but there is hope."

"Throughout the class, we will be reading from a script," the woman wearing the pastel smock says. "Most of you probably haven't experienced this format, but the reason we do this is to ensure we deliver the information in this course completely and accurately. We strive to be consistent in our message wherever this course is offered."

When I've taken classes on how to be an effective trainer, I learned that we shouldn't read from a script. We should talk naturally to make a connection with our students. But I can understand why NAMI would want their facilitators to follow a script. The facilitators aren't trained counselors or medical personnel, but they have personal experience. Each person's experiences are different, though, so it's important to provide consistent information from professional experts for people who want to learn more about mental illness and where they can find help.

Keep an open mind, Charlotte says. *This will help you.*

The twelve weeks fly. Each week, I gain new insights that help me feel empowered. Although there are many unknowns about mental illness and why it affects each person differently, at least I now understand this. The students in the class grow more comfortable sharing their experiences each week, and we feel like we're no longer alone. We can talk to others who relate to what we're going through without worrying whether we'll be judged or will receive unhelpful advice like, "They're just going through a phase," "They'll come around," "They have to buck it up and move on," or we're not doing enough to help our loved ones.

During a support session, a student says, "I hate to say this, but I wish my husband had cancer instead of mental illness. People react to cancer differently. They're sympathetic. They bring food to help the family. They offer rides to and from appointments. They help in other ways to ease the family's burden. But when someone has mental illness, it's different. People are afraid and they avoid us."

Caregivers are shunned because of the stigma that our loved ones will become violent and attack or kill someone. Most people with a mental health condition are never violent and don't harm anyone. It's more likely they'll try to harm themselves when they're in crisis, depending on the situation. But reports of violence stemming from mental illness are featured on the local and national news, so to viewers without first-hand experience, it's easy to assume that everyone struggling with mental illness is dangerous. Will perceptions ever change? Outside support groups and classes like Family to Family, mental illness is a topic few want to talk about. I think about what I can do to spread the message, but with all the struggles I'm going through, where would I even start?

Take one step at a time, Charlotte says. *The day will come when you can pay it forward, but for now, you must focus on yourself.*

During these classes, I learn that mental illness can be inherited, and the conditions can manifest differently. Is this what happened with Tom? His mother suffered from depression, so it's likely, but his brothers don't have any symptoms. His father didn't, either.

In the sections of the course where we learn about the types of mental illnesses, their symptoms, and treatment options, the facilitators mention a condition called *anosognosia*. I've never heard of it, but apparently it's common in people who suffer from bipolar disorder and schizophrenia. Anosognosia is a neurological condition where people are not aware they have symptoms of a mental illness. Their brains cannot distinguish fiction from reality. The more I learn about it, the more I wonder whether this is why Tom believes he's fine and I have "a problem."

I also learn that I can't force Tom to go to counseling or get treatment. No one can unless he's a danger to himself or others. If this happens, the program lasts only two weeks, which isn't enough time to accurately diagnose a condition and provide any lasting results. Often it takes years to find the correct diagnosis and establish an effective treatment program. It's a difficult and frustrating path for patients and caregivers alike, but for those who continue the quest, they eventually discover solutions.

Tom needs to make this choice on his own. All I can do is stand by and support him, but I need to take care of myself first. Betty, my doctor, and my counselor have said this many times, so this is another strong reminder to nurture myself physically and mentally.

The best ways I can support Tom is to listen to him and try to understand how he's feeling. I need to understand his fears, how stressful it is coping with his perceived threats from people trying to hurt him. And I can try to help him understand that I will listen to him, but because he doesn't trust me, will he believe me? Probably not, but I can continue trying. And I can continue hoping if the real Tom is listening deep down, someday he will decide to seek help on his own.

An Encounter with the Police
Massachusetts, March 2004

When Tom and I were students at the University of Oregon and he had written assignments for his classes, I typed his papers. Over the years, his typing skills barely improved. Whenever I watched him use the hunt-and-peck method with his two index fingers, I took pity on him and offered to help. He always gladly accepted until he started taking classes at NYU.

But since I left him, he wants me to type his papers again. I don't understand this sudden change, unless he thinks it's a way he can stay connected to me. If he's worried about my knowing what he's doing, wouldn't he be concerned about me reading his assignments while I type them? That's why he didn't want me to type his papers for his classes at NYU.

I agree on one condition: I won't do it at the apartment in Waltham. He can send his handwritten pages to me via eFax, a cloud-based facsimile service, then I'll type the papers and email them to him. He has a printer to print them out. This system was working well for his first three assignments, but then he calls me with a different request.

"Can you come over after work and type a paper for me?" he asks.

"Fax your pages to me, and I'll finish it as soon as I can," I reply. "When can you send them?"

"I don't have time," he replies. "It's due on Thursday, before class starts."

It's Tuesday afternoon at two-thirty.

"Have you started it?" I ask.

"Yes. I will have some pages ready for you when you arrive."

"All right," I say. "I will see you at seven-thirty."

What are you doing? Charlotte screams at me from the back of my mind.

I'm going to Waltham tonight to type a paper for Tom.

He can type his own papers. You're enabling him. What happened to the boundaries you set?

I can make an exception one time, can't I? I'm not doing it again.

When you bend the rules, Tom will convince you to bend them more. You're feeling guilty for leaving him again, aren't you?

What if I am?

Stop it! This is not your fault. Have you forgotten the conversations with your counselor about this? Why do I have to keep reminding you?

The counselor and I talk about this in some of our sessions. Through her questions, she steers me to the same conclusion: This is not my fault. I can't fix Tom's condition. The only person who can take care of Tom is Tom. He needs to acknowledge he needs help and begin his own journey to recovery.

She also steers me to another point about guilt: Women tend to put other people's needs above ours and don't take care of ourselves. Even when we practice self-care, we work it around others' priorities instead of setting boundaries for ourselves. That's because we feel guilty about affecting their schedules, their wants and needs, etc.

But I've made a commitment already, I say to Charlotte. *I can't cancel.*

Don't do this! It's not safe to go there tonight!

What could possibly happen? I'm not having sex with him again. I'm only typing a paper.

On the way to my apartment in Acton after work tonight, I see a red fox running in the woods a few yards from the shoulder of the road. They're often visible in the winter and early spring when they're looking for food. Foxes and wild turkeys. Often the turkeys stop in the middle of the road and block traffic while they decide which way to go, but the foxes always keep a safe distance from the cars. If only I could be like the foxes and keep my distance from Tom...why is it so hard?

At my apartment, I freshen up, change from my office clothes into jeans and a sweatshirt, and check on the cats' food, water, and litter box. Both cats are sleeping, TC curled on the bed and Tiger lying on his back on the couch with his front paws tucked against his chest and his back legs spread wide. His shape reminds me of an upside-down flying squirrel wearing a heavy fur coat. I laugh at him, but he doesn't move. Either he's in a deep sleep, or he's ignoring me—most likely the latter.

At seven-thirty, I knock on the door of the apartment in Waltham. I have a key, but I don't use it. With Tom under stress from writing this paper, he might accuse me of snooping on him again.

There's still time to turn around and walk away, Charlotte says.

I'm here now. I need to finish this.

It's not safe to be here tonight!

Tom opens the door a crack, peeks through, and smiles at me. He opens the door wider and stands back while gripping the knob, allowing enough space for me to pass in front of him, and shuts the door behind us.

The blinds in the living room are closed. Two small lamps shine through the darkness at one end of the couch and at the desk. Papers are scattered all over the couch, the footstool, and on the desk.

I sit at the desk and open Tom's laptop. He pushes some papers from the end of the couch closest to the desk to the middle and sits in the empty spot. I turn around and face him.

"What do you have ready to type?" I ask.

"Here's one page," he says. He rips the page from a tablet on the footstool and hands it to me. I look at the yellow sheet with Tom's handwriting in black ink on the blue lines. Only one paragraph with three sentences.

"This is all you've done? Do you know what time it is? I can't stay up all night. I have to be at work at seven-thirty in the morning."

"I'm working on it," he says.

I type the paragraph and wait for more pages while fuming inside. Tom shuffles the papers and turns pages in his textbooks, searching for words.

"I haven't finished because they've been following me again," he says. "Someone tried to contaminate me today."

You can't stay here, Charlotte says. *You must stop feeling guilty. You can't help him. Please listen to me! I'm here to help you.*

"Tom, you know what my work schedule is," I say. "I need to get some sleep. I can't focus on my job without a good night's sleep."

I pick up my keys from the desk and stand. "Fax it to the office tomorrow, and I'll finish it during my lunch hour and email it to you."

Tom gets up and snatches the keys from me. "No. You're staying here until I finish writing this paper!"

He stands in front of me, his back to the apartment door, glaring at me like a caged tiger trying to escape.

Fear grips me. Charlotte is right. I can't stay here, but now I can't leave without help.

I grab the receiver from the phone on the desk and dial 911.

"Nine-one-one. What's your emergency?" a calm female voice says in a slightly bored tone.

"My husband is…"

Tom yanks the receiver from my hand and slams it onto the phone base.

"Why did you do that?" he yells at me. He throws the keys at me. They ricochet off my arm and land on the floor. I pick them up and drop them in my pants pocket.

I look up at Tom. His eyes are burning through me. I'm afraid to move.

Someone pounds on the door. Tom turns, facing the direction of the sound, and freezes while I walk around him and open the door. Two Waltham police officers are outside dressed in uniform. The officer closest to me is my height with light brown hair and hazel eyes. He's a couple of inches shorter than his dark brown-haired, brown-eyed partner standing behind him.

"We got a call about a disturbance," the light brown-haired officer says. "Can you step outside and tell me what happened?"

I follow the officer a few feet away while his partner enters the apartment and starts talking to Tom. I watch the officer with Tom through the open doorway.

"My husband tried to take my car keys away from me," I say to the officer with me. "We're separated. He's extremely paranoid."

"Are you living here?" the officer asks.

"Not anymore. I have an apartment in Acton."

"Why are you here tonight?"

"He asked me to type a paper for him. He's a student at the Harvard Extension School. The paper isn't ready, so I asked him to fax his pages to me tomorrow and started to leave. That's when he took my keys away from me."

Then I see the officer with Tom walk outside, down the hill and around the corner to the back of the building toward the entrance of the apartment below. Tom must have told him about the person he believes is in there monitoring him, but that apartment has been empty since I upgraded my lease a year ago.

Tom's disclosure to the officer is a cry for help. This is the first time he has shared this story with anyone else.

At last! Tom's journey to recovery can start tonight because of my call to 911.

When the officer returns from the empty apartment, he stops at his partner's side, looks at me, and says, "Stay here. We'll be right back."

They walk far enough away so I can't hear their conversation. Tom stays in the apartment. He's standing in front of the desk, staring at his laptop and rubbing his chin.

The officers return a minute later, and the one who questioned me says, "There's nothing you can do here tonight. We think it's best for you to go home and get some rest."

That's it? They're not taking Tom in for an evaluation?

The thought crushes me. My spark of hope for getting some help for Tom has been snuffed out with a short conversation. Through my shock and sadness over this, I remind myself that if they hadn't responded so soon, the outcome might have been much worse. I should have listened to Charlotte.

I'm sorry, I say to her. *You were trying to protect me. You always have my back.*

She doesn't respond. She knows I learned my lesson the hard way. From now on, I will listen to her.

I nod and thank the officers. They walk me to my car and wait for me to leave. The last time I see them is in my rearview mirror, when they're in the patrol car heading toward the police station.

I don't know if Tom finished the paper. I don't call him. He'll have to figure it out on his own.

The next time he contacts me is a week later by email. "I want to talk to you," he wrote. "Can we meet before class on Thursday night?"

"I am not coming to the apartment anymore," I reply. "I will meet you at the entrance to the Harvard Square station at six-thirty."

This is my new boundary: We'll meet in a public place.

After we meet at the station, we walk to Dunkin' Donuts, buy a drink and snack, and sit at a two-top table facing each other. Then Tom announces, "I'm going back to Seattle."

Tom Returns to Seattle
New England, Spring-Summer 2004

My cell phone rings while I sit at my desk eating lunch: a smoked turkey sandwich and banana from the deli at Donelan's, a supermarket nearby. The caller ID displays Don's office number.

I pick up.

"Hi, Cheryl," Don says. "I thought you should know I got a call from Overlake Hospital this morning. Tom went to the emergency room, complaining he was contaminated."

Tom's delusions about contamination obsessed him constantly before he took off to Seattle at the last minute. "I'm volunteering for the summer," he said that night we met briefly at Dunkin' Donuts in Harvard Square, but he wouldn't tell me what he would be doing or for whom.

He left Massachusetts almost three weeks ago. His spontaneous trip puzzles me because he didn't want to talk about Seattle after we moved to the Northeast. Why is he returning now? And how can he afford to go there without a job? Is he drawing out money from his 401(k) from his former sales job? He wouldn't have enough left from his student loans to cover this and he won't get any more financial aid if he doesn't take any classes in the certificate program this summer. He left for Seattle before he finished spring semester, which could affect his eligibility for future aid if he didn't hand in his final assignments before he left.

On one hand, I'm relieved Tom is gone, but on the other, I'm upset because he decided to volunteer instead of getting a job to help me wash away the rising tide of bills. Sometimes I wonder whether he really went to Seattle, or he returned to New York City where he can hide in plain sight. The latter is more believable because with his paranoia, he would be attracted to a place where no one would notice him unless he drew attention to himself. He would stand out too much in Seattle. But according to Don's news, Tom is indeed there; otherwise, he wouldn't have visited an emergency room in Bellevue today.

"What happened?" I ask Don.

"They ran a series of tests, which didn't show any signs of contamination. The doctor on duty told Tom he was okay, but he needed to see a psychiatrist. Tom got mad and left."

None of this surprises me, except the part where Tom went to the emergency room. He doesn't trust anyone, so it doesn't make sense he would go there to be checked. Maybe he felt sick and believed he needed medical treatment, but he didn't get the results he wanted. In his mind, counseling isn't the solution. I don't know what will convince him to get counseling. My leaving him didn't change his mind, so will anything else sway him? Knowing what I know now, probably not. He will have to hit bottom before he can rise again. It's uncertain how far he needs to fall and for how long, or if he will ever land.

"How did they get your number?" I ask Don.

"Tom listed me as an emergency contact," he says, "so they called me as soon as he left the hospital."

"He doesn't want anyone talking to me, obviously. He's covered on my insurance."

I don't know why I mentioned the insurance to Don. Maybe it's because I thought it would be one less worry for him.

I'm concerned about how Don feels about my leaving Tom, but Don hasn't told me it was a bad decision or I should return. Instead, he stands by me from three thousand miles away and calls whenever he hears from Tom. I didn't expect this after my first phone conversation with him about Tom's condition in December. I didn't ask him to support me and won't ask him why he's doing it now. Don has always been the one who circulates news about the family, when necessary, so he probably feels it's his responsibility to keep me informed.

"Tom hasn't mentioned the contamination during our conversations," Don says.

"He started talking about it after Tiger was diagnosed with

diabetes and the vet prescribed insulin shots. It got worse after Tess passed away."

"I don't understand it," Don says. "How can he believe someone is doing this to him? Why would anyone do this? It's impossible."

"I know. It doesn't make sense to me, either. I understand it's coming from the paranoia, but I don't know what triggered it. Maybe it's because of the insulin shots. He wouldn't touch the bottles and needles—not even the boxes and bags they come in. I buy the supplies and give the shots to Tiger. But Tom is in Seattle now, so I would think he would forget about it. There's no logic in his behavior anymore."

"He said he was volunteering for an organization called Star something...I can't remember the full name. He said the organization helps kids."

My nephew and niece, Julie's children, loved Tom. When we visited them, he would play with them like he was a kid for hours. They would romp around and chase each other with squeals of delight. My eight-year-old niece's favorite game was "riding the horse." Tom would drop to his hands and knees, she would climb on his back and ride around the living room on a rainy day. She laughed the entire time Tom "trotted" around the room. Her brother, a toddler, would watch, sucking his pacifier with his blue eyes wide in fascination.

The only time Ron brought his family to Coos Bay to visit during a holiday, Tom acted the same with Ron's daughter and son. They filled the house and yard with happy squeals and laughter.

Before Tom's paranoia set in, he would have been a great father, but we decided not to have children until we could buy a house. When we were younger, many managers of apartment complexes wouldn't rent to anyone with children, but the laws have changed since then.

We stopped talking about having children after we realized we would never be able to afford a house in Seattle. Real estate prices rose so fast there in the nineties with the booming economy and the demand for housing, we couldn't qualify for a large enough loan despite two incomes and a good credit record. But now when I think about how much money we've spent on Tom's endless education, we could have saved enough for a large down payment, which would have qualified us for a loan that would have covered the balance.

In hindsight, I'm glad we didn't have children. I don't know how I could take care of them now when I'm fighting to survive. We'd probably be living in a tent or my car, or the Massachusetts Department of Children & Families would have taken them away from me. And there's the chance they could have inherited Tom's mental illness. I couldn't bear to see my children struggle like Tom has.

I launch my web browser and search for non-profit organizations for children in Seattle with "star" in the name. The first hit in the results shows Starlight Children's Foundation in Redmond, Washington, which helps seriously ill kids.

"Does Starlight Children's Foundation sound familiar?" I ask Don.

"That's it," he replies. "He was there for only four days, He left because he thought someone was interfering. I asked him why anyone would interfere, and his reply was someone was following him constantly. I said there's no reason anyone would follow him."

"How did he respond?"

"He went into a long rant about how someone is following him, bugging his phone, and trying to contaminate him. I said that this is impossible because no one is interested in what he's doing. Then he accused me of being involved."

That's the first time Don mentioned Tom believing he was part of "the conspiracy."

"He blames me, too," I say. "Why does he think you would do anything like this? You wouldn't."

"I'd never do anything like that."

Tom's quitting over his suspicions doesn't surprise me, but the length of his volunteer stint makes me wonder why he even bothered to go to Seattle. Is this really why he went? He lasted at the volunteer position in Waltham for almost three months before he left for the same reason.

But why is Tom now blaming Don for snooping on him? Maybe it's because the emergency room doctor said he needed counseling. Tom thought Don had talked to the doctor before the diagnosis was finished. In Tom's confused mind, it would have been more likely he'd accuse me instead of Don. Maybe Tom has shifted his focus because Don is now located closer to him than I am.

"Do you think he would come to Coos Bay?" Don asks. "Nancy's condition is worse, and I don't want anyone upsetting her."

"I doubt it," I say. "He doesn't talk about Coos Bay anymore."

"I will keep you updated if I hear anything else," Don says. "If Tom asks about you, what should I tell him?"

"He probably won't, but if he does, I think it's best to say that you aren't in contact with me. If he knows, he'll probably stop calling you because he'll believe you and I are plotting something against him. I know this doesn't make sense, but neither does Tom's behavior anymore."

I don't want Don to lose his connection with Tom. If Tom loses his trust in Don, then Don will never hear from him again.

"Okay, that's what we will do," Don says. "I'll talk to you later."

Five days later, a few minutes before lunchtime, Don calls from his office. "Tom showed up at my office early Saturday morning," he says.

"I'm so sorry," I say. "I can't believe he did this."

"There's no need to apologize. It's not your fault."

"What happened?"

"We sat and talked for about an hour. At first, he talked about some people who were following him. I asked him why he thought he was being followed and who these people are, but he couldn't answer my questions."

All of this is familiar territory to me, but it's new to Don. I could tell by the tone in his voice that navigating this conversation was as frustrating to him as it has been for me.

"I needed to go home and check on Nancy. I said he could go with me, only if he agreed to stop talking about the people following him."

"Did he do it?"

"He did. We had a nice conversation with Nancy for about a half hour."

"I'm surprised he could hold it together for that long. He doesn't here."

"After we left the house, I offered to take him to the cemetery to visit Mom and Dad's graves. He agreed."

"How did he react when you were there?"

"He was quiet. He just stared at the graves. After we left the cemetery, we returned to my office, and he left. I haven't heard from him since."

"Did he tell you where he was going after he left?"

"No. I assume he returned to Seattle."

We're silent for a few seconds. I wonder where Tom is now. He could be anywhere.

"Cheryl, I want you know that I didn't know how bad this was until I saw it for myself," Don says. "I'm sorry you've had to go through this. I wish there was something I could do."

"Thank you, Don, but there's nothing you can do. Tom must make that decision for himself."

A week later, an agent from the apartment management office in Waltham calls.

"Hi, Cheryl," she says. "I'm calling because I haven't received the rent for this month. Tomorrow is the tenth."

Tom should have paid the rent before he took off to Seattle. I kept the lease after moving out so he would have a place to live. Tom is probably expecting me to pay the rent while he's gone. It's time to set another boundary, and this one will have bigger consequences.

"I'm sorry, I don't have enough money to cover it," I say. "Tom and I separated in January, and I moved to Acton. He stayed, and he should be paying the rent now. I hoped we could resolve our differences, but now it appears we can't. I need to give a thirty-day notice."

"I'm sorry to hear that," the agent says.

"Is it okay if I apply my deposit to this month's rent and I'll pay the rest before the end of the month? I don't have enough money to cover the balance today, but I will after my next paycheck."

"That will be fine," the agent says. "Can you fax your notice to me today?"

"Yes. I will take care of it this morning."

When I'm finished, I dial Tom's cell number. The call goes straight to voicemail, and I hang up. I'm tired of talking to his voicemail. He'll see my number on his phone log, so if he wants to talk to me, he can call me back. He should have taken care of the rent before he left. Now he'll have to figure out what he'll do next, like get a job.

The next day at noon, I'm sitting in my car, preparing to make a few phone calls before a trip for takeout. When I start to dial a number, my phone rings. A toll-free number that looks familiar displays on the caller ID.

"Hi, Cheryl," the friendly voice says on the opposite end of the line. "It's Crystal from the bank."

She's calling from the bank in New York, where Tom and I had a joint checking account. I closed the account after we separated in January and opened a new one in only my name at a bank in Massachusetts. Why would she call me now?

"I wanted to make you aware of a past-due balance on your credit line."

"What credit line? I don't have a credit line with you or any other bank."

"You are Cheryl Landes, correct?"

"Yes."

"Is your husband's name Tom Landes?"

"Yes."

"Tom opened a credit line when you had a checking account here."

"How could he open a credit line without my knowledge and permission?"

"It isn't required with a joint account. Either one of you could open a credit line, but the account would be in both names."

I recall Betty's advice about spouses having separate bank accounts and regret I didn't pull the plug sooner. What other financial surprises are waiting for me?

"The past-due balance is eight hundred dollars," the agent says. "It has been outstanding for more than ninety days. I can take payment in full over the phone today."

"I can't pay in full today. I'll have to make payments."

"The best I can do is split the balance over two months. Can you pay four hundred dollars today?"

"No. The earliest I'll have it is on Friday. That's the best I can do."

"That will be fine. Call me on Friday and I'll take your payment over the phone." She gives me a different toll-free number with her extension.

This conversation with the bank becomes a launching pad for more calls from collectors for other bills I didn't know we had. Soon I'm letting some regular bills slide for a month to pay these new bills, then let the new bills slide the next month to catch up on the others. How could Tom get credit when he hasn't worked for so long? I try calling him again about these new bills, but all I get is voicemail. He never calls me back.

Soon the amount of money owed exceeds my income. I'm getting fewer editing and indexing projects because of the continuing consolidation of the publishing companies and more work being outsourced offshore. I begin applying at temporary agencies that hire secretaries, clerks, and laborers in hopes I can find odd jobs in the evenings and on weekends. The first one is a three-week assignment for a call center in Marlborough, a half hour's drive from the office, from six to nine weeknights.

At the beginning of our shifts, the supervisor gives each worker a list of phone numbers to call. The numbers are for student leaders on college campuses. When someone answers, we read a simple script: "We have a great opportunity for your organization to raise some money. Would you like to hear more about it?" If they say "yes," we forward the calls to another person who describes the offer. No one tells us what the offer is.

After a few days on this assignment, I notice when I cross off numbers from the list after a contact says, "do not call me again," they reappear on a fresh list the supervisor gives to me at the beginning of my next shift. One night, a frustrated but friendly student leader says she received three calls from us during the past week and every time, she asked to be removed from the list.

"Every time I talk to someone and they ask me to remove their name from the list, I cross it off and make a note to delete it," I say. "I'm sorry this is happening. I will make another note for my supervisor tonight."

"Thank you," she says. "Do you know what they're trying to sell to us?"

"No. They never shared this information with us."

"They want us to encourage students on our campus to apply for credit cards," she says. "They say they'll give us a commission for every application the students fill out. My organization is not encouraging students to go into debt. They'll already have a heavy enough burden from their student loans when they graduate. They don't need to add credit card bills to the pile."

It's easy to do, and I applaud her for discouraging this. Tom and I overburdened ourselves with credit card debt to cover his classes and workshops for his failed career change. It's convenient, and when

The Best I Can Do

someone isn't careful, the balances add up quickly.

I want to share my experiences with this student leader but don't because someone would overhear me. After listening to her comments, I don't want to continue this assignment. I feel creepy, trying to sell something that brings trouble to a lot of people, but I need the money to pay toward my own credit card bills.

From this conversation until the end of my assignment, I go through the motions of calling the numbers on my list but don't encourage the student leaders who answer my calls to be forwarded to the next level. By then, most of the people on my list have been contacted at least three or four times by different call center workers and are tired of hearing from us. I apologize to them but know my supervisor will never remove them from the lists regardless of how many notes I make, but I still cross off their numbers with the note, "Please remove."

While I'm working at the call center, I'm also cleaning out the apartment in Waltham. I don't have anywhere to keep our belongings because there's no space in the storage unit we have a mile away. So, I donate everything I can to the Goodwill and Salvation Army. Anything they don't accept, I offer to the neighbors or throw it away. The next-door neighbors, two freshmen students from Bentley University, score enough furniture from me to outfit their living room and kitchen, along with a TV I can't use. They're shocked that I offer so much to them but elated about their good fortune.

They repeatedly ask me, "Are you really sure you want to do this?"

My reply is always, "I'm sure. I can't take it with me, and I'm happy I can give it to someone who can use it."

It's true, although I was especially sad about giving away the beautiful maple dining table and chairs I bought while I was in college. Globe Furniture let me make payments for two years until I paid the balance in full. I worked extra hours at my fast-food job at Taco Time during my freshman and sophomore years at Eastern Oregon University in La Grande to make the payments on time. It was the first time anyone gave me credit to buy anything. Despite now having to let the dining set go, I'm thankful that someone else will use it and take good care of it. These guys seem to be the types who don't take anything for granted—a hunch from Charlotte.

After I finish cleaning out the apartment and turning in the keys to the rental agent, she says, "Tom called me a week after I called you to pay the rent. He was disappointed that you gave notice, but I said that even if you hadn't, it would have been too late. By then, we would have served the eviction notice."

When I'm finished at the apartment, I drive to the storage center to grab a few items from our unit and pay the bill. I try to insert the key in the lock, and it doesn't fit. Why? We've used the same lock on the unit since we started renting it in September 2003.

I stop at the front desk, where a tall young man with black hair is on duty.

"My key isn't working for our storage unit," I say. "Is there any way you can let me in?"

"What's your name and unit number?"

"Cheryl Landes, unit 107."

He looks up the unit number in the database.

"What name is on the account?"

"My name and my husband's, Tom Landes."

"I don't see your name here."

"That's not right. Both of our names are on the account. We included both names on the application to rent the unit last fall."

"Tom must have removed your name from the account."

"How is that possible? Wouldn't he have to get permission from me first? He hasn't."

"Well, your name isn't on the account now, so I can't let you in. Even if your name were on the account, I still couldn't let you in because the rent is past due. If the rent isn't paid by May fifteenth, we'll block access to the unit and auction off the contents."

I want to scream, but it won't help. When will this end?

"The contents aren't all his. I have stuff in there, too."

I don't have many items I want to keep in the unit, but a few things have sentimental value. There's a gold Sarah Coventry necklace with rhinestones that Grandma wore. Mom gave it to me after Grandma died. There's a toy stuffed skunk I've had since I was four. I thought Grandma gave it to me, but Mom said my favorite great-uncle gave it to me before we moved from California to Missouri. There's also an ice-cream soda mug with a picture of an old-fashioned soda counter popular in the drugstores decades ago that the same great-uncle bought for me at a dime store on the square in downtown West Plains during one of his visits to Missouri with his wife. And there are dozens of antique postcards Tom and I collected over the years that I don't want to lose. Tom won't have any interest in them now.

Tom must have taken my name off the account during one of his delusions, when he thought I would do who knows what.

"You need to contact him and make arrangements. And while you're at it, tell him the rent is past due."

"I can't reach him. He's gone for the summer and isn't returning my calls."

"I'm sorry, but I can't help you. Have a nice day."

Have a nice day…right.

As soon as I return to the car, I call Tom and receive the voicemail again.

"Tom, I just went to the storage place and found out the rent is past due. They also told me that you took my name off the account. Why? I want to remove my stuff and need you to let me in. Call me back. And call the storage place and pay the rent. It's your bill now."

Tom never returns my call.

The call center assignment helps me pay off one small bill. A few days after it ends, the same agency calls me. "The receptionist at a jewelry store in Chestnut Hill is on maternity leave for two months, and they need someone to fill in until she returns," the recruiter says. "She works nights and weekends. Would you be interested?"

I accept the assignment. It's unlike any other receptionist job, where I worked at a front desk, welcoming visitors, answering calls, providing information, and dispensing coffee, tea, and water to guests waiting to meet with someone. At this one, I'm sitting in a storage room behind a wobbly gray metal desk, answering the phone and taking messages for the salespeople on the floor. It feels like I'm toiling in a cave, but I try to stay optimistic. The hours fit perfectly around my full-time job, and the work is helping me pay off a few more bills, but when I think I'm starting to get ahead, more calls come from the collectors.

You need to protect yourself financially, Charlotte says one night during my shift at the jewelry store.

How in the world can I do that? I can barely make ends meet now, and I don't know what else I'll run into. The collectors are going after me, not Tom.

That's exactly why you need to protect yourself.

But again, how can I do that? These collectors will harass me until they get what they want.

You need to file for a legal separation. It will protect you from the creditors.

I don't want to end my marriage, although in reality, it has ended. A legal separation wouldn't mean my marriage is completely over; it means there's the option that Tom and I could reconcile if he decides to get help and commits to recovery, but that's up to him.

Finding an affordable lawyer is a challenge. Whenever I call the offices specializing in family law for information, the receptionists ask how many assets are involved. They won't accept me as a client because of the amount of money we owe and the only asset is my car—a depreciating asset on a lease. I sense they also don't want to take my case because of Tom's mental illness. Most of the lawyers charge a retainer up front, ranging from three thousand to six thousand dollars. I don't have that much money and don't want to pay up front because I can't control how they will spend the money.

Finally, I find an office in Newton that handles cases like mine and charges an hourly rate. One hundred twenty-five dollars an hour is high for me, but I'll have to find a way to pay it. In the long run, if something can be done to protect me financially, the money will be well spent. I'll have a better chance of getting back on my feet.

Melanie, the lawyer, is a petite woman with dark brown hair, hazel eyes, and a creamy complexion. She's probably in her mid-thirties and wears just enough makeup to blend in with her skin so it looks natural. She's dressed in a navy blue suit covering a white button-down blouse. Her office is bright and welcoming with large windows stretching across two perpendicular walls, white oak furniture, walls painted in a cream color, and a powder blue carpet. Potted plants thrive on top of the bookshelves, in the windowsills, and in the corners next to the windows. Outside, maple trees line the perimeter of the parking lot.

When Melanie greets me, she's soft-spoken yet confident. I sit in one of the guest chairs in front of her desk and summarize my situation and what I want to do.

She sits behind her desk and looks at me thoughtfully until I mention the legal separation; then a solemn look crosses her face. "I can help you if you want to work with me," she says. "However, I need to inform you that you cannot get a legal separation in

Massachusetts. The only options you have are to get a divorce or remain married."

Now what do I do? I ask Charlotte while staring at my hands folded in my lap.

Get the divorce, she replies.

It's so final. Do I really want to do this?

You must break the ties. Tom isn't getting any better. You need to protect yourself. This situation won't improve until you help yourself. You need to put yourself first. There's nothing you can do for Tom anymore.

"If you need time to think about it, I will understand," Melanie says.

I look up at her. "No, I don't need any more time. I want to move forward with the divorce." Saying those words crushes me, despite my knowing it's the right decision.

Melanie gathers a pile of forms, slides them into an envelope, and hands it to me. "Fill these out as best you can. Let's schedule an appointment next week to review them and answer any questions you may have."

The forms take a few hours to fill out. It feels like I'm telling the story of my marriage in fields and checkboxes: When and where we married, our assets, our liabilities (what we owe), where we last lived before we split up, and why I want to get a divorce. When I finish, the information on paper looks neatly organized for such a complicated situation.

When I'm commuting to work and appointments, I hear ads on Magic 106.7, a radio station in Boston, about a debt consolidation service. "Do you have more than ten thousand dollars in credit card debt? Get relief by consolidating your credit card balances into one convenient monthly payment. With our program, you can even pay off your balances faster. Call us or visit our website today!"

At first, I'm skeptical about whether a service like this can help me pay off the credit card bills faster, but after hearing the ads multiple times, I look up the company's website, followed by other debt consolidation agencies, all of which provide the same information. They all work with people who have charged ten thousand dollars or more on credit cards. Testimonials from previous clients praise the companies for helping them get out of debt. Then I look for information about whether these programs are effective. Overall, the answer is "yes." I also learn there are three different programs.

The first is a debt consolidation loan, where I'd apply for a loan through a bank or credit union for the balance I owe, pay off the bills, and then make monthly payments to the bank or credit union. The second is a debt management plan, where a non-profit credit counseling organization helps people who owe unsecured debt like credit cards get their balances under control. A counselor works with each borrower and the credit card companies to develop an affordable repayment plan. Then the borrower sends the monthly payment to the credit counseling organization, and the organization distributes the money to the credit card companies, minus a fee to the organization that's built into the plan. The third program is a debt settlement, where the debt settlement company asks the borrower to stop payments directly to the creditors. Instead, the borrower makes monthly payments to the debt settlement company, which sets the money aside in an escrow account. When the borrower is far behind on their bills, the debt settlement company tries to settle the balances for less than the amount owed.

As I look through these options, I rule out the debt consolidation loan and debt settlement immediately. My credit isn't good enough to qualify for a loan. The debt settlement would make my credit worse. The debt management plan would be the best option because I can work on paying off the bills I have without going deeper into debt.

The organization advertising on the radio seems to offer the debt management plans, but I decide to wait to contact them until talking to Melanie again.

I'd thought about filing bankruptcy but quickly dismissed this idea. When I've accepted job offers, the companies hiring me run credit checks in addition to the background and reference checks. A bankruptcy on my credit reports would be an automatic rejection. I don't understand why these companies require credit checks when I'd never handle money on the job, but this is their policy.

At my next appointment with Melanie, she reviews the forms, clarifies some information, and says she will file the paperwork with the courthouse. "Middlesex County is very slow, so I do not know when we will hear from them."

I'm not surprised about the county's speed because at the office, Human Resources sometimes waits two to three months for a background check to clear when they're hiring a new person. I'm relieved the divorce process is at least moving forward but sad at the same time about being forced into this. Tom still hasn't called me since he left for Seattle, so I haven't talked to him about this.

I ask Melanie about the debt consolidation service.

"It can help you pay down your credit card debt," she says.

I agree with her, Charlotte says. I didn't fight back this time because I learned my lesson. She knows what she's doing.

I also tell Melanie about the storage unit. "We can get a court order so you can retrieve your belongings," she says. "I can take care of this today."

The next day, I call a counselor at the debt consolidation service during my lunch break and ask her to explain the program to me. "The program is for unsecured debt, which is any money you owe that does not have assets set up as collateral. The most common debt consolidated through our program is credit cards. We work with clients who owe ten thousand dollars or more."

"I want to consolidate my credit card debt," I say.

"When you enroll in our program, any credit card accounts in your debt consolidation program are closed. You cannot use them anymore. We work with these credit card companies to develop a payment plan that you can manage. You will make one payment directly to us each month, and we distribute the money to each credit card company. You payment includes a monthly fee for us to manage this service. Usually, your monthly payments will be less than what you're now paying separately to each credit card company, and you can pay off the balance faster."

"How do I make the payments?"

"We do not accept checks, so you have two options: a money order or an automatic monthly withdrawal from a bank account. If you choose the first option, you need to mail the money order to our office in time to arrive by the due date. If you use the second option, the money will be deducted from your account on the day the payment is due."

Go for it, Charlotte says. *This will give you some relief, and you can start paying off some more bills that don't qualify for the plan.*

"I'd like to enroll," I say to the counselor.

"Great! While we're on the phone, I need to get some basic information from you. Then I will email some forms for you to fill out and sign. You can fax them back to me." She gives me the fax number.

After the paperwork is processed, the counselor tells me that my payments will be reduced to two hundred thirty-five dollars a month and I will pay off the balance in three years. I select the monthly automatic withdrawal and set it up for the twentieth of the month.

When I hang up, Melanie calls. "I have the court order to access the storage unit," she says. "You can pick it up at any time."

"I'll stop by after work today," I say. "Thank you again."

"I'll leave it at the reception desk."

My next stop after Melanie's office is at the storage company. When I show the court order to the person on duty, he says, "I can't let you in."

"Why not? This is a court order signed by a judge!"

"I can't let anyone into a storage unit if their name isn't on the account."

This is ridiculous. I'm not giving up.

"I'd like to speak to a manager," I say.

"He's not here."

"When will he be back?"

"I don't know."

I don't believe him. He doesn't want to deal with this, so he's trying to shoo me away like an annoying fly.

"Is there another place where I can contact him?"

The man sighs. "Give me your phone number. He'll call you when he's back."

I write it on the piece of paper the man hands to me but don't expect to hear from the manager. This isn't stopping me from accessing the storage unit. I'll find another way.

When I'm at home, I look up the storage company's website and find a phone number for their headquarters. It's closed now, so I will call them tomorrow.

I'm on the phone with them as soon as they open the next morning. "How can I reach the manager of the Waltham store?" I ask. "I have a court order to access a storage unit."

"We can't release that information," the receptionist says. "You can stop at the store and ask to talk to him."

"I tried that already."

"I'm sorry, I can't help you."

"Is there another manager I can talk to there? I don't have much time before the contents are auctioned off. My husband removed my name from the account, disappeared, and stopped paying the rent. He's mentally ill."

The receptionist's voice softens. "I'm so sorry. I can forward you to the district manager. He's available now."

She transfers my call, and the district manager picks up. I explain the situation.

"I don't understand why they didn't let you in when you have a court order," he says. "I'll talk to the store manager about this. He'll call you today and schedule an appointment to let you in. Bring the court order to your appointment."

Less than ten minutes later, the manager in Waltham calls. We set up the appointment for two o'clock tomorrow afternoon. "Ask for me when you arrive," he says.

The manager is at the counter when I arrive. I show the court order to him, and he drills the lock to break it apart. He opens the door to a messy unit. It wasn't like this when we moved the boxes in here; everything was stacked neatly and organized. But now, dirty men's pants and shirts are strewn over the boxes in the front of the unit, along with several white plastic garbage bags tied shut.

I recognize the clothes; they're definitely Tom's. Why is he storing dirty clothes and garbage here? Maybe he believes the clothes are contaminated and the garbage is "evidence" he gathered to prove his claims. This seems far-fetched, but it's the only answer that makes sense to me.

"How long do I have to finish removing my belongings?" I ask the manager.

"Two days are the longest I can allow."

"That will be enough time. Thank you."

The postcards are easy to find; they're in a safe on one side of the unit. The safe is the size of a mini refrigerator used in campers, hotel rooms, and college dorms, easily weighing one hundred pounds. I manage to move the safe to the cart by "walking it"—rotating the base with every step. Fortunately, the bed of the cart is six inches from the floor, so I'm able to lift the safe high enough to shuttle it to my car. Lifting the safe from the cart into the back of my car is a bigger challenge, but I finally muster enough adrenaline to finish the job. When I'm done, I sit on the cart to catch my breath.

The other items take longer to find. While I go through each box,

I quickly learn that some no longer contain the items that match the labels on the outside. What was Tom doing in here?

By closing time that afternoon, I find Grandma's rhinestone necklace and tuck it away in my backpack. I also find the photo album with the pictures of our wedding from the professional photographer. I'd forgotten about it, but I'm glad it's still here. Despite our crumbled marriage, I want to preserve the happy memories.

I place the album on the cart, along with a thick polyester-filled maroon comforter we bought at JCPenney in Seattle one unusually cold winter. I might need it.

When the storage company closes, I stop by the counter to ask when I can return tomorrow. "I've retrieved a few things but am still looking for the rest," I explain.

"Any time we're open," the man behind the counter replies. "I'm here all day."

"I'll be here when you open in the morning. Thanks again."

The next day, I'm in the unit until an hour before closing, searching for the two missing sentimental items. I finally find the toy skunk in a box of Tom's jazz albums he collected from Time Life before we started dating. We played them for hours before and after we married. I didn't know much about jazz music before meeting Tom, but I fell in love with it the more I listened. The slow, complex rhythms and harmonies of the instrumentals, and vocals of raw, deeply emotional stories pulled me in. No other type of music expresses the experiences of life and love, happy and sad, the way jazz does.

I never find the mug. I remember packing it when we moved from Staten Island. Where did it go? I've searched every box, but I don't have time to look again.

Let it go, Charlotte says. *You have many beautiful memories of your great-uncle and aunt. Be grateful for those.*

Be grateful for what I have.

That's right.

My next appointment with Melanie is a week later, when she says, "I need to take a leave of absence for medical reasons. I don't know yet when I can return. I'm sorry."

"I'm sorry you aren't feeling well," I say while asking myself, *What will I do now?* Her partners aren't accepting new clients.

I don't ask for a referral. Instead, I accept this as a sign that I shouldn't move forward with the divorce.

Don't stop now, Charlotte says. *You need to protect yourself financially.*

You know how hard it was to find Melanie. Where will I find anyone else who's willing to represent me?

You will. Don't give up.

I decide to wait. There's too much to deal with right now.

Cheryl Landes

Reconnecting with Nature
Maine, Summer 2004

I'm standing on the dock at Odyssey Whale Watch on a sunny June morning in downtown Portland, Maine, watching the crew prepare the boat for our trip. A cool gentle breeze blows across the harbor and plays with the short hairs in my dark brown braid. They work themselves free and tickle my forehead, ears, and neck.

Two seagulls coast the air currents at the edge of the dock between the boat and DiMillo's On the Water, a restaurant housed in a retired ferry. They land side by side on the railing at the end of the dock.

This is my first attempt to reconnect with nature since Tom and I separated. I miss the long walks and watching sunsets, sunrises, and wildlife. They soothe my body and soul, and I need this more than ever. I'm still seeing the counselor once a month, but talking to her isn't the same as being comforted in the great outdoors.

It's also my first trip to Maine. Except for a weekend leaf-peeping trip to Stowe, Vermont, the fall before Tom and I separated, I've never explored New England beyond Massachusetts. I've driven a lot through Connecticut on weekend trips to and from Staten Island, but my only stops were to eat dinner and refill the car's tank with gas.

"All aboard," the captain announces over the public address system. I hand my ticket to a crew member at the boat ramp, climb the ladder to the top deck of the boat, and sit on a bench on the starboard side. The temperature feels warmer here—likely in the high seventies.

The air is cooler from the wind after we're underway, but it's still pleasant enough to shed my jacket. It feels good to be at sea, smelling

The Best I Can Do

the salty air, feeling the wind brush my skin, watching the gulls, and bouncing on the swells. I recall memories of walks on the Oregon Coast with Tom, strolls along Alki Point in West Seattle, and ferry rides across Puget Sound. We never went on whale watches in the Northwest, although there were several to choose from in Oregon and Washington. Tom never expressed interest in them, but when an orca swam into Hood Canal and hung out there for two weeks, we took a ferry from the Fauntleroy terminal in West Seattle to the Kitsap Peninsula one Sunday morning to watch him.

An hour after we're underway, the captain announces, "There's a school of dolphins at twelve o'clock. Looks like they're ready to give us a show."

I rush to the bow on the lower deck for a closer look, where the dolphins turn somersaults in the water. When they surface, their gray backs and fins glisten in the sun. Some swim around the boat, others continue the somersaults, and a few swim in smaller circles in front of the bow. I love watching them play and wonder if they know how much joy they're giving me and the other passengers.

Forty-five minutes later, the dolphins gather in a V formation in front of the bow and swim east. "They must have spotted a school of fish," the captain says. "Lunchtime!"

We continue searching for whales for the next hour and a half but come up empty. The captain turns the boat around for the trip back to Portland.

"We're disappointed you couldn't see any whales today," he says. "That happens sometimes when we're out here. We never know what they're up to.

"Because we didn't see any whales, we'd like to offer you a free voucher for a future trip. Stop by the office after we dock, and they'll take care of you. This is our thank-you for joining us today. We hope to see you again!"

It's a gracious offer and appreciated, but I'm not disappointed about not seeing any whales today. The dolphins' performance lifted my spirits.

I descend the ladder and find a quiet place in the aft starboard corner of the lower deck to relax and enjoy the view. I'm not looking forward to returning to the stress in Massachusetts.

A few minutes later, a petite woman and boy approach, both wearing matching navy blue windbreakers and blue jeans. The woman appears to be my age, with short, straight light brown hair. The boy's hair color matches hers. He's probably eight or nine years old.

They stop when they see me. The woman says hello, and we start chatting about the dolphins' antics. A couple of minutes into the conversation, they sit on a bench across from me.

"Are you alone?" the woman asks.

"Yes," I reply. "I travel a lot by myself."

"Oh dear, I'm so sorry," she says. "Aren't you afraid to travel alone?"

"I have two choices," I say. "I can stay at home and wonder what it would be like to explore different places. Or I can go and enjoy myself."

She smiles. "Well, I truly admire you. We traveled a lot before my husband died two years ago. After he died, I was scared to travel alone with my son. I was afraid something would happen to us."

"I'm so sorry about your husband."

"He died suddenly. We miss him."

"I understand. My husband disappeared this spring. He went to Seattle, and no one has heard from him for two months."

Why did I open up to her so easily? It took a long time to gather the courage to talk about Tom to my closest friends and Don, and I haven't told Mom yet. I know she'll worry too much. Why should she worry when there's nothing she can do to help me or Tom?

I haven't heard from Don since Tom left Coos Bay, so I know Tom hasn't talked to Don recently. Don always calls me after Tom calls him. Reporting Tom's disappearance to the police is useless, as I learned from my experiences in Waltham.

Maybe it's more comfortable to share our struggles with strangers because we'll never see them again.

"Oh, dear," the woman says. "That must be horrible!"

"He's very paranoid. He doesn't trust anyone anymore."

"That's so sad. Is there anything anyone can do to help him?"

"No. I tried, but no one can help someone who doesn't want it."

We stare at the ocean for a while, lost in our thoughts. Mine return to Tom. Will he ever be capable of asking for help?

"Is this your first whale watch trip?" I ask.

"Yes," she replies. "We started doing some things we haven't tried this summer. It was time to move forward."

She looks at her son and smiles. "This is our second trip. We tried whitewater rafting two weeks ago. We take turns choosing our trips. He chose whitewater rafting, and I picked whale watching."

"I've always wanted to go whitewater rafting. What's it like?"

"We went to The Forks and floated the Kennebec River. We were nervous at first, but when we were in the water, we had so much fun." She smiles. "The guides reassured us that we could do it. We're planning another trip before the season ends."

She wraps her arm around her son's shoulders and pulls him into a sideways hug. He grins and blushes.

"The name of the outfitter is Northern Outdoors. You should go there."

I pull a pen and tablet from my backpack and write down the name. "Thanks! I'll check it out."

By then, the boat is anchored at the dock, and we wish each other well.

During my ninety-minute drive to Massachusetts, I think about the woman and her son, her husband's death too soon, and her newfound bravery to explore with her son. I think about her admiring me for my courage to travel alone, and it reassures me that although I have many challenges ahead, I have the strength to make it through.

That you do, Charlotte confirms.

On my next payday, I book a rafting trip on the Kennebec River through Northern Outdoors. During the safety briefing before we put into the river, I consider backing out when one of the guides say, "Our trip starts over an eight-foot waterfall." Images of Niagara Falls flash through my mind, followed by Multnomah Falls in the Columbia River Gorge. I want to scream and am surprised I don't.

You can do it, Charlotte says. *You're here, aren't you? You can't leave now.*

Why not?

It's only an eight-foot waterfall, not six hundred twenty feet like Multnomah Falls. You've wanted to do this for a long time, and you drove more than four hours to get here. Do you really want to give up now?

So, I exaggerated the height, but it's still a waterfall!

Would these guides go over it if it weren't safe? Would the company they work for let them?

I suppose they wouldn't.
No, they wouldn't, so get out there and enjoy yourself!

When we're in the rafts, we listen to the guide shout commands on when to paddle and when to stop while we sail over the waterfall. When we're at the bottom, all seven of us still safe in the raft, we raise our paddles and cheer. We made it! And I'm hooked. Why didn't I do this sooner?

During the workweek, I look at maps for trails to hike and browse the web for other outdoor adventures. One Saturday, I drive to Freeport, Maine, for a Walk-On Adventure at L.L. Bean's flagship store. For twenty dollars, I can learn how to kayak in two hours—something else I've never tried. The rafting trip gave me confidence to try more new experi-ences.

These mini-workshops showcase L.L. Bean's products, but there isn't any pressure from their salespeople. The products sell themselves. When we finish the lesson, I'm sold, but I can't afford a kayak and don't have anywhere to store one. I can always sign up for kayak tours when the budget allows—something to look forward to on my journey to recovery.

After that, I focus on hiking because it's less expensive. I choose different trails every weekend in the White Mountains National Forest in New Hampshire. I hike trails to waterfalls and sweeping views, through pine and maple forests, and in wildlife refuges. The more trails I finish, the more I crave.

Then I discover a website for Baxter State Park in Maine, seventeen miles north of Millinocket. It's a seven-hour drive from my apartment. The climb to the top of Mount Katahdin in the park intrigues me. At 5,269 feet above sea level, it's the tallest mountain in the state and where the Appalachian Trail starts or ends, depending on which direction one is going. I'm ready for the challenge after tackling so many emotional mountains in my life.

One day when I'm meeting with Todd, our conversation wanders to hiking and I mention Baxter State Park. He takes his family on hiking trips a lot.

Todd's hazel eyes light up and he smiles. "That's my favorite place to hike in Maine! Are you hiking to the top of Katahdin?"

"Yes. I thought I'd take the Hunt Trail, the last leg of the Appalachian Trail."

"I recommend using the Roaring Brook Trail. It's shorter and easier to navigate. Usually we climb the mountain on Roaring Brook and take the Cathedral Trail back.

"You need to arrive early because everyone wants to hike Roaring Brook. The rangers limit the number of people on each trail to the top of Katahdin. You should arrive at the gate at least an hour before it opens."

I make a mental note: *The gate opens at five a.m. Arrive by at least four.*

"I hope you enjoy your trip," he says.

I reserve an inexpensive hotel room for two nights in Millinocket and use some paid leave to take a half day off on Friday. When I arrive in Millinocket that evening, I'm reminded of the small logging towns on the Oregon Coast. Millinocket was once a logging town, too, but the mills are long gone. It now attracts folks who want to go whitewater rafting on the Penobscot River, fish, or hike Baxter State Park. In the winter, it's a popular place for snowmobilers.

The next morning, I arrive at the park's south gate at exactly four o'clock. At least twenty cars are lined up in front of me. When the gate opens, an attendant asks each driver which trail they want to hike. By the time it's my turn, no spots are left for Roaring Brook. The driver in front of me took it, so I ask the attendant to recommend the next best option.

"I'd suggest climbing the AT (Appalachian Trail) and coming back on the Abol Trail," he said.

"OK. I'll take the AT."

He places a sticker on my windshield indicating my trail choice, and I'm off to begin my adventure.

After signing the registry at the trailhead, I follow a dirt trail along a stream through a pine forest. Forty-five minutes later, the trail becomes steeper. Soon, I'm scrambling over rocks and boulders and keeping watch for the blue splotches of paint that guide me forward. I wasn't expecting a self-taught crash course in rock climbing, but that's what I'm doing as I continue up the mountain. My pace slows to a crawl—literally—because there's nowhere to walk. Why on Earth would anyone call this a trail?

When I finally reach Katahdin's peak, I see the blue-green tint of the surrounding hills and mountains and a thin layer of clouds hugging some of the valleys. A few steps away, I spot a cairn, a monument of stacked rocks someone probably built to celebrate their climb. There isn't much vegetation at this elevation—just random scraggly plants that are too stubborn to give up in the bare dirt and rocks.

The Abol Trail starts on dirt covered in loose pebbles and jagged rock chips. This should be an easier hike, although it will be a steep descent at an almost forty-five degree angle.

I'm expecting to arrive at Katahdin's base in two or three hours. Then I can walk the two miles to my parked car and head back to the hotel in Millinocket. It's four-thirty, about three hours until dusk. If it gets dark before I reach my car, I have a headlamp filled with fresh AAA batteries in my day pack.

While descending the mountain, I look at the scenery. I'm still above the tree line, where there's a beautiful panorama of the hills and mountains in the distance. Suddenly, I slip on some loose pebbles and fall flat, like someone grabbed my shoulders and shoved me straight down into a chair. I feel something snap in my lower back and wonder whether my tailbone broke. The sharp pains shooting up my spine slow my pace, but I must keep moving to finish the descent by nightfall.

As the pain increases, every step takes more effort. Now I take more breaks to ease the pain as much as possible while the sun begins sliding toward the horizon. With each step, each break, it's becoming clearer that I can't make it down the mountain tonight. Because I'm still above the tree line, there isn't much I can use for shelter, and I'm equipped only for a day hike. I find a pile of large rocks surrounding a flat rock on three sides that's usable as a chair and bed. This area creates a cubby big enough to partially protect me for the night.

I sit on the flat rock and look for extra clothes in my backpack. There's only a pair of shorts and my sweatshirt. When it gets colder, I'll slip on the sweatshirt and pull the shorts over my head for a hat. I'm scared about spending the night here. Although I've camped many times, I had a tent and I wasn't alone. My cell phone doesn't have a signal, so I can't call anyone for help. If I could, would anyone try to help me this late in the day? Probably not because it isn't safe to climb the mountain at night.

I watch the sunset, snap a few pictures of the view, and think about the happy times when Tom and I watched such colorful displays together. The only time I remember us watching the show from a peak was when we rode the tram to the top of Grouse Mountain for dinner during a trip to Vancouver, British Columbia.

There's no pain as long as I don't move, so I sit as still as possible until the stars twinkle in the velvet sky. With no light pollution up here, I can see hundreds, maybe thousands, of them. I try to focus on the beauty instead of my dilemma.

The sharp pain returns while I curl into a fetal position on the rock and try to sleep, using my backpack for a pillow. I nap off and on but wake up every time a breeze brushes against my exposed skin. Sometimes I shiver, then squeeze myself into a ball as tightly as possible, grimacing from the pain triggered by the movement.

The temperature must be in the forties tonight. It's quiet, but as darkness continues, my worries shift from being here overnight to whether I can contact anyone for help in the morning. For now, Mother Nature is taking care of me with this partial makeshift shelter.

At twilight, I slowly sit up, gazing at the gray overcast just before the sun begins to rise over the horizon. So far, there's only dull pain. Maybe I can finish the hike this morning.

I sip some water, pack my shorts hat in my backpack, and stand. When I pull my backpack over my shoulders, stabbing pain in my lower back takes my breath away. I try to ignore it and walk a few feet, groaning all the way. There's no way I can walk the rest of the way to my car in this condition.

I look at my watch. It's five-thirty. The attendant started letting people through the gate a half hour ago, so probably in about two hours, hikers will be passing me on the trail. Hopefully someone has a phone with a signal who can call for help.

I return to the flat rock, sit, and wait while the pain subsides to dull pulses, then stops.

At seven-thirty, a young man and woman appear, and I ask them if their phone is working. They check the signal, but no bars register. I thank them and they continue up the mountain.

The next party arrives fifteen minutes later—a man and two women in their twenties. They wear well-worn, sturdy hiking boots, shorts, ball caps, and short-sleeved T-shirts with stuffed day packs slung over their shoulders. Their choice of clothes and tanned skin indicate they spend a lot of time outside.

"Hey!" I yell to get their attention.

They stop.

"Do you have a phone that works here? I fell yesterday a few yards up the trail and spent the night here. I think my tailbone is broken."

One of the women pulls her cell phone from her day pack, flips it open, and the signal registers five bars. She hands it to me, and I call 911.

After I report my situation and give an approximate location, the dispatcher says, "I will have a search and rescue team hike up to check on you. It will take at least a couple of hours, so please stay where you are."

"I'm in too much pain to move," I reply.

I hand the phone to the woman, thank her, and give her an update. "We'll stay with you until they arrive," she says. Her companions nod.

In the meantime, we chat. I learn that they're guides for Northern Outdoors, here for the summer to take guests on whitewater trips along the Penobscot River. We talk about our outdoor adventures, which makes me forget about the pain in my back and my struggles in Massachusetts.

When the search and rescue team arrives, they assess the situation and decide it's best to call a National Guard helicopter from Bangor to fly me to the hospital. Although I'm complaining about my tailbone, they don't know the extent of the damage. They're afraid if they slip and fall while carrying me in a litter off the mountain, they'll make my injuries worse and get hurt in the process. The fewer people who need to be rescued, the better.

They call in the request from a portable radio, and forty-five minutes later, a black helicopter hovers over our spot. By then, I'm lying on my back, covered in blankets in a litter and strapped in so tightly, I can't move or feel any pain. The helicopter pilot lowers a cable, and one of the rescue team members grabs it and hooks it to a ring on the strap around the middle of the litter. Another team member gives a thumbs-up to the pilot, who slowly pulls me into the sky.

At one point, the litter tilts and I'm hanging upside down while the helicopter ascends slowly. My eyes widen, and I wonder whether the cable will break. An attendant watching through the open helicopter door notices my position and signals to the pilot to lower me back on the ground. The search and rescue team on the ground adjusts the litter so it's horizontal, and the pilot tries again.

He's successful this time.

After the attendant pulls the litter through the helicopter door and places it on the floor, I fall asleep. I awake when we're landing on the helicopter pad on the roof of the Millinocket Hospital. In the emergency room, a doctor takes an X-ray, which reveals a cracked tailbone.

"You'll be sore for at least a month," he says, while he injects medication into my butt cheek to ease the pain. "This medication will wear off in four hours. Take ibuprofen when you need to."

A park ranger drives my car to the hospital, and he's in the waiting room when I'm discharged. He hands the keys to me and asks me to sign some paperwork. Another ranger, who followed him, gives him a ride back to the park.

The medication wears off five miles north of the exit to Augusta. I pull off, find a hotel for the night, take two ibuprofen, and crawl into bed. While lying there, I think about the hike and promise myself I'll try again next year using the Roaring Brook and Cathedral trails. I've conquered too many challenges to give up on Katahdin, and now that I know the obstacles facing me, I will be better prepared.

And I will continue hiking and enjoying the outdoors in other ways as much as I can. The sounds of waterfalls, river currents, ocean waves, and singing birds reach deep into my soul and comfort me. My walks through forests, along beaches, and in gardens and parks relax and rejuvenate me. Nature sustains me, and I need her more than ever.

I also have a renewed determination to tackle the other obstacles in my life. I will emerge victorious on the other side.

Yes, you will, Charlotte says. *You're doing your best, and I'm rooting for you!*

More Financial Struggles
Massachusetts, Fall 2004

Tom returns to Massachusetts in September, three weeks after my fall on Mount Katahdin. He calls during my lunch break and asks me to meet him at Dunkin' Donuts in Harvard Square after work.

"I should be there by five-thirty." I hope to learn what he has been doing all summer, but will he tell me?

When I arrive, he's sitting at a two-top table near the counter, sipping a cup of Dr. Pepper. From here, he reminds me of my real husband, relaxed in his short-sleeved gray sweatshirt, khakis, and a pair of white Reebok running shoes.

He smiles when I sit across from him.

"How was Seattle?" I ask. I don't ask a more detailed question because, depending on his mood today, he might not share anything. Just because he looks like my real husband doesn't mean he's thinking like him.

"It was great," he replies.

Was it really? Based on Don's two reports, it couldn't have been.

I wait for him to continue. I want to ask him about the volunteer position, but he'll believe I'm snooping again.

Tom glances over his left shoulder, then says, "The volunteer position didn't last long. Someone interfered."

Here we go again. I'm not responding because he'll blame me.

He glances over his shoulder again. He believes someone is stalking him, but no one is paying attention to us.

"Are you going back to the extension school this fall?" I ask. There isn't any other reason he'd return to Massachusetts.

"I don't know yet. Probably." He glances over his shoulder again.

Classes have started already, so he probably enrolled in a class or two if he's still eligible for financial aid. He won't give me a straight answer if I reword my question, so I change the subject.

"Did you get my voicemail?"

"Yes."

"Why didn't you call me back?"

He glances over his shoulder again. When he shifts his gaze to me, he doesn't reply.

I don't bother repeating the question. He won't answer.

"Do you need to talk to me about something?" I ask. "I'm wondering why you asked me here."

He looks at me but doesn't answer.

"Surely there's a reason you asked me here," I say. This conversation is frustrating. I spent an hour and a half commuting here to find out he won't talk to me because he believes someone is watching us. We could go somewhere else to talk, but he'll assume we'll be followed.

He glances over his shoulder again while I stand and sling my backpack over my right shoulder. The dull pain in my tailbone returns, a reminder it's still healing.

"I've got to go. I have a lot of meetings tomorrow, and I'm under the impression you're waiting for someone."

He watches me leave with a confused look on his face.

On payday, I log into my bank account to verify the direct deposit. The landing page shows a negative balance of twenty dollars. How can I be overdrawn when my paycheck was direct deposited this morning?

I look for the direct deposit. It's listed in the transaction activity. Then I skim the rest of the transactions and find duplicate automatic withdrawals from the debt consolidation service, both from today.

Why would they withdraw two payments on the same day?

I call. "The first transaction didn't go through," the counselor says, "so we tried again. The other one was successful."

"But my account shows two transactions, and both are deducted from my balance," I say.

"The other one should drop off in a few days."

"But if the first transaction wasn't successful, only one should show on my account. How can the other one drop off when it appears the amount was deducted from my checking account?"

"It will be credited. Keep an eye on your account, and if the transaction doesn't drop off in five business days, call us back."

This doesn't make sense. Are they now automatically doubling my monthly payments? They can't without my permission.

My next call is the bank. "They're two separate transactions, and we're covering both of them," the customer service representative says. "You need to make a deposit to cover the overdraft as soon as you can."

"Can I dispute one of the charges?" I ask. "I didn't authorize two withdrawals from this company in the same month."

"Yes, I can take care of it," she says. "I will reverse the overdraft fee as well."

I call the debt consolidation service again and reach a different counselor. "Your account shows only one payment for this month," he says. "I don't see another payment being processed."

"I can't afford double payments," I say. "How will you ensure this doesn't happen again?"

"We don't make more than one withdrawal a month. If a payment doesn't go through, we try again, but only once."

"This isn't reassuring to me after my experience this morning. I'd like to stop the automatic withdrawals."

"You realize if you do, your only option is to make your payments by money order every month. They might not arrive on time."

"Please cancel the monthly withdrawals."

The counselor places me on hold to complete the cancellation, but the experience makes me nervous and wary. What if the cancellation isn't processed? What if they double-dip next month? I can't afford another mistake.

During my lunch break, I stop at the bank, close out my account, and open a new one. If the debt consolidation service tries to make an automatic withdrawal next month, they can't because they don't have my new account number.

I'm also worried about mailing money orders after the conversation with the counselor today. I can send the money orders by certified mail or priority mail, but what if the agency claims they didn't receive them? I'll have proof of delivery, but they're delivered to a post office box. How long will my money orders wait there for someone to pick up the mail and process them?

Would it be better to use a different debt consolidation agency? The one I'm using now is a small agency in Massachusetts. Would a larger agency provide more options for making payments? Can I break a debt consolidation agreement after committing to one?

After work, I research these questions online. I can't find information on breaking an agreement, but there's a lot of information on debt consolidation agencies. I read their websites carefully, check their ratings through the Better Business Bureau, and pick a national organization with the highest rating to call tomorrow.

The payment options are the same: automatic monthly withdrawals and mailing a money order. For the money orders, the counselor recommends sending them a week before the due date to ensure the payments are processed on time. She says I can set up a due date that fits my budget. Although I'm still nervous about sending payments by money order, I decide to take the risk.

The next day, I cancel the agreement with the Massachusetts debt consolidation agency and set up an agreement with the other one. The amount of my monthly payments don't change.

Calls from collectors continue, but the new ones are for Tom. I don't ask how they got my number but tell them they called the wrong number. When they ask where they can find him, I say, "I don't know." I really don't know, but I wouldn't tell them even if I did.

One time when Don calls me, he says he's receiving calls from collectors looking for Tom.

I laugh. "It's ironic they call a lawyer. Wouldn't they be afraid you'd sue them?"

Don laughs. "They hang up when I tell them."

Speaking of lawyers, you need to find another one, Charlotte says after this conversation with Don. *It's time to finalize your divorce.*

She hasn't mentioned this since Melanie went on medical leave.

Why are you reminding me now?

The collectors aren't giving up, are they? You need to protect yourself financially.

Where will I find another lawyer? I can't afford a retainer.

Contact Melanie's office and ask for a referral. They have a lot of connections.

How can I manage this with my other bills right now?

You'll manage. You can't afford not to do this.

I haven't moonlighted since the assignment at the jewelry store ended last spring. I still check in with the agencies, but the answer is the same: "The only openings we have are nine to five, Monday through Friday." No freelance work is coming in from the publishers, either, despite regular follow-ups with my contacts. If I hire a lawyer again, I'll need a second job. It will help me pay off the other bills faster, too.

One afternoon while running errands, I pass the ski area near the office. It's now September, so it won't be long before people will return for ski lessons, skiing, and tubing. There's a restaurant here, and they'll need servers for the season. I haven't worked as a server since college, but how hard can it be to start again? I think of the cliché of riding a bicycle: Once you learn how, you'll never forget.

Before applying, I schedule a meeting with Todd to tell him what I'm doing. "It will not interfere with my work here," I say. "I will work in the evenings and on weekends."

"I trust you," he says. "Thank you for sharing this with me."

Throughout my struggles, I've always kept up with my work at the office. Todd knows I won't let him down.

The next day, I take a late lunch break and stop at the ski area to fill out an application. Leonardo, the restaurant manager is there, so he interviews me after I finish.

"You don't have any recent experience serving," he says after reading my application. "Are you sure you want to do this?"

"I worked full-time as a server in different restaurants for six years during college," I say. "The skills are the same, no matter where one works. Although it has been a long time, I will not have any problems returning to an efficient routine."

"Okay, you're hired. You'll have a four-week training period, where you'll receive a regular minimum wage, and you can keep any tips you receive. After that, we'll assign you to a section and pay you the minimum wage for a server. We cash out at the end of each shift, so you'll receive the tips you earned before you leave."

Currently in Massachusetts, the minimum wage for servers is two dollars thirty-five cents an hour, but my tips will more than make up for it.

"That's great! When can I start? I'm available now."

"We'll open on October first for the Halloween events. We're having an orientation on September thirtieth at four-thirty. I'll review the shifts with everyone then."

"I'll be there!"

My next item on the to-do list is calling Melanie's former office.

"I was a client of Melanie's before she went on medical leave," I say to the receptionist. "I'm looking for another lawyer to handle my divorce and am wondering if anyone else there can recommend someone who charges by the hour. I can't afford a retainer."

"Melanie is back part-time," the receptionist replies, "but she isn't accepting any new cases right now. Would you like to leave a message for her?"

"No, thanks. I'll send an email. Thank you for letting me know."

I've read about people defending themselves in divorce cases. Maybe Melanie can provide advice on an hourly rate if I do this. It doesn't hurt to ask.

"Hi, Melanie," my email begins. "I heard you're back in the office and am writing to ask if you could work with me as a consultant. I'm thinking about representing myself for my divorce, but I need someone who can give me advice while I work through the process. I know you're working only part-time and you aren't taking new cases, but because I'm a former client, I thought I'd ask about this. Please let me know if this is possible. Thank you."

She replies the next day with, "I do not recommend representing yourself. Your situation is too complicated. You need a good lawyer to represent you, but unfortunately, I cannot continue working on your case. However, I know someone who can. She specializes in family law and has more than twenty years of experience. I will contact her. Someone from her office will call you."

That call comes two days later from Kaitlyn's office. Peg, her assistant, schedules an appointment for next week.

Kaitlyn is my height with short curly brown hair and hazel eyes, wearing a brown pantsuit and white blouse. She holds the door open while I walk into her office, then motions to a chair in front of her desk.

"Have a seat," she says while she sits in a brown leather swivel chair behind her oak desk. A yellow legal tablet and a file with my name on the tab are side by side on top of a writing pad in the center of her desk. She opens the file and grabs a pen from a clear glass cup next to the phone.

"Melanie filled me in on your case," she says. "She filed the paperwork, but no one knows what happened to it after she went on medical leave. I have copies, so I will follow-up with the courthouse."

I nod.

Kaitlyn pages through the information in the file, then looks up at me. "Does your husband have a permanent address? I don't see one here."

"I don't know," I say. "When we see each other, he wants to meet at a Dunkin' Donuts at Harvard Square. He's a student at the Harvard Extension School."

"We need a physical address to serve the divorce papers."

"I don't know if he's staying in one place. He's constantly afraid someone is following him."

"We'll contact Harvard and ask for his school records."

"Will they release them? I thought those records are private."

"They should accommodate us under these circumstances."

Kaitlyn pauses while thumbing through the pages, then looks at me again. "Does Tom have any assets?"

"Only a 401(k) from his former employer. The last time I saw a statement, which was more than a year ago, it had a balance of two hundred fifty thousand dollars."

"Do you have any details about the account, such as the account number and where the account is held?"

I give Kaitlyn the name of the company that administers the 401(k), then say, "I don't have the account number, but I have his Social Security Number."

"That will help. I can request the records with his Social Security Number. If we can get a freeze placed on the account, then we can negotiate for part of the balance in the settlement."

"If I could get enough money to cover the bills from our marriage, that would help a lot."

"I will ask for half the balance. You deserve it."

She asks a few more questions, then asks Peg to schedule our next appointment in two weeks. "By then, I should know about the status of your paperwork."

Everything seems to be falling into place. Maybe this nightmare will end soon.

It doesn't. A week later, I pick up a call from a New York area code. A debt collector is on the line from one of the credit card companies in my debt consolidation program.

"I'm calling because your payment is ninety days past due," she says.

"My payment isn't late," I reply. "I have been making my payments on time every month through a debt consolidation service."

A week after I mail the payments to the debt consolidation service, I call to verify they received the money order and the payment was posted. They don't provide online access to accounts, so this is the only way I can check. So far, according to the counselors I talk to, all my payments have arrived on time and posted before the due date. So, how can this credit card payment be three months overdue?

"My records show you're past due."

"Are you receiving my payments from the debt consolidation agency?"

"Yes, but you're still past due."

"How is that possible? You agreed to those payments."

"It doesn't matter. We can collect whenever we want, and that's why I'm calling."

"But you signed an agreement, and there aren't any clauses in it about this. I read it."

"We can still collect whenever we want."

How can they get away with this?

After this call ends, the phone rings again. It's a collector from another credit card company in the program who says I'm three months past due on my payments. Our conversation follows the same pattern as the first call.

A collector from another credit card on the debt consolidation plans calls a day later, and the conversation repeats.

What will I do now? I can't make monthly payments to the credit card companies and the debt consolidation service. I shouldn't have to; that's why I'm in the debt consolidation program.

After hanging up from the last call, I dial the debt consolidation service. The counselor's response isn't what I expected.

"They can collect whenever they want," he says.

"So, you're telling me the agreement isn't valid?"

"I'm not saying that. I'm saying if the creditors in the program want to collect, that's up to them."

"If they're not willing to abide by an agreement they signed, then why am I in this program?"

Silence.

"Well, that answers my question. This program can't help me pay off my debt. I want to terminate this program."

"All right. It will take a couple of minutes, so I'm placing you on hold."

The counselor didn't try to change my mind. That says a lot!

I thought Charlotte advised me to do this. Did I misunderstand her? Melanie said debt consolidation could help me pay off my credit cards, too. I did my research before contacting the first debt consolidation service. Maybe I overreacted when I canceled the first program. Would it have worked if I gave it another chance? Maybe my desperation overshadowed my ability to make a rational decision. This experience taught me how easy it can happen when someone feels trapped.

Now I need to find a way to work directly with the credit card companies to pay off the balances. Hopefully I can earn enough tips from my job at the ski area to catch up, then make the rest of the payments on time.

At my next appointment with Kaitlyn, I talk to her about this.

"Have you thought about filing for bankruptcy?" she asks.

"Yes, but I can't. If I need to look for another job in my field, the employer will run a credit check after I accept their offer. A bankruptcy on my record would be an instant disqualification."

She nods. "It doesn't make sense why they'd do this when you aren't handling money."

"I don't get it, either. What's interesting is when I applied for the server job at the ski area, no one mentioned a credit check. They only wanted personal references."

Kaitlyn shakes her head. "Well, keep paying what you can to the credit card companies. They won't stop calling you, but at least you're showing that you're making a good-faith effort."

"I haven't heard from the courthouse yet about the status of your paperwork, but I will continue checking. Middlesex County has a tendency to be slow."

A week later after I return home from work, I hear a knock on my door. Ernie is standing on the other side, and I invite him in.

"This will only take a moment," he says. "I wanted you to know I'm raising the rent one hundred dollars a month, effective November first."

That's seven hundred fifty dollars a months, a hefty increase I can't afford. I had a feeling this was coming. Since the daughter of my neighbor across the hall left two months ago, I'm the only female tenant. Ernie has hinted a few times lately that he wants to return to an all-male house. Raising the rent is the easiest way to kick me out, because he doesn't have any legal grounds to evict me. I've always paid my rent on time and am a well-behaved tenant, as are Tiger and TC.

I scour the newspapers and websites for apartments at my current rent or less but come up empty, so I start searching for rooms. On craigslist, one that sounds promising is listed in a bordering town at one hundred fifty dollars a week, but there's one problem: no pets are allowed. Maybe I can manage to board Tiger and TC until I can find a more permanent place to live. The boarding house I've used is owned and operated by two veterinary assistants, so they can take care of Tiger's shots if his blood sugar levels spike and he needs insulin again. For the past two months, they've leveled off.

Jenny, a co-owner of the cat boarding house, and I make arrangements to board the cats for two weeks with the option to extend. I don't tell her about my situation; she doesn't need to know.

Manny, the house owner, has two rooms for rent in the basement. "The other tenant works full-time," he says. "He has lived here for six months and is very quiet. You'll share the bathroom at the end of the hall.

"The rent is due every Friday," he continued. "If you're interested, I need two references."

He shows the room to me. It's the size of my current bedroom, furnished with a bed, desk, chair, and fluorescent desk lamp. The lack of windows doesn't bother me because I'll be here mostly to sleep. This will do until I can find an affordable apartment.

But work is slow at the ski area because it's too warm to make snow. Many nights, I leave my shift with less than twenty dollars in tips. More collectors are calling. So, three weeks after Manny allows me to move in, I must choose between paying rent and keeping my car. I need a car to commute to work, so the room must go.

Hitting Bottom

Massachusetts, Fall 2004-Winter 2005

After the debacle at the cat clinic in Brighton, I switched vets. The new one is in his early sixties, of medium build, with short gray curly hair. Every time I see him, I think of Dr. Dolittle—especially after the time he walked down the hallway of the animal hospital with a macaw perched on his left shoulder and a smoky gray Persian cat tucked under his right arm. The macaw didn't seem concerned that a cat was riding along, and the cat wasn't eying the bird as a meal, so I've concluded this vet has invisible powers to maintain harmony in the animal kingdom.

Tiger and I come here every other week for blood tests to monitor his diabetes. When I brought Tiger to his last appointment, his glucose levels were bouncing around more and the vet increased the insulin by a half unit. I'm hoping his readings have stabilized but wonder whether the stress from moving into the boarding house is causing the spikes. Jenny said he seemed to be feeling better when I picked him up for his appointment today.

I'm dreading this checkup because I'm talking to the vet about finding someone to adopt the cats. They need a stable, permanent home. I don't want to let them go, but I don't know when I can get back on my feet. It's not fair to them to wait for me in a boarding house.

When Tom wanted to adopt a cat a year after we married, I hesitated. My biggest fear was becoming attached to another cat and having to let it go. After Grandma died, Bubby wouldn't let me keep Charlie, my powder gray tabby cat. That's when I promised myself I'd never go through that experience again. But after many conversations with Tom, where he reassured me we'd never abandon the cat, I agreed to adopt Tiger from the Seattle Animal Shelter. Now, almost fifteen years later, I'm here at the vet's office, about to break my promise to not only Tiger, but also TC, my special companions who have brought joy to my life, even during the darkest times.

Of all the struggles I've gone through since leaving Seattle, this is the most agonizing decision I've made. But what else can I do? Tiger and TC can't live in a car. It will be tough enough for me.

The vet has many connections in this community, so he should know some kind humans who will take good care of an elderly diabetic cat and a shorthair tabby who loves all creatures and humans, except young children. TC still has traumatic memories of his torture from the boys running wild in our West Seattle neighborhood before we adopted him. During the rare occasions he sees or hears a child under the age of six, he runs away and hides.

The vet's assistant walks into the waiting room, holding a file. "Tiger Landes," she calls.

We exchange greetings, then she escorts us to the exam room. She leaves the file on the counter, and the vet arrives a minute later.

"Hi," he says, unlatching the door of Tiger's carrier. "How's Tiger today?"

"He has been okay," I say. "I haven't noticed any change in his behavior since our last appointment. His water and food intake are normal."

The vet removes Tiger from the carrier, checks Tiger's vitals, and draws blood for the next round of tests.

"I need to talk to you about the cats," I say. I dread this conversation but need to get it over with.

"Sure," the vet says.

"My husband and I separated, and I'm struggling with a lot of debt from our marriage. I can't afford a place to rent anymore, so I need to live in my car for awhile. I can't keep the cats with me. I don't want to let them go, but I don't have any other options."

"I'm so sorry," he says. "I'm on the board of the local Humane Society. We can find a good home for them."

"I would appreciate it," I say, still wishing I didn't have to do this.

"Leave them here, and I'll see what I can do."

"Thank you," I say, and leave as fast as I can before I start crying.

The current starts as soon as I'm in the car.

After I pick up TC, I drive back to the vet's office. Before we go in, I pull TC from his carrier and hug him for a long time. He rubs my face and softly purrs while tears stream down my cheeks.

"I'm sorry, sweetie, but I have to say good-bye," I say. "The vet is looking for a nice home for you and Tiger. I don't want to leave you, but I have to live in my car now. I love you, and I will miss you so much. I will never forget you."

I don't have much to load into my Honda CR-V—a few clothes, a laptop, blankets, a pillow, and the futon cushion I kept after moving from Brighton to Waltham. The futon cushion is thin enough to fold in half and fit perfectly in the SUV after I fold up the back seat. The space is long enough to stretch out when I position myself diagonally from the back of the front seat to the tailgate.

Every night, I look for a different place to park and sleep. It needs to be well lit, in a safe location, and quiet. I rotate nights at three rest areas north and west of Boston, the parking lot at the office (behind the building after everyone is gone for the night), Walmart parking lots, and other lots that allow overnight parking. Occasionally I park on the street in a residential neighborhood and sleep with my face completely covered so if someone peeks through the windows, they'll see a big pile of blankets. I don't want to spend consecutive nights in the same location because I don't want anyone to recognize my car and challenge me.

Over time, I notice how many people have the same lifestyle, especially at the rest areas and in the Walmart parking lots. Like me, they sleep for seven or eight hours, get up, freshen up and change in the restroom, and leave for their jobs. They've had bad breaks and are doing whatever they can to survive. And like me, they're on this journey without calling attention to themselves or asking for anyone's sympathy. We keep to ourselves because we're embarrassed and ashamed.

Through this dreary experience in the middle of winter, I remind myself to be grateful because my circumstances as a homeless person are better than most. I have shelter, thanks to my car. I have access to a microwave and refrigerator at the office, where I can heat food and store leftovers. I eat a lot of Asian food because I can buy soup and a dinner entrée and make it last for two or three days. I'll eat the soup and a few bites of the meal at the restaurant, then take the rest with me. After everyone leaves the office for the day, I take a shower in the restroom across from the company's fitness center.

Although the cold weather is a challenge as a car occupant, it's a blessing at the restaurant at the ski area. Now I sometimes make enough money from tips to rent a room at the Motel 6 in Leominster for a night or two. Those nights are like heaven—sleeping in a bed and taking a shower whenever I want. I dread returning to my car after checkout but am thankful to have it for shelter and a reliable mode of transportation, which allows me to commute to my two jobs.

I don't eat meals at the ski area because the employees don't get discounts. It's much cheaper to eat at the Asian restaurants. Even if I could get a discount, I can't stretch the meals as far because the portions are smaller. Occasionally when the cooks make a mistake on an order, the servers will split up the food and munch on it between trips to take care of our customers. Leonardo doesn't care because the food would have to be thrown out.

Tom periodically emails with requests to type papers for his classes at the Harvard Extension School. Lately he has been sending handwritten pages through a cloud-based fax service, and I type them into Microsoft Word and email the files to him. I wonder where he's staying but never ask because he wouldn't tell me. Then one night, he asks me to meet him at the McDonald's across from the Park Street T station at Boston Common to type a final project for a business class. After we order a Dr. Pepper for him and coffee for me, we walk to a suite he's renting at a Hyatt nearby. The only way he can afford this is by withdrawing money from his 401(k).

I tell him about my homelessness, why I'm homeless, and ask for his help. He ignores my plea.

Two months after I move into my car, my cell phone rings during my lunch break and displays the animal hospital's name on the screen. Tiger and TC's former vet is on the line.

"I'm calling about Tiger," he says. "He's here at the hospital."

Am I hearing him correctly?

"Tiger is there?" I ask. Wouldn't he have been adopted by now?

"Yes," the vet says. "I boarded your cats in hopes you could find a place to live soon."

I never anticipated this, but I'm grateful for his generosity.

"Tiger isn't well," the vet says. "I don't expect him to last much longer. If you want to see him, you should come now."

"I'll be right there."

The vet leaves Tiger in an exam room at the end of the hall. As soon as I arrive at the animal hospital, he escorts me there and closes the door behind us. "His system is shutting down from complications from the diabetes," he says. "I'm doing all I can to keep him comfortable, but he's in a lot of pain. I'll leave you two alone; take all the time you need. Let me know what you want to do when you're ready."

Tiger stands on the white tile floor at the foot of the exam table. He has shrunk to the size of the eight-month-old kitten Tom and I adopted from the Seattle Animal Shelter.

When Tiger sees me, he chatters in a delighted voice. I kneel in front of him and rub between his ears. A couple of tears slide down my cheeks.

"Hi, sweetie. I'm happy to see you, too. I've missed you so much." I choke on my words.

Tiger purrs loudly and turns slow circles while rubbing against my knees. I rub gently between his ears and along the length of his back and tail. His movements take a lot of effort. He's losing his two-year battle with diabetes, and I can't prolong his suffering. My heart breaks to see him this way.

The vet charges twelve dollars for the procedure. I stand at the side of the table in the exam room, where Tiger lies in a pile of soft blankets, and gently rub his head between the ears while the vet injects the solution. Tiger doesn't flinch when the needle penetrates his skin.

After the procedure, the vet says, "I have a few patients coming in for long-term care, so I won't have enough room for TC to stay here any longer."

"I'm still living in my car," I say. "I'll check with the boarding house. Maybe we can make some arrangements until I can find a place to rent."

"I know the owners there, and they can probably help," the vet says. "I wish you the best."

"Thank you for everything you've done. It means a lot to me."

I stop at the cat boarding house an hour later. Jenny stands behind the counter, looking at the booking schedule on the calendar pad on the desk. She must have driven here directly from her veterinary assistant job nearby because she's wearing her sea-green scrubs, which complements her short, curly gray hair. Her business partner is another assistant at the same clinic.

Jenny greets me in her mild Boston accent while I place TC's carrier on top of the counter. She inserts an index finger through the bars on the door and rubs his nose.

"Hi, TC. How are you today?"

TC squeezes his eyes in contentment.

"Where's Tiger?" she asks.

"The vet put him down today. His system was shutting down because of complications from the diabetes."

"I'm so sorry. He was such a sweet kitty." Jenny continues rubbing TC's nose.

"I stopped by tonight to ask if I could leave TC here for a while," I say. "My husband and I separated, and now I'm living in my car. I can make weekly payments on the boarding until I can get back on my feet again."

Jenny stops rubbing TC and looks at me with concern. "I'm so sorry you're going through this."

She studies the calendar pad on the desk for a minute, then looks up at me again and says, "We have a tiny empty mother-in-law apartment at our house. It has a separate entrance. You're welcome to stay there until you can afford to pay rent. TC is welcome, too."

"Are you sure you want to do this?" I ask, examining her face for clues on why she would offer temporary rent-free shelter to TC and me.

"I've been through tough times and am grateful for the people who helped me," she says. "I want to pay it forward."

"Thank you," I say. "I appreciate your generous offer."

She writes on a notepad, then tears off the top sheet and hands it to me. "Here's the address and directions. The door is unlocked. You're welcome to come whenever you like. I'll stop by later and drop off the key."

The apartment is an extension on the back of a two-story Victorian house tucked away in the woods along a sharp curve of the Assabet River in Stow, a twenty-minute drive from the office. The gravel driveway ends at the entrance. I pull the screen door open and turn the knob of the door behind it, which opens to a room measuring approximately three hundred fifty square feet. Indoor-outdoor carpet the color of oatmeal covers the floor, and a sliding glass door is on the opposite side of the room—perfect for TC to watch the world go by. Along one wall is a tiny closet, large enough to hang the few clothes I have, and a mini-kitchen, complete with sink, cabinets painted white above and below the sink, a small gas-powered stove with an oven, and a dorm-sized refrigerator. A bathroom with black-tiled walls and floor connects to the living area and has the basics: toilet bowl, sink with a cabinet underneath, medicine cabinet, and walk-in shower.

It's the perfect stepping stone on my journey to recovery.

Since we reunited, TC's demeanor has changed. When I get ready for work in the morning, he watches my every move and tries to follow me when I walk out the door. After work, he runs up to me, chattering and rubbing my legs as if I'm a long-lost friend. Then he follows me everywhere I go. When I sit on the folded futon cushion, which doubles as a couch, he sits next to me, as close as he can. Part of his body touches me at all times, like he thinks as long as he can feel the warmth of my body, he's safe.

He misses Tiger, and he's afraid you'll abandon him again, Charlotte says.

Poor TC! My heart fills with sympathy and my mind with guilt for leaving him for more than two months. I don't know how I can convince him that I'll never leave him again, nor with my shaky situation, know if I can even renew this commitment to him. I do know I couldn't bear to part with him again. But I can try to make up for lost time by giving him a lot of love. I pick him up, hold him, and rub his head and chin with my chin. Soon, he's purring and rubbing me back.

Talk to Jenny about TC, Charlotte says. *She might have some ideas for comforting him.*

Ideally, I should adopt another cat to keep him company, but now isn't the right time.

Don't push that idea aside. Talk to Jenny.

How can I manage two cats when I'm struggling to take care of myself?

You'll find a way. There are many lonely kitties out there who need love as much as you do. And the one who chooses you will love you more than you can imagine. Think about TC. He chose you and Tom, and he has loved you through every struggle. It hasn't been easy for him, either.

The next day after work, I stop at the boarding house, where Jenny is on duty again.

She smiles when she sees me walk in. "How's everything going?"

"Great, except I want to talk to you about TC. He isn't himself since we reunited."

"I noticed him moping behind the sliding glass door a couple of mornings when I've been working in the yard," she says. "He must be taking Tiger's death hard."

"I think he is. Tiger never warmed up to him, but TC still enjoyed his companionship."

"I have an idea. We have a cat boarding here, who's stayed with us for six months. The family had to move out of state when their daughter was diagnosed with cancer. She's getting treatment there, and they're living in an apartment complex that doesn't allow pets. They've asked me to look for someone who can take care of the cat temporarily, until they can return to Massachusetts. Right now, they don't know how long they'll be gone.

"The cat is a twelve-year-old female. Would you like to see her?"

"Sure."

Jenny leads me into the back room and stops in front of a wall of boarding cubes. She points to the top left cube, where a gray and white cat is curled on a braided throw rug next to her food and water dish. The cat looks up at us with her blue eyes.

"This is Maggie," Jenny says. "She's a friendly girl."

"Hi, Maggie," I say.

Maggie walks to the door of her cube and sniffs the air between us through the stainless-steel bars.

Jenny opens the door and reaches in to stroke Maggie's head, shoulders, and back. Maggie stands still, soaking in the attention.

I stretch my fingers on my left hand and slowly move the tips toward Maggie's nose so she can sniff them. It's the proper way to introduce myself to a cat. After she finishes, I gently rub her chin. She rubs back.

"She likes you," Jenny says.

"She'd probably like TC, too," I say.

"What do you think about introducing them? Bring TC here for a couple of days, and I can let them out at the same time and see how well they get along."

When cats board here, Jenny and her partner let them out of their cubes for a half hour in the morning and again in the evening to roam around the boarding room, play, or just hang out. They only allow one cat out at a time, unless a customer is boarding more than one from the same household.

"That's a great idea! I'll drop him off after work tomorrow."

When I put TC in his carrier, his eyes look at me with a sad curiosity. I read his silent message as expecting I'm taking him somewhere again and will not return.

"Sweetie, I know you're afraid with all you've been through," I say. "Today, I have a surprise for you, and it's a good surprise. Jenny and I want you to meet someone. We think you'll like her."

TC's expression doesn't change. He's probably skeptical. If I were in his situation, I would be, too. After all, why would he trust me now? I've abandoned him twice. How does he know I won't do it again?

"I'll bring you home in a couple of days. I hope you understand I'm not abandoning you again."

His sad eyes widen, followed by a heart-wrenching "meow."

I rub his nose with my finger. "I'm not leaving you again, I promise. I hope you can regain your trust in me."

The next day after work, I call Jenny at the boarding house. "They're getting along well," she says. "I think they'll be great companions."

I stop by the following night to pick up TC.

"I talked to Maggie's owners again today, and they've changed their minds," Jenny says. "Instead of asking someone to take care of her temporarily, they believe it's best for Maggie if someone adopts her. They don't think it's fair to have her live with someone for a while and then take her back, and they don't know when they'll have a place where she can be with them again."

I agree. "That would be the best for Maggie."

And TC, too. He would be devastated if his new furry friend is taken away from him.

"They paid her boarding in full today," Jenny says. She pulls a folder from a file drawer under her desk and hands it to me. "These are her medical records. They adopted Maggie when she was six months old."

I open the file and scan the records. I've never seen anyone keep such detailed vet records for so long. This family genuinely loved Maggie, and they must be agonizing over their decision to let her go.

"I haven't let them out yet tonight," Jenny says. "Let's do that so they can spend a little time together before you take them home."

Jenny removes Maggie from her cube and gently lowers her onto the floor, followed by TC. They stay hunched in their separate spots for a minute, then TC walks over to Maggie and tries to sniff her nose. Maggie hisses at him, warning him that he's too close. TC backs up a step, hunches, squints his eyes, and looks at her as if he's asking, "Why did you do that?"

"TC has a lot of confidence," Jenny says.

I nod. Any other cat would have hissed back or cuffed Maggie, which probably would have triggered a scuffle. TC just wants to say "hello" to her.

Neither Maggie nor TC move. They're hunched with their eyes halfway closed. Both seem to be lost in their own thoughts.

"I think they'll be fine," I say. "Maggie is allowing TC to get closer to her than Tiger ever did."

After I release Maggie from the carrier inside the apartment, TC and I sit on the futon cushion and watch Maggie sniff every inch of the apartment, gathering kitty data about her new surroundings. After she acclimates herself, she lays at the foot of the futon cushion with her paws tucked underneath her and looks at TC and me for a minute. TC matches her pose, looks at her and squeezes his eyes—a clear sign he's content with her. Maggie closes her eyes, and neither cat moves as they quietly enjoy each other's presence inches apart.

Tonight, TC has relaxed for the first time since we reunited. I'm comforted knowing he will have company while I continue working long hours and Maggie has a home. I silently vow to do whatever I can to ensure our tiny family will remain intact.

A month later, Kaitlyn calls with news that the courthouse lost my divorce paperwork. When I ask how she found out, she says, "It was taking them longer than usual to respond, so I contacted the clerk's office. They couldn't find any record of the papers being filed. I refiled and asked them to expedite the process, but because they're slow, I don't know when I will hear from them again."

Cheryl Landes

Tom Becomes Homeless
New England, Spring 2005-Winter 2006

Occasionally, I still see Tom. Since the cold, snowy night I typed the last paper for him at the Hyatt in downtown Boston, he asks me to meet him at Dunkin' Donuts at Harvard Square on evenings when I'm not working at the ski area. The last few times I've seen him, he constantly looks over his shoulder as if someone is listening to our conversations. It's hard to talk to him this way because I don't know if he's really listening to me, so I never stay long. Often I wonder why I go there when I can't have any focused conversations with him.

One night, I disclose that I've filed for divorce, and he responds with a blank stare. After a minute, he asks, "Why are you doing this?"

"I don't want to but have no choice. I need to protect myself financially. I can't continue paying all the bills you're running up."

His reply is glancing over his shoulder. When looks at me again, he doesn't ask me to reconsider. He only looks at me with the same blank expression.

In March and April in New England, the cold grip of winter and the warmth of spring fight a battle, and this year, it's fiercer than usual. Just when it seems spring will prevail, another snowstorm arrives and dumps a foot or two of snow over a twenty-four-hour period. While I'm looking forward to warmer weather, I'm also grateful for the snow because it keeps the ski area open longer. More extra hours means I can pay off more bills. I'll still struggle when the ski area closes for the season, but at least I've made some progress.

Things will continue to improve, Charlotte says. *You need the break to take care of yourself.*

When the ski season ends, I return to hiking. I've missed being outside, where I can enjoy the peacefulness of the woods, the soothing flow of the rivers and cascading waterfalls, the waves crashing on the beach, the sweeping panoramas through a clearing, and the music from the birds.

During my lunch breaks at the office, I walk in the Acton Arboretum and find other trails nearby where I can walk again after work. Every weekend, I pick a different location on a map, go there, and hike. Those random points take me to waterfall trails in New Hampshire, wilderness areas in Maine and Vermont, and eventually to some mountain peaks. My first is Hedgehog Mountain near Freeport, Maine, followed by Mount Chocorua in New Hampshire, Camel's Hump in Vermont, and Mount Washington, also in New Hampshire.

Mount Washington is the most challenging. At 6,228 feet, it's the highest peak in the Northeast and the most topographically prominent mountain east of the Mississippi River. It's also well-known for its unpredictable weather. One minute, the sun is out, and the next, the mountain is covered in clouds. The weather ranges from chilly to frigid regardless of the season, and the wind is persistent.

My hike to the Mount Washington summit is sort of last-minute because I'm monitoring the weather forecasts for the most ideal conditions. On my chosen weekend, I leave the office early on Friday to check into an inexpensive hotel near the Tuckerman Ravine trailhead. Early the next morning, I'm on the trail. The sun shines the entire way, and the view is the clearest I've ever seen from the summit. This isn't my first time to the top; the other trips were by car on the steep, windy Auto Road.

The temperature is in the mid-thirties as I stand at the end of the trail and soak in the view of the Presidential Range and other hills and mountains in varying shades of blue and purple. The wind bites the exposed skin on my face while I continue admiring the view and bask in my achievement.

The sun is just starting to set when I return to my car. I drive to a restaurant nearby and treat myself to a steak dinner and chocolate cake for dessert. It has been a long time since I've treated myself to a steak, so I eat it slowly, savoring every bite. It might be a long time before I can splurge on another one.

This hike boosted my confidence to tackle Mount Katahdin again. I'm determined to successfully climb it after my mishap last year. Two weeks later, I arrive at the south gate of Baxter State Park at three-thirty in the morning to ensure a spot on the Roaring Brook Trail. My earlier arrival paid off.

The Roaring Brook Trail is a combination of dirt and rocks, but there's far less scrambling over boulders than the Hunt Trail. In four hours, I'm at the end of the trail, absorbing the panorama and snapping pictures with my tiny Kodak digital camera next to a weathered sign marking the summit. Two men behind me on the trail stop to enjoy the scenery and offer to take my picture. When I look at it on the screen, my smile is the brightest I've seen in a long time and I look relaxed. That's exactly how I feel. Nature has restored me. Now if I can restore myself financially…

One afternoon while I'm at the office, Kaitlyn calls my cell phone with an update. "I have good news and bad news. The good news is I managed to get Tom's current address from his school records. He has a post office box in Waltham, so we will serve the divorce papers by mail. Also, I was able to contact the financial services firm where his 401(k) is located, and they provided information about his account. The bad news is the balance is thirty-five hundred dollars."

Tom blew almost two hundred fifty thousand dollars in a year! How could anyone spend that much money in such a short time? This is not like the original Tom, who was great at managing money, investing, and keeping abreast of financial trends. His goal was to invest for the long-term and never overreact to changes in the markets.

"I don't think it's worth trying to freeze his account," I reply. "At this rate, what's left won't last much longer."

"I agree," Kaitlyn says. "I'm sorry to have to share this news."

I'd hoped to get enough money from the divorce settlement to pay off the debt, but that's no longer possible. Now the only thing I will receive is the divorce, but it will protect me from Tom's creditors. Although the money from the tips at the ski area helped me pay off a few small bills, I'm still struggling with massive credit card debt. Currently three card balances are with different collection agencies. The other one has not been turned into collections.

After I ended the agreement with the last debt consolidation service, I set up monthly repayment plans with the collection agencies. But collectors still call every other week, asking me to increase my monthly payments or pay in full. My response is always the same: I can't. I have no wiggle room in my budget.

One day, a collector actually listens to my story with some empathy. When I'm finished, she asks, "Has anyone ever mentioned there's another option that can get you out of debt faster?"

"No," I say. "What is it?"

"We can negotiate a smaller balance, and it won't affect your credit rating."

"I've never heard of this. How does it work?"

"We can reduce the balance by fifty percent if you can pay it in full."

"That would help, but I don't have enough money to pay a lump sum. Monthly payments are all I can manage."

Charlotte cuts in with, *You can pay a negotiated balance in full by withdrawing money from your 401(k).*

I don't want to tap into it. What will I use for retirement?

If you reduce the debt now, you'll have more money to save for the future.

"Maybe I can, but I need to check on something first," I say to the collector. "How long will this offer last?"

"I'd advise accepting it as soon as you can," she replies. "I don't know when these terms will change."

The next morning, I stop by the comptroller's office. He listens with compassion, then says, "You can request a hardship withdrawal, "but you will pay a ten percent penalty for early withdrawal, and the money you withdraw will be taxable."

I call the other collection agencies, ask about negotiating a payoff balance, and both collectors say they can offer the same terms. My 401(k) will cover the total for all three cards with two thousand dollars to spare. I can leave the remaining funds in my 401(k), build up the account again, and increase my contributions as I pay off the other bills that aren't in collections.

The comptroller approves the paperwork the next day, and the money is transferred to my checking account three days later. After the funds post, I call the collection agencies to finish the arrangements. They ask me to pay with cashier's checks. I send the checks Express Mail through the US Postal Service and call after the deliveries to confirm receipt. They verify the balances are paid in full, and I will receive statements in the mail showing the accounts are paid in full. The statements arrive a week later.

Finally, I'm free of one burden!

After I stop working at the ski area, I start attending free and inexpensive networking meetings through STC and other high-tech professional organizations. On one Saturday, I go to a conference hosted by the Connecticut chapter of STC. One of the speakers is a career-life coach named Sharon. During her presentation about work-life balance, I start thinking about making some changes in my life, and Charlotte encourages me to *go for it*.

At the end of Sharon's presentation, she offers a free half-hour coaching session for the forty people who attended the conference, so I schedule a phone appointment with her in hopes she can give me guidance about my idea. Charlotte encourages me again to *go for it*.

Sharon is friendly, empathetic, and approachable during her presentation, and she's the same during our conversation three days later. She listens intently while I briefly tell her about my situation and my idea:

"I'm homesick. I want to return to Seattle and resume my life there. The work I do as a technical writer can be done from anywhere, and I've wondered whether I could work for my employer from Seattle. I've worked remotely for other companies and it went well, but I don't know whether my current employer will allow me to do it. I love my job and don't want to quit, but I want to go home."

One person at the company works remotely two days a week, but she has a different manager. No one works remotely full-time.

"Have you thought about asking your manager?" Sharon asks.

I hesitate before replying, "No." She makes it sound so simple.

"Why not?"

"What if he says 'no'?"

"But what if he says 'yes'? You won't know until you ask him."

It's that simple. Just ask.

Charlotte jumps in with, *She's right. Ask him.*

"Okay, I'll do it," I say to Sharon.

"Great! Let me know how it goes."

After the meeting at Dunkin' Donuts where I mentioned the divorce, I never see Tom again. A month later, Don calls, asking me where Tom is. He says he hasn't heard from Tom for six weeks. I tell Don about my last conversation with Tom and explain why I made this decision. He listens quietly, then says, "I understand, and I want you to know that regardless of your decision, you will always be part of the Landes family." His words comfort me.

Don ends the call with, "If I hear from Tom, I will contact you."

Four months pass before Don calls me again. "I just got off the phone with Tom. He called me from a pay phone in New York City. He said he is living on the streets now."

Tom is homeless after depleting his 401(k). After my last call with Kaitlyn, this thought persisted in the back of my mind. I've hoped he would stop the reckless spending and find a job, but he's no longer capable.

"I asked him if he has shelter," Don continues. "He said he has been sleeping in subway stations and riding in subway cars until the police catch him. Then they make him leave."

I remember the homeless people who hung out in the subway stations when I lived in New York and shudder at the thought of Tom being there, but there's nothing Don and I can do. Knowing someone we love is in this state and knowing we can't help them is one of the most agonizing experiences we can endure. According to the system, Tom must make his own decisions, but his choices, which are based on his fears, are harming him and placing him in danger. As he continues spiraling downward, I wonder if he will ever be able to recover.

Cheryl Landes

The Proposal

New England, Spring 2006

I return to Baxter State Park this morning, not to climb Katahdin again, but to take some long walks and think about how to ask Russ about working remotely from Seattle. This is another bold move for me. Working three thousand miles away—will he think I'm crazy? I can write from anywhere. The only times I need to be in the office are to work with the electrical boards in the training room when there are updates to the software, which happens once or twice a year.

Russ, the Vice President of Marketing, became my manager after a department restructure. The entire department now reports to him. Todd is still there and has the same title as the Director of Marketing. Russ knows about Tom because I shared the high-level information with him. He has been supportive and understanding so far.

I stop at the main gate on the south side of the park to pay the seventeen-dollar entrance fee for out-of-state residents and tell the ranger on duty which trail I plan to hike. "I'm going to Roaring Brook for the Moose Walk."

The ranger hands a red sign with large black letters spelling, "MOOSE WALK," to me to hang from my rearview mirror. "This lets the other rangers know you're not climbing the mountain," he says. "When you leave the park, drop it in the box at the gate."

The mile-and-a-half trail along the southeast shore of Sandy Stream Pond is flat. The grasses growing out of the water remind me of the bogs on the Oregon Coast. Pine trees, some with the tops snapped off from lightning strikes, line the shore. It's a sunny, cloudless day, which reveals clear views of Mount Katahdin above the trees.

I take my time, stopping to watch birds fly overhead, admire the views of the mountain, or when movement catches my eyes through the trees. I linger at one spot where a moose stands belly deep in the water, grazing on the tender blades.

I decide the best approach is to be direct with Russ and have a solid justification for why I want to return to Seattle. It's time to move on with my life, but I love my job. Seattle will give me a fresh start from losing Tom to mental illness.

When I arrive at the office on Monday morning, I open my calendar in Microsoft Outlook and glance through my meetings for the week. I click the New Appointment button, enter Russ' name in the To field, and browse the times he's available. My mind hesitates; is this a good time? Is this really a good idea?

Don't hold back, Charlotte says. *Talk to him today. This is the perfect time, and he has availability on his calendar this afternoon. You can do this!*

She's right. What am I waiting for? Nothing is keeping me in Massachusetts except for this job. I love my job, but I can enjoy it from Seattle, too. And I can move forward there in the place I call home. There are too many bad memories in Massachusetts of Tom's mental decline and our marriage falling apart.

I select the one-thirty to two o'clock time slot. Russ will be settled by then after his hour-long lunch break.

My mind balks at the Subject field. What should I enter here? I don't want to give anything away before our meeting, so finally, I choose one word, "Proposal," and click the Send button.

Russ' acceptance of my meeting invitation lands in my inbox within minutes after he arrives at the office at nine o' clock. Now I'm committed. This feels like the right thing to do.

For the rest of the morning, images of returning to my old neighborhood fill my mind while I edit a marketing brochure. I'm walking in the Admiral District of West Seattle on a sunny spring day, with a gentle breeze rustling through the pink and white blossoms on the ornamental cherry trees in full bloom. I stop in front of a restored 1920s Tudor-style home to watch a hummingbird drink nectar from a feeder hanging from a branch of a pine tree.

Everything will be okay, Charlotte says. There's that line again. How many times has she said this and everything has turned out okay? I've lost track.

Her words reassure me that whatever happens this afternoon, it will be the right path to follow.

When I walk into Russ' office at one-thirty, he looks up from behind the monitor and smiles, exposing the dimples in the middle of his cheeks. He's wearing a long-sleeved white button-down shirt, and his thick, neatly-trimmed brown hair covers his head like a cap.

His windowless corner office contains his desk on one side and a long cabinet on the other, both oak-stained, and two chairs with periwinkle cushions for visitors in front of the desk. Piles of papers are stacked neatly on top of the cabinet and on one side of his desk. A flat-screen computer monitor is on the opposite side of the desk, near the wall. A five- by seven-inch photo of his wife and two children is in a silver frame under the monitor stand.

"Have a seat," he says, while motioning toward the chairs in front of his desk.

"Thank you for taking the time to meet with me today," I say.

Russ swivels his computer monitor toward the wall so we have an unobstructed view of each other. "So, what's this proposal you want to talk about?" he asks. The curiosity shows in his brown eyes.

"You're aware of the situation with my husband," I say. "I'm homesick and would like to go home."

Russ' eyes widen, and his jaws tighten. "Are you leaving?"

"No. I'd like to work remotely...from Seattle. Most of my work can be done from anywhere. I've worked remotely several times before starting this job, and I've always been more productive from my home office."

Russ looks at the ceiling while rubbing a corner of his square chin for a few seconds, then shifts his eyes back to me.

"My wife is a writer," he says, "and she works from home. I've noticed she gets a lot done when she's there and the kids are in school."

"My research for the manuals is mostly online, logging into our test system to use the software and writing the steps. For the marketing and training materials, I can schedule phone conversations with the subject matter experts, if needed, or send questions by email."

We hear an alert from Russ's inbox. He glances at the screen, then looks at me again. "I think this can work. We'll have to come up with a plan."

"I will outline one by the end of the week."

"Great. I'm looking forward to seeing it."

My heart soars. It's the perfect day. I can finally go home, and I don't have to quit my job. I can enjoy the best of two worlds on opposite sides of the country. The deal isn't sealed yet; I must create a workable plan that Russ will approve. He said "yes" already, but the plan must convince him that I will be successful. I can start over, personally that is, in a place where I have friends and am closer to family. I can have a real life again, away from the sad memories. Returning to my old neighborhood will rekindle memories from the happy days Tom and I lived there, but it's a place of healing—a place of natural beauty that will comfort me.

Tom will always be part of my life through my memories. I still hope he can get the help he needs to recover from his paranoia, but based on Don's reports, he's far beyond that point. Now he's delusional every time he calls Don.

"Some days, I can't hold an intelligent conversation with him," Don says with a sad tone in his voice when he calls me with updates.

I know Don isn't implying that Tom is stupid. It's his way of saying he can't have a regular conversation with Tom because Tom can't stop talking about his imaginary followers and the contamination. Don still struggles to make sense of this behavior.

Yes, today is the perfect day. I'm going home soon. I can't wait to tell TC and Maggie tonight. They won't say anything, but TC will probably ask for a hug and head rub. TC is going home, too. Maggie has never been to Seattle or flown on a plane, as far as I know. How will she handle the trip?

When I arrive at my apartment after work, TC and Maggie are hunched in front of the sliding glass door, watching a giant snapping turtle lumber across the backyard. This turtle often walks across the backyard instead of following the river. There were a lot of snapping turtles in the rivers in the Ozarks, where I grew up, but I never saw them come out of the water and didn't know they would, so whenever I see this one, I wonder whether it's an outlier. That's often how I feel—like someone who doesn't fit in—especially after everything I've experienced with Tom's mental illness during the past ten years.

You are loved for the way you are, Charlotte says. *Don't try to be different.*

Tonight, I don't have any desire to change myself. My talk with Russ today renewed my confidence. I don't know why I haven't been more confident during my slow recovery from my troubles with Tom. Maybe it's because things didn't work out the way I wanted. Maybe it's because I still wrestle with thoughts of being a failure because I couldn't help Tom. But through it all, I've found resilience, strength, and tenacity—traits I never acknowledged until the counselor helped me embrace them before our sessions ended last fall—but I still need reminders from Charlotte. She always delivers.

TC runs to me as soon as I open the door and props his front paws on my right calf. I pick him up, and he rubs his head vigorously on my chin and cheeks. "I'm happy to see you, too," I say, "and I have some good news. We're going home to Seattle."

The volume of TC's purr rises while I carry him to the futon cushion and lower him on top of it. I sit between him and the pillow propped against the wall. Maggie ignores us, immersed in watching the snapping turtle. I wonder why she's fascinated by a snapping turtle, then remind myself that cats are curious about everything.

TC stands next to me and watches me boot up my laptop and log in. "Hey, TC," I say while scratching him between his ears, "would you like to help me with a project? I need to create a plan for my boss on how I'll work with him remotely after we go home to Seattle. Surely you have some ideas."

TC rubs my upper arm and shoulder with his head and purrs loudly.

"Thank you for your support," I say. "You've inspired me already."

He curls into a ball next to me and purrs until he drifts into a cat nap. Maggie continues to absorb the view outside.

I open a new document in Microsoft Word and start organizing my thoughts, from ways to communicate effectively at a distance to the hours I plan to work. I'll work my regular East Coast hours, which means I need to rise at four o'clock every weekday morning. I'm a morning person, so this won't bother me. The other nice part is my workdays will end at one o'clock in the afternoon, so I'll have plenty of time to enjoy walks in the neighborhood, read a book, run errands, finish some personal projects, and play with TC and Maggie (if they want to).

Two hours later, I'm done proofing the final draft. I send the file to my work email. In the morning, I'll read it one more time before forwarding it to Russ for approval.

It's hard to sleep tonight because of the excitement. I'm thinking about the details to finish before leaving Massachusetts—looking for an apartment in Seattle and finding a place to store anything I can't carry in my car until I can afford to move it. I don't have much, but there isn't enough room to carry everything in my car. Then there's the question of when to move. I want to go as soon as possible, but I need to give a month's notice on the apartment here. And I need enough money to pay a deposit on an apartment in Seattle, which is equal to one month's rent.

Plus, I need to fly TC and Maggie from Boston to Seattle, so that's another expense I need to prepare for. Driving cross-country would be tough on them. TC wouldn't complain because he's always happy to hang out with me, but he would be uncomfortable.

Since Tom and I adopted TC, he has doubled in size and weight, from eight to sixteen pounds. He was small enough to fit comfortably in a carrier under the seat in front of me when we flew from Seattle to Newark, New Jersey, to live on Staten Island, but now, he must ride in cargo with the other animals. He'll love hanging out there—he's never met a critter he doesn't like, even when they don't care about him—but I'm concerned about his well-being during a six-hour flight. I need to learn more about this and make a mental note:

Research information about animals flying in the cargo hold, talk to the vet, and read the airlines' rules for checking animals. And find a direct flight so TC isn't transferred to the wrong plane. I don't want to lose him!

There are also the expenses for gas, food, and places to sleep during my cross-country drive. I'll buy non-perishable snacks, like trail mix, and treat myself to grocery store delis as much as possible. I can nap at rest areas and sleep at truck stops. Gas prices I don't have as much control over, but my CR-V gets good mileage for an SUV—twenty-seven miles per gallon on the highway.

You can do this, Charlotte says. *It's time to start a new life.*

She's right...I can do this. Now I need to wait for Russ' decision.

The next morning, I'm rested despite my erratic sleep patterns throughout the night. *Everything feels right about this,* I think while showering, dressing for work, and finishing the final touches in the bathroom. As soon as I turn on the water to brush my teeth, TC and

Maggie race into the bathroom and jump on opposite sides of the sink. Maggie loves to drink the running water from the faucet, and when TC discovered her obsession after I adopted her, he decided he likes it, too.

Now, every time I'm in the bathroom and run the water, they're fighting over who can drink first. Sometimes they compromise with Maggie drinking directly under the faucet and TC lapping at the bottom of the stream, but there isn't enough room for two cats to jockey for position on this tiny sink. Somehow they make it work; cats have an amazing ability to expand and contract in proportion to their curiosity and determination, which I'll never understand. But after adding a human who's trying to use this sink into the mix, it's impossible to drink or clean anything. The only solution is for me to push them off the sink, which results in one or more reactions: They sit on the floor on opposite sides of me, staring at the running water with longing in their eyes, they jump on the sink and try to drink again, or TC will leave and Maggie will try again.

I always laugh at their antics. Sometimes I think if the original Tom were here, he would laugh, too. He never met Maggie, but he loved TC and Tiger. Those two boys brightened his days as much as mine. I push the memories aside and continue getting ready for work.

As soon as I arrive at the office, I download the plan from my inbox, read it one more time, then forward it to Russ. I'm on edge waiting for his feedback but am elated at the same time. I'm expecting him to approve it but keep telling myself not to get my hopes up. It's easier to expect the least from an outcome than to believe it will happen and be disappointed. This doesn't make sense because of my optimistic feelings and Charlotte reassuring me that I am returning to Seattle and will work remotely for this company. Where did my confidence from yesterday go?

Russ walks in at his usual time while I'm editing a sales bulletin for a new product announcement. When he passes, he smiles and says, "Hello." I return the greeting, watch him disappear into his office, and wonder whether he'll see my message. I try to concentrate on the sales bulletin through my suspense of waiting for his answer.

Two hours later, an email from Russ displays in my inbox. The subject line reads, "Do you have a few minutes?" He didn't write any words in the body of the message.

I walk into his office and sit in one of the guest chairs.

"I just read your plan," he says. "Nice job."

"Thanks," I reply. "Is there anything you want to change or add?"

"No. It looks perfect. I think this will work."

I want to jump up, squeal with joy, and give him a bear hug, but instead, I take a deep breath, smile, and say, "Thank you. You don't know how much I appreciate this."

"Glad to help. I can't imagine how hard this has been for you."

After work, I start searching online for an apartment in West Seattle. While browsing the ads, I think about the building where Tom and I lived the first two years after we married. It's in a convenient location and close to the parks and viewpoints I love. I know the building well and loved living there, so I'm comfortable signing a lease sight unseen.

The building has one-bedroom and large studio apartments. At seven hundred fifty square feet, the studios are more than twice the size of my current apartment—plenty of space for TC, Maggie, and me. Each apartment has a floor-to-ceiling window, which will give TC and Maggie hours of viewing entertainment.

I look up the name of the apartment building and find openings. During my lunch break the next day, I call the management office.

"We have a studio available on the first floor," the manager says. "It's seven hundred fifty a month. If your application is approved, we'll need a last-month deposit equal to one month's rent."

That's one hundred dollars more than I'm paying now, but with careful budgeting, I can manage. The cost of living in Seattle is lower than Massachusetts, which will help, too.

"I'd like to fill out an application," I say. "My husband and I were two of your original tenants, so I'm familiar with the apartments. We lived in 409 for two years."

The manager faxes an application to me an hour later. *The plan is starting to fall into place*, I think while filling it out. The reality of returning home is sinking in.

In the meantime, I find a storage company that ships people's belongings in containers for a fixed fee. They drop off the container for two days while it's filled, then pick it up and deliver it to the preferred destination. They'll give me two days to unload it.

My application is approved a week later. I schedule a move-in date, give notice to move out of my apartment in Massachusetts, and make an appointment for the storage company to drop off a small container. When I finish loading the items I don't need for my cross-country drive, it's only half full. I ask the storage company to store the container for me until after I'm settled in Seattle. They'll charge a monthly fee, which is almost half the cost of renting a traditional storage unit.

The pieces are falling into place, except for the status of my divorce. Kaitlyn hasn't heard from the Middlesex County Courthouse since she refiled the papers seven months ago and asked the clerk to expedite them.

One day when we're talking on the phone, I ask, "Would I be able to refile in Washington State after I move there? It isn't where Tom and I last lived together, but the process should move faster. I can get a legal separation there."

"It's up to you," Kaitlyn says. "Middlesex County is slow, but usually it doesn't take this long to schedule a hearing. If you can reach a resolution sooner in Washington, I'd advise you to proceed."

Although my financial situation is improving, I still need a divorce or legal separation to protect myself. Calls continue to come from collection agencies and letters arrive in the mail about bills Tom accumulated and hasn't paid. The recent ones are from after we separated. There's a six-hundred-dollar bill for damage to a car Tom rented. A dentist on Staten Island is trying to collect for a past-due bill. A bank where Tom had a checking account sent a collection notice because he overdrew six thousand dollars. Why would any bank allow someone to overdraw that much money?

When I show the letter from the bank to Kaitlyn, she says, "This bank has a reputation of allowing people to accumulate high overdraft balances. I don't understand it, either."

I've stopped answering the phone when I see an unfamiliar number. Kaitlyn says collectors can't force me to pay bills that aren't in my name, but this doesn't stop them from trying. But I still worry about whether they could garnish my wages, seize my tiny savings account or what's left of my 401(k), or do something else that could cause havoc in my life.

They can't go after you, Charlotte reminds me when I worry about this. I know she and Kaitlyn are right, but it's hard to be reassured when I'm scared of another setback. I've had too many resulting from Tom's reckless behavior.

Sometimes when I'm not paying attention, I accidentally pick up calls from familiar area codes. Collectors often mask their numbers from local area codes to entice their targets to answer.

Whenever this happens and someone asks for Tom, I respond with, "You have the wrong number."

Then they ask, "Are you Cheryl Landes?"

I have no idea where they find my phone number. It's unlisted.

"Yes."

"I'm calling for Tom Landes. I need to talk to him about an urgent matter."

They're also poor listeners. Didn't they just hear me say they have the wrong number?

"Tom disappeared a year ago. No one knows where he is."

"Do you know how I can reach him?"

"No. He disappeared. No one knows where he is."

"I'd like to leave a message for him."

"Don't you think it's pointless leaving a message when I can't give it to him? I've told you twice he disappeared, and no one knows where he is. What parts of 'disappeared' and 'no one knows where he is' don't you understand?"

That's when I hear, "Thank you for your time" and a click, or they just hang up. I always let them end the call first. If I do, they'll call me back. When they do, I never hear from them again.

The Hearing

Massachusetts and Seattle, Summer 2006

TC flew once when he was small enough to be a carry-on from Seattle to Newark, New Jersey, via Phoenix, seven years ago. He handled that flight well, despite the long distance and a wait on the tarmac in Newark for forty-five minutes after landing until a gate was available for the plane to park. When other passengers discovered a cat was with me, several commented, "He handled the flight better than most of the humans."

When I check in TC at the Alaska Airlines ticket counter at Logan International Airport in Boston, he seems to take everything in stride. He looks around through his carrier door with the usual cat curiosity. The agent adds plastic ties to the carrier to ensure it doesn't fall apart during the flight. A Golden Retriever checked in for the same flight is waiting to board in a large carrier at the end of the conveyor belt. The agent transfers TC to the same location. Both animals point their noses in each other's direction and sniff the air.

After I finish checking in, I stop at TC's carrier and rub his nose through the bars of the carrier door. "I'll see you in Seattle," I say. "Everything will be okay."

He closes his eyes while I rub his nose, enjoying the attention. When I remove my finger, he meows at me.

"It's okay," I say. "We'll be home soon."

Maggie counts as one of my two carry-on bags. I don't know how well she'll handle a flight, because this is her first time as far as I know.

I carry Maggie to security for screening, which means removing her from the carrier so it can be sent through the X-ray machine. I hold her tight while walking through the metal detector. She doesn't squirm, thankfully, because her senses are in overload mode.

I retrieve the carrier on the other side and repack Maggie. Then we continue the journey to the gate for our flight.

After we board the plane, I stow Maggie under the seat in front of me. She turns around in her carrier a few times to get comfortable and finally curls in a loose ball. She sleeps most of the flight, except for meowing briefly during takeoff. I'm surprised she doesn't say anything during the descent because the pressure bothered TC when we flew the last time. He didn't fuss too much, though.

Although the flight to Seattle is uneventful, I think about TC in the cargo hold and hope the temperature isn't too hot for him. When I called Alaska Airlines with questions about traveling with checked animals, the agent assured me that the animals are placed in a climate-conditioned section of the space. Being close to the friendly dog will reassure him.

After we land and Maggie and I reunite with TC at the baggage claim office, he looks tired but happy to see us. His expression translates to, "Are we there yet?"

I rub his nose again through the door. "Hi," I say. "We're almost home! No more plane rides today."

We take a shuttle to my new apartment in my old neighborhood, the Admiral District of West Seattle. The neighborhood is a fifteen-minute drive from downtown, on a small peninsula that overlooks Elliott Bay with beautiful panoramic views of downtown Seattle and the Olympic Mountains on a clear day. The neighborhood is full of parks and Alki Beach, and anything we need is within walking distance. And now that I'm telecommuting full-time, my office will be in my apartment.

Tom and I lived in the same apartment building for the first two years of our marriage. Our one-bedroom apartment was on the fourth (top) floor, which had a fantastic view of downtown Seattle from our floor-to-ceiling living room window. I loved to sit in a chair in front of the living room early in the morning and look at the city lights while sipping a cup of coffee. On rare rain-free mornings behind the skyscrapers, the sunrises painted a beautiful canvas of red, orange, and yellow above a purple silhouette of the Cascade Mountains.

Now I'm on the first floor in a large studio apartment, so there's no city view. It doesn't matter. I'm home and can start my new life in the city I love.

I make arrangements with Connie, TC's former catsitter, to check on him and Maggie once a day until I return to Seattle. Then I fly back to Boston for two days to wrap up the rest of the moving details before starting the cross-country drive.

Back in Massachusetts on the way to the office, I stop at the UPS Store in Acton to check my mail. It's mostly the usual pile of bills and junk flyers, except for one envelope with a return address from the Middlesex County Courthouse. I open the envelope and find a notice for my divorce hearing, which is scheduled six weeks from today.

This is good news, but it throws a wrench into my plans. I moved out of my apartment in Massachusetts already, and I have a reservation for only two nights at the Motel 6 in Leominster. With the catsitting expense, I can't afford to stay there any longer, buying another plane ticket is out of the question, and I don't know anyone well enough in Massachusetts who will let me stay with them temporarily. So, I'll car camp until the hearing ends, then drive to Seattle.

While I was in Seattle, New England's weather switched from winter to summer, which isn't unusual here. Now the daily highs are in the 90s and accompanied by high humidity, so sleeping in my car is miserable. When I was homeless in the winter, I could always add extra blankets and curl up in a tight ball to conserve body heat and stay reasonably comfortable. Staying cool in this heat isn't possible unless I run the air conditioner in the car constantly, which drains the battery or the gas tank, depending on the type of power I use.

By the fourth day, I'm exhausted. Yvette notices when she sees me in the office that morning.

"You look terrible," she says. "I hope you don't take that as an insult."

I shake my head.

"Is everything okay?" she asks.

Yvette is among the few people in the office who know about my personal life. I chose the people I confide in because I can trust them. They don't feed information into the grapevine.

She and I work closely with the training manager. Two years after I started working here, she transferred out of Human Resources into a new role that reports directly to him. I help him create the training materials for his classes.

"I am," I say. "I've been living in my car for a few days. It's hard to sleep because of the heat."

"You're staying in your car? You shouldn't do that."

"I finally received news about my divorce hearing. It's on August twenty-fourth. I need to stay here until it's over. If I try to reschedule it, I don't know when it will be. Middlesex County is slow."

"Well, you're not staying in your car. You can stay at my place until the hearing."

"I appreciate your offer, but I can't impose on you."

"It's okay. I *want* you to come."

Swallow your pride and do this, Charlotte says. *You can't stay in your car for another five and a half weeks in this heat.*

"All right. Thank you," I say.

After work, I follow Yvette to her condominium, where she sets me up in her spare bedroom. During my stay, I help her as much as I can with food, cleaning, or anything else I can think of. I'm gone a lot, too, because I want to finish some big projects at the office before the cross-country drive.

On August twenty-fourth, I meet Kaitlyn in the courthouse foyer a few minutes before nine o'clock, when court starts for the day. After walking through the metal detector at the entrance, we enter a dreary room resembling an auditorium. The walls are gray, exposed concrete with no pictures or decorations. We sit four rows from the front and wait for our case to be called.

The bailiff announces, "All rise," as the judge enters the courtroom. She's an attractive middle-aged woman with dark brown skin, short black curly hair, and a frown on her face.

Kaitlyn instantly notices the judge's demeanor and shifts in her seat. She turns to me and says, "She's having a bad day already. This isn't good."

I watch the judge call and hear the cases before ours and wonder what will happen. Will she approve my divorce so I can finally go home?

Some people in the back corner of the courtroom start a conversation that's too loud for the judge's liking. She warns them twice over a fifteen-minute period. The second time, she says, "If I have to warn you again, I will have you removed from this courtroom."

Kaitlyn shifts in her seat again and turns toward me with a worried look on her face.

Then we hear, "The next case is Landes versus Landes. Would the plaintiff and defendant come to the stand?"

Kaitlyn and I approach the bench and stand in front of the judge.

The judge looks at us. "Are you the plaintiff?" she asks.

"Yes," Kaitlyn replies. She motions toward me and says, "This is my client."

"Where's the defendant and his attorney?" the judge asks.

"They are unable to attend," Kaitlyn says. "The defendant's attorney has another court appearance today. He sent this letter to me to give to you, along with his regrets."

Kaitlyn hands the letter to the judge, and the judge reads it. The letter states that Tom has not been cooperative with the attorney, and the attorney is acceptable with the judge granting my divorce and any other terms I want.

The judge is angry about Tom's attorney's absence and fines him five hundred dollars.

Then Kaitlyn says, "Your Honor, in light of the defendant and his attorney's absence, we would like to request that the hearing be completed today."

"Granted," the judge replies. "Proceed."

The hearing is simple. In front of the judge, Kaitlyn verifies where Tom and I last lived together before we separated and that I indeed want a divorce. When she finishes, the judge says, "I hereby grant Cheryl Landes a divorce. Case dismissed."

My marriage to Tom is officially over after almost eighteen years. I have a range of feelings, from relief and sadness to guilt and regret. I'm relieved another battle has ended and I am safe from the collectors who are after Tom. I'm sad our marriage ended like this. I still feel guilty because I couldn't help him, although there's nothing I can do. And I regret allowing us to move to the Northeast to pursue a career change for Tom that was destined to fail. But would things have been different if we stayed in the Pacific Northwest? That's a question I'll never be able to answer.

Kaitlyn walks me to my car and hugs me after I open the door on the driver's side.

"Thank you for everything," I say. "I couldn't have done this without you."

"You're welcome. I'm glad I could help. Good luck."

I start the drive to Seattle. After more than six and a half years that feel like an entire lifetime, I'm finally going home.

Home Again

Pacific Northwest, September 2006-September 2009

I take my time driving to Seattle along a route plotted on MapQuest through Vermont, upstate New York, Ontario, the Upper Peninsula of Michigan, the Northern Plains, and the Rocky Mountains. The farther I drive, the more I relax. I'm on the way home, and I can stay this time.

On the Friday before Labor Day weekend, almost a week and a half after leaving Concord, I arrive in Seattle while the sun sets behind the Olympic Mountains. I cross the West Seattle Bridge and take the exit to Harbor Avenue for my first glimpse of the lights reflecting in Elliott Bay from the skyscrapers downtown. I'm not ready to park at the viewpoint but it will come soon. It's time to reunite with TC and Maggie and begin my new life.

Moving back to the neighborhood where Tom and I lived and renting an apartment in the same building where we settled after our wedding may not make sense, and I think about this on the way there. Compared to all the other places I've lived, this is my favorite, and that's why I chose it. From the first time Tom showed this neighborhood to me when we were engaged, it felt like home.

Everywhere I look, I will be reminded of the memories from the ten years we lived here together. There are many happy moments among the sad ones, but by reliving these memories, I can heal. My outdoor adventures in New England provided temporary respite, but the stress always waited for me when I returned to my tiny apartment in Stow. There will be stress in Seattle because I'm still paying off bills and taking care of other details from my dead marriage. But overall, my positive outlook from returning to the Pacific Northwest will help me move forward in a familiar place.

When I arrive at the apartment, TC and Maggie stand in the hallway staring at me as if I'm a stranger. How could they forget? Maybe they're surprised because they expected Connie to walk through the door instead of me.

"Hey, there, I'm finally home! I missed you!"

I squat and extend the back of my hand in front of their noses—the proper way for a human to introduce, or reintroduce, themselves to a cat. They accept my offer by sniffing my fingers. When TC is sure it's me, he begins rubbing my hand. Then I rub between their ears, and they squeeze their eyes in enjoyment.

"Let's see what Connie said about you," I say. "I hope you behaved while I was gone."

Connie left her notes on the kitchen counter. I read her daily briefs, one sheet for each week. Nothing earth-shattering happened while I was gone. Connie's entries praise TC and Maggie for their outstanding behavior.

The holiday weekend gives me time to unpack and get organized. I don't have much to put away, but it feels good to empty the boxes and my suitcase. I don't have any furniture yet, except the futon cushion from my old apartment in Stow.

My weekday routine quickly falls into place: Get up at four in the morning, eat breakfast, log into my employer's computer at four-thirty, take a half-hour break at nine o'clock while my coworkers in the Northeast are at lunch, and log off at one in the afternoon. Then I walk in the neighborhood for an hour and return to play with TC and Maggie when they aren't sleeping. On clear days, I often go on another walk after an early dinner to enjoy the sunsets from the viewpoints on the bluff. On weekends, I treat myself to long hikes on trails outside the city.

Gradually I furnish the apartment with a desk from JCPenney and a desk lamp, round maple table with two chairs, two bookshelves, and a rocking chair. During a conversation with Lily, she offers a couch and double-size futon cushion and frame she and Larry no longer use, and they deliver them on a Saturday morning. All are in excellent condition.

Life feels like it's returning to normal again.

Lily, Betty, and I resume our periodic long lunches at a new restaurant centrally located for us—the Bahama Breeze at Southcenter

Mall. I also reunite with other colleagues in the Seattle area, and we meet for coffee or lunch.

When Tom and I were students at the University of Oregon in Eugene, we had a mutual friend, Emily, who was also a regular customer at the 7-Eleven where I worked. Before Tom and I married, we'd meet up with Emily and my roommate for movie nights at Emily's apartment on weekends when we weren't working or in classes or on holidays when everyone was in town. We rented stacks of video cassettes from Blockbuster, assembled a smorgasbord of snacks and sodas, and stayed up all night. Usually we were in town on New Year's Eve, so our movie night became an annual tradition for greeting the new year.

We lost contact with Emily after moving to the Northeast, so I'm excited to reconnect with her. I begin visiting her on weekends whenever I can, and we resume the New Year's Eve movie watching tradition at her house in Springfield. Now, though, we never make it through the night, thanks to age creeping up on us, but we manage to cross the line from the old year to the new, when we toast each other with champagne glasses half filled with sparkling apple cider.

Don calls whenever he hears from Tom. His reports aren't as frequent and are mostly the same. Tom is still homeless, he's in Manhattan, and his conversations with Don are primarily about the people following him in his mind. But during one conversation four months after my return to Seattle, Don shares some new details.

"Tom got a job," he says.

I never expected to hear those words in a sentence again. Hope swells in my head and heart that Tom is actively seeking help.

"What's he doing?" I ask.

"He was a clerk at Radio Shack," Don says.

He *was* a clerk. What happened this time?

Before I can ask Don, he continues. "He worked there for two weeks, then stopped showing up. He said someone was interfering with his job."

My bubble of hope bursts. The cycle continues.

"He was living in a subsidized apartment for three months," Don says. "I encouraged him to apply, and his application was accepted."

"Where is he now?"

"He's back on the streets. He was kicked out of the apartment. When I asked why, his answer was vague, but from what I could gather, he didn't follow the rules."

We'll never know, but I can guess that Tom probably reacted inappropriately to one or more of his delusions, which violated some of the landlord's policies and triggered his eviction.

I've accepted that Tom will never change. The longer he's alone on the streets, the less chance he will be capable of understanding he needs help. That's because the longer a condition like his continues untreated, the worse it gets. His paranoia prevents him from making rational decisions because of his inability to trust anyone. At this point, he will live the rest of his live as a homeless man, and there isn't anything anyone can do to bring him back.

Don says he started sending Tom two hundred dollars a month and set up an inexpensive mobile plan so Tom could stay connected. Tom stopped using the cell phone on my account a long time ago. I don't know if he lost it, threw it away during one of his delusions, or it was stolen. Before Tom received the new mobile phone from Don, he called Don collect from pay phones, but phone booths are becoming harder to find because of the growing demand for cell phones.

"How can you get money to him when he doesn't have an address or a bank account?" I ask.

"I send a wire to the Western Union at Grand Central Station," Don replies. "Tom and I set up a date and time when he will pick up the cash."

"I'm surprised he agrees on a date and time when he's afraid someone is following him," I say.

"So am I, but he always shows up," Don says. Apparently the need for cash temporarily overpowers Tom's fears.

Despite my acceptance that Tom won't change, I'm sad that I can't help him find a path to recovery. Often I still feel guilty, but Charlotte reminds me that it's not my fault.

You did the best you could, she says.

Don also updates me on Nancy's condition, which is worsening. During one of our conversations, I ask if it would be okay if I visit briefly during a weekend trip to the Oregon Coast.

We set up a time early Saturday evening. Nancy is sitting in the hospital bed Don rented in the family room, her back propped up with pillows. She wears a wig with loose light brown curls, similar to her natural hair color and style. Inky, a solid black cat they rescued from the alley behind Tess and Al's home, is curled at the foot of the bed, sleeping. She doesn't move throughout our conversation.

Despite her condition, Nancy's face glows and she smiles the entire half hour we visit. She doesn't talk about her struggles. We talk about the weather, what's happening in town, Don's and my work, and Don's office remodeling project on the bottom floor of his parents' house.

Nancy was a nurse her entire career, and I wonder how she's really holding up. She will never share her feelings in front of anyone, except when she's alone with Don. She remains strong while fighting this losing battle—a battle that started more than seven years ago.

Don and Nancy are still very much in love after almost twenty years of marriage. This is the type of love I expected to share with Tom for the rest of our lives. Mental illness took that away from us. I still love Tom, but even if he's capable of remembering me now, his paranoia probably continues to prevent him from trusting me. Can he remember the life we lost?

Before I leave, Don asks if he can speak to me privately in the den. He doesn't want to disturb Nancy.

When we're out of earshot, he says, "I just want you to know that Nancy and I do not hold any hard feelings about your decision to leave Tom. We understand why you made that choice."

"Thank you," I say. No more words would come. It's the second time Don said this but with different words, and I wonder whether he feels guilty for not believing me the first time I told him about Tom's condition. Like me, Don also struggles because Tom isn't getting the help he needs, but Don knows there's nothing he can do, either.

That's the last time I see Nancy; she dies six months later. At her memorial service at the Episcopalian church in North Bend, Don leads the service and plays a piano tribute to her—a movement from a favorite Beethoven symphony. I'd never heard him play until then, although Tess told me he learned in school. His performance was passionate and flawless. Tears well in my eyes while thinking how hard this service must have been for him, but it was his way of saying good-bye to Nancy and expressing his love for her.

A year after my move back to Seattle, there are changes at my employer. A large corporation that bought us out before I started working there is inserting its tentacles deeper into our daily operations. Until last year, we were protected, thanks to the president of our subsidiary. I don't know how he managed this for more than five years because the corporation is known for buying out companies, laying off everyone as fast as possible, and taking control of the products they want and discarding the rest.

When the president's latest three-year contract ended, upper management wouldn't renew it. Instead, they transferred him to Europe and assigned a long-timer from the corporate office to oversee our subsidiary. Within a month after he arrived, he laid off ten percent of the workforce, which is a lot for a site with one hundred people. Russ was among the casualties, so now I'm reporting to Todd again. Then three months later, four people were laid off, and four more quit and were not replaced.

At the same time, our workloads increase—not only because of the cutbacks, but also because of heightened expectations from upper management. Soon I'm doing the work of four people, and the never-ending volume of work confines me to my apartment. Eighty-hour weeks become common, and some weeks, I work as much as one hundred hours. As a salaried employee, I'm not eligible for overtime.

When I can sleep, I'm never fully rested. My body is always on high alert. I skip meals to finish projects, and when I stop to eat anything, my choices usually aren't healthy. When I take food and bathroom breaks, I feel guilty. I miss my daily long walks, but I'm afraid if I go out, I'll miss an urgent request or will fall farther behind. There's no way to keep up because as soon as I finish one project, three or four more are added to the list. My shoulders and back are stiff and sore constantly, and the shooting pains in my right arm and hand never stop from heavy use of my mouse for desktop publishing.

One night, I take a break to refill the cats' food and water dishes and clean out the litter box. TC appears as usual, but there's no sign of Maggie. I find her peeking out from under the couch with blood oozing from her mouth.

"Maggie, what's going on?" I ask. "Are you all right?"

Her weary blue eyes stare at me.

I gently tilt her head, then lift her lip to find the source of the blood. I can't see it because the blood covers her gums and teeth.

Maggie doesn't move. If she were feeling better, she would have run away and hid.

We rush to the twenty-four-hour animal hospital, where the vet, a woman in her mid-thirties with shoulder-length hair the color of a wheat field, runs a series of tests. I wait in the exam room with Maggie for the results, gently stroking her fur. She crouches on the stainless-steel table with her eyes half closed and dried blood on her lower lip and chin.

When the vet returns with the results, she says, "I'm afraid I have bad news. Maggie has mouth cancer."

Why didn't I notice this sooner? Why am I even asking myself this question? It's obvious—I've been so busy with work, I missed Maggie's signals that she isn't feeling well. I feed her and TC well, they have ample water, and I clean their litter box every day, but I'm not giving them the full attention they need.

"Is there anything that can be done?" I ask and brace myself for the answer. Maggie is fourteen, so would she recover if she can be treated?

"It's in her jawbone and a section of the bone above her teeth," the vet says. She raises Maggie's upper left lip and points to a dark red spot in the middle of the gumline. My mind cringes at the sight while I struggle to contain my emotions. How much pain is Maggie in? I wish she could talk to me.

"We can't remove the cancer from the jawbone, but we can remove this section of bone," the vet continues. "If we do, Maggie will lose four teeth, and we don't know if the cancer will spread. At her age, she might not survive the surgery."

I don't ask the vet about the price of the operation because I can't bear to watch Maggie suffer, even if she makes it through the procedure. Her life would be prolonged, but she'd struggle eating and be in a lot of pain. Even if the cancer could be removed from her mouth and didn't spread, the cancer in the jawbone has progressed too far. She doesn't deserve this.

"Whatever we do, she will suffer too much," I say. "I can't allow her to go through this."

"I understand," the vet says. "I'll give you some time alone with Maggie."

After the vet leaves and closes the door, I gently stroke Maggie's back and between her ears while struggling to hide my tears from her.

"It's okay. Everything will be all right." I repeat a few times. Maggie begins purring, and I wonder whether it's painful.

"You're a sweet, beautiful kitty, and I love you very much. I don't want you to suffer anymore. I'm sorry you're going through this."

I don't want to put her down, but it's the best choice for both of us. I can't hide the tears any longer.

Maggie stops purring a minute later, but I continue stroking her. She looks at me briefly with her tired eyes, then turns away.

It's time. I tell the vet we're ready and stay with Maggie until her breathing stops and she's at peace.

At home, TC watches me with a puzzled look when I place the empty carrier on the floor near the bed. I pick him up and carry him to the bed, where I sit and lower him onto my lap.

"I have some sad news, sweetie. Maggie isn't coming home. She was very sick."

TC's green eyes widen. I hug him while he rubs my face and chin.

"Let's go to bed. I don't know if I can sleep tonight, even though I'm exhausted. I'll try not to disturb you too much."

When I stretch out, he crawls on the pillow and cuddles against the top of my head. He's asleep on my chest when I awake the next morning.

After Maggie's death, I schedule an overdue appointment for an annual checkup at Dr. Reynolds' office. The petite woman with shoulder-length brown hair, pulled back into a ponytail, was my primary care physician before I moved to New York. She transferred to another clinic while I was gone, but it was easy to find her again through my insurance provider.

This morning, she walks into the exam room, smiles at me, and asks how I'm doing. When I open my mouth to reply, I begin sobbing and cover my face with my hands to hide my tears. Where did this come from?

Dr. Reynolds stands in front of me, holding my chart and watching me with her brown eyes.

When I can regain some composure, I say, "I'm sorry. I'm exhausted. I'm working a lot of hours lately," followed by a description of my routine.

"You can't continue doing this," Dr. Reynolds says. "I'm placing you on medical leave immediately."

"But I can't go on medical leave! I have four manuals to write for new product releases by New Year's Eve." That's only four weeks away, and I know it's humanly impossible to finish them, even if I could work around the clock the rest of the month.

"I don't care how much work you have. It can wait. You're getting some rest!" She grabs a pad from the counter and starts writing.

I know she isn't mad at me. She hears stories like mine constantly from overwhelmed employees in the high-tech industry. They spend most of their time in meetings during business hours, so the only time they can focus on their projects is in the evenings and on weekends.

She hates how companies mistreat their employees and don't give a damn. When these companies wear out someone, they can find a willing replacement with promises of promotions and other incentives they'll never receive.

Dr. Reynolds hands the note to me, and I read it. Her directive is effective today, with a return-to-work date of January second.

I dread relaying the news to Todd. Although he has supported me for six years, he's losing control with the changes from corporate. Like the rest of us, he's in constant fear he'll be laid off or fired. It's not a good time to look for another job, thanks to the worsening economy.

When I call him, he says, "Do what you need to do."

For the next four weeks, I sleep most of the time, usually with TC curled next to me. But no matter how much I sleep, I never feel rested. I worry about the growing pile of projects and what will happen after my medical leave ends. The president won't like my missing deadlines for four major product releases on December thirty-first. Why would anyone decide to release products during the holidays when most of their customers are on vacation?

When I return to work on January second, Todd schedules my performance evaluation. The news isn't good; he places me on probation.

"I'm sorry to do this," he says, "but my hands are tied."

The message is clear: The president is upset about my medical leave, and probation is his retaliation. Todd must follow his orders or risk being fired. To compensate, Todd makes my goals to pass probation easy, so I'm able to complete them before the three-month deadline.

But my health doesn't improve. Soon I'm back to the long work weeks and struggle to finish my projects. The requests continue piling up. I'm in physical therapy three times a week to strengthen my right arm, but with the demands on my body, it's only maintenance. My physical therapist begs me to quit my job every time I see him.

"I can't afford to quit," is my standard reply. "How will I find another job in this economy?"

"You can't keep up this pace," he says. "You're killing yourself."

Three months later, during another meeting with Todd, he says the president asked him to place me on probation again. "The paperwork will be ready tomorrow," he says. "I'll schedule a meeting to review it."

It's time to resign, Charlotte says. *Listen to your physical therapist: You're killing yourself. Things will not improve if you stay there. If you don't quit, you'll be fired. It doesn't matter how hard you work; the company doesn't want you there anymore. You must take care of yourself.*

Betty agrees with the physical therapist during one of our phone conversations. "The company doesn't care about your dedication and your contributions. Even through this is their fault, they see you as a liability and want to avoid a lawsuit. If you don't quit, they'll find a way to fire you."

I can't sleep tonight from worrying about what I'll do. Fighting this losing battle isn't the answer, but now isn't a good time to find another job with unemployment rising nationwide from the Great Recession. What probation goals will Todd assign this time? The president probably wants Todd to be tougher on me to make me fail. Is continuing worth the effort, when it's likely I'll be fired in the end—all because I can't manage a workload that's impossible for any human to maintain?

Charlotte is right. My best option is to leave, but am I ready? My financial situation has improved slowly, but a prolonged setback could send me back to living in my car. If I don't leave, I'll probably kill myself from overwork, like the physical therapist says at every session.

I think about when I was the happiest in my career, when I freelanced full-time during the last four years Tom and I lived in Seattle. My schedule was flexible most of the time, and I could enjoy life when Tom wasn't delusional. I wasn't stressed from overwork. When my calendar was booked full of assignments, I could turn down new projects. And I was paid for every hour I worked.

Go for it, Charlotte says. *It's the best way to get your life back.*

I write a brief resignation letter with a generous five-week notice, schedule a meeting with Todd for nine o'clock Eastern time tomorrow morning, and email my contacts at the placement agencies in Seattle.

Todd accepts the resignation. His prolonged silence after he reads the letter tells me he regrets my leaving, but he understands my decision. "I wish you the best," he says, then offers to be a personal reference.

Recruiters from the agencies send me to several interviews for long-term contracts at three tech companies. Three weeks after my resignation, Microsoft delivers the first offer for editing marketing materials, and I accept. This one-year, full-time contract is remote, with monthly meetings onsite for content releases.

The four-week break between my old job and the first day at Microsoft helps my body start to recover, as does a regular schedule after the contract starts. I can enjoy a healthy breakfast before work, relax in the evenings, and take the weekends off. I resume my daily walks, and my energy slowly returns.

But the contract doesn't last as long as expected. The recession is affecting everyone, including Microsoft, which was immune from economic downtowns since its founding. In January 2009, the company announces its first mass layoffs in its history, and my contract is among the casualties.

Two weeks later, a consulting firm who works directly for Microsoft hires me for a five-week research contract, but it ends abruptly after two weeks. When the owner of the consulting firm delivers the news to me in a private meeting, he said he was forced to lay off half his staff and all the contractors. Microsoft is his only client.

After my second layoff, tech work dries up. I scour the job boards every day and call the agencies twice a week. I apply for secretarial and clerical jobs but am constantly turned down. When I ask one recruiter about the rejections, she replies, "They say you're overqualified. As soon as you get an offer for an opening in your field, they believe you'll leave."

"But these jobs are only temporary," I say.

"Yes, but they're trying you out for permanent roles. They don't want to take any chances on new hires if they can avoid it."

My unemployment isn't enough to continue covering my expenses. The only way I can survive is to move into my car again and find another home for TC. My heart breaks over parting with my sweet buddy again.

Talk to Emily, Charlotte says.

Emily has two cats, a male tabby named Calvin who looks like TC and a gray and white female named Princess. Calvin's demeanor is like TC's—a friendly, happy kitty who takes life in stride. During some of our visits, Emily said she believed Calvin and TC would make great playmates. Princess isn't a socialite; her focus is on food. Emily rations meals twice a day to prevent Princess from gorging herself and gaining too much weight.

I ask Emily if TC can stay with her until I can get back on my feet again, and she agrees. When I drop him off at her house, TC and Calvin greet each other and within seconds, they disappear into Emily's bedroom. I hug Emily and start the drive back to Seattle, thankful and relieved that TC has a loving, safe, comfortable place to stay until I can afford a home for us.

Cheryl Landes

Homeless Again

Pacific Northwest, Utah, and New England,
Fall 2009-Winter 2012

Rain pounds the windshield of my Honda CR-V while I sit in the driver's seat, watching the waterfall. For the past week, I've been parking in a Walmart lot in Lynnwood, Washington, trying to figure out what to do next. In this current job market, I'd have a better chance of finding a grain of sand in a jar of brown sugar than a lead for a technical writing contract. The high-tech economy in Puget Sound is a vast wasteland.

I'm considering a return to New England, where Massachusetts' diverse economy is faring better—not much better, but at least it's better. Yesterday when I checked email using the free Wi-Fi at the closest McDonald's, I found an announcement from the Boston Chapter of STC about a meeting in November on the topic, "Tips for the Job Search." The presenter is one of the chapter's most popular speakers. Maybe I can reunite with my colleagues out there and get some leads or referrals.

That meeting is two months away, though. What will I do in the meantime? Staying here isn't changing anything.

Maybe I should follow the asphalt river from coast to coast. I have some income from unemployment, and I can keep my commitments to job searching along the way. My checks are direct deposited, so I don't have be anywhere at a certain day or time. As long as I continue keeping good records of my applications and contacts and meet the minimum weekly job search requirements, I won't have any problems if the Washington State Employment Security Department challenges me.

Go, Charlotte says. *You'll find work there.*

The Best I Can Do

Early the next morning, the sun finally breaks through the clouds after hiding for two weeks. Hopefully it will guide me until I reach the dry side of the state, east of the Cascade Mountains. Then it will stay with me for most of my journey.

I cross the Cascades to Cle Elum and Ellensburg, and through the Yakima Valley and northeastern Oregon, stopping at viewpoints for short breaks. After entering Idaho, I park at the first rest stop with a view of the Snake River, sit at a picnic table to eat dinner—a hot dog, chips, and soda I bought at the convenience store at the Stinker truck stop in New Plymouth—and watch the sunset paint shades of orange and deep purple on the water while wondering why the truck stop owners named their business after a skunk.

From there, I continue driving long after dark on I-84 through southern Idaho, then exit onto I-15 South. After crossing the border into Utah, I find another rest area and stop there for some sleep on the thin futon cushion folded in half in the back of my CR-V. I have the comforter I rescued from the storage unit in Waltham, a pillow that cradles my neck well, and extra blankets. There's a slight nip in the air in this high desert, but the comforter keeps me warm. I'm a pro at car camping now because this is the third time I've been homeless in the past four years.

I awake four hours later, when streaks of orange, red, and yellow break through the navy blue sky. I grab a change of clothes and a small zip-top bag of toiletries from my suitcase and change and freshen up in the women's restroom. There's no showers here, so I'll look for one at a truck stop farther down the road.

Two hours south of Salt Lake City, I exit onto I-70 toward Colorado and start thinking about where I'll spend the night. Another three hours later, I see a sign for Arches National Park—a place I've always wanted to visit, and now I can if the entrance fee is affordable. Hiking there would be the perfect gift to myself for my birthday, which is tomorrow.

I stop at a McDonald's for a dollar meal of a cheeseburger, small fries, and soda and to check messages on the free Wi-Fi. There's nothing in response to my job applications again. I look for new postings on Indeed.com, but the search results display only jobs I've applied for. Then I search the tech job boards, which show the same openings.

Don't be discouraged, Charlotte says. *Keep moving forward.*

Why does she make it sound so simple?

After dark, I park along a street in a nice neighborhood and bury my body under the covers so if anyone peeks through the window, they'll see a big pile of blankets. Steam will cover the windows from my breathing, but no one will notice anything unusual there, either. All the car windows on this street will fog up because it's a chilly night.

The next morning, the sun's rays break through the trees, a clear sign that another nice day is on the way. Can I celebrate my birthday with some hikes through the park? What a treat that would be!

At the entrance to Arches National Park, the sign delivers good news—the admission is ten dollars. I can manage this.

When I pay at the gate, the ranger hands the receipt to me and says, "This is good for seven days. You can enter as often as you want during that time as long as you show us this receipt."

Happy birthday to me!

The landscape is more beautiful than I imagined—bright rusty red rock formations of all sizes everywhere I look. The cottonwoods with their white trunks and yellow leaves at peak fall color stand out against the rocks under a blue sky free of clouds.

During the next two days, I take advantage of every second of daylight in the park, hiking as many trails as possible and saving Decoration Arch, the landmark I want to see the most, until the end. I time my hike along that steep 1.6-mile trail for the Golden Hour, where I sit on the ground and watch the sunset from the panorama framed by the curve in the red rock. I want to stay here forever, but I must move on in the morning.

From there during daylight hours, I stop long enough to fill the tank with gas, grab cheap eats at either convenience stores at the gas stations or fast food restaurants to use the free Wi-Fi to check emails and the job boards. At night, I sleep at rest areas or in parking lots at the truck stops. In the Missouri Ozarks, I take a break for a week to visit cousins I haven't seen for years, then continue driving to New England.

After arriving in Massachusetts, I spend my days in libraries, reading and surfing the Internet for local openings and emailing colleagues that I'm back. If I can reconnect with enough people, I'll increase my chances of finding some work.

"If you have time, would you like to meet for coffee?" I ask.

"It's my treat." That's all I can afford to offer on my limited budget. Several accept my invitations.

At night, I sleep in familiar parking lots, rest areas, and service areas. The slow economy has brought more people here who are struggling, just like me. There's now a term for this type of living, I learn from my reading at the library: *vehicular residency*.

A week after returning to New England, I find a message in my inbox from Victoria, a former coworker. "Why don't you come to my house for coffee on Saturday morning? We can chat while watching the birds in our backyard.

"If you need a place to stay, we have a spare bedroom. You're welcome to stay here as long as you need to."

I accept her offers.

Victoria and Marty, her husband, live in a two-story, four-bedroom house at the end of a cul-de-sac in a quiet neighborhood west of Boston. The homes along this street are built on large lots with neatly landscaped yards and asphalt driveways ending at two-car garages. On Victoria's side of the street, a dense forest of maples, oaks, and pines thrives at the edge of the backyards.

When I arrive, Victoria hugs me. She's slightly taller than me, with short curly auburn hair and green eyes.

"Come in, come in," she says and escorts me to the family room. "Have a seat wherever you like. The coffee's almost ready. Would you like cream and sugar?"

"Cream will be fine, thank you."

"I'll be right back. Make yourself at home. Marty is out of the country on business for three months, so we have the place to ourselves."

I sit at one end of a brown leather couch, where there's a view of the bird feeders on the deck through the sliding glass doors on the east side of the room. Cardinals, blackbirds, and sparrows take turns pecking the seed in the trays. A chubby red squirrel munches on the seed the birds drop on the deck.

During our conversation, Victoria says, "I started a new contract at a start-up near the Cape two weeks ago. They're talking about hiring a second technical writer. If you're interested, I'd be happy to refer you. It would be fun to work together again."

A week later, I start the contract. Victoria and I take turns driving to the office on the days we work onsite. When we aren't working, we hang out in the living room, chatting and surfing the Web on our laptops; reading; walking Chloe, her standard poodle, in a nearby park; and laughing at the antics of her cats.

Daisy is a clumsy short-haired light gray tabby who never shows any embarrassment over her mishaps. Her most bizarre accident happens one evening when she jumps into a large empty cardboard box and somehow manages to flip it upside down, trapping her inside, when Victoria and I aren't looking. Her sister, Kiki, a medium-haired brown and black tabby, loves to sit at my feet and stare at me with her big green eyes as if I'm a rock star. I imagine her swooning over her favorite guitarist from a front row of a stadium.

Chloe likes to share the couch with me. Her definition of "sharing" is to stretch as far as she can, which leaves me a cramped space at one end. She doesn't ask for attention; she only wants to hang out or nap. When she's asleep, she often rolls on her back with all four legs in the air or props them against the back cushion of the couch. On warm days when I wear shorts, she likes to sit on the floor next to me and lick my calves. When she does this, I joke with Victoria that I have the cleanest legs in town.

Hanging out with the cats and Chloe brings much joy, but it also makes me miss TC even more, despite knowing he's happy having Calvin as a companion and Emily takes good care of him. I feel guilty that my financial situation caused me to break my promise to him yet again.

As the weeks pass, my friendship with Victoria grows stronger. We discover several interests in common, from our deep love for animals to reading books.

Tom has become a distant, sad memory. I haven't received any updates from Don since my return to Massachusetts until he calls one afternoon, worried about Tom.

"I haven't heard from Tom for two months," he says. "I've tried calling several times, but he doesn't answer. I'm afraid something has happened to him."

Horrible thoughts fill my mind. So many things could have happened to Tom: hypothermia from sleeping outside, he was hurt and unable or afraid to get help, he was arrested for loitering, he was in crisis. If he's in crisis, he's so frightened from his paranoia that he's hidden somewhere until he feels his pursuers are gone. This heightened fear could last days, weeks, months, even years.

There's another scary option: Tom passed away. He could have been killed by a mugger or died from hypothermia, pneumonia, or other health problems from being homeless for so long. I try to push those scenarios out of my mind.

"I'd like to ask a favor," Don continues. "Would you research private investigators in New York City and find out how much they charge?"

I agree to do it, and Don asks if I can find some candidates by Friday. After our conversation ends, I begin worrying about what will happen if Don hires one and Tom is okay. Will a PI searching for Tom and finding him feed into his paranoia? Suddenly his fantasies would become reality. But how would he ever discover someone is really looking for him? PIs are discrete and wouldn't contact Tom unless Don asked, but that could jeopardize Tom staying in contact with Don. He might vanish forever, and then if something happened to him, no one in the family would ever find out.

My search online turns up a dozen PIs in New York City that specialize in missing persons cases, and after further research, I narrow the candidates to six and email them. Two call to provide general information about how they handle cases like Tom's and their rates, which I forward to Don.

Two days later, Don calls again. "Tom called me this morning. He's okay."

"Did he say where he was or what happened?"

"No. I asked, but he wouldn't tell me."

My contract at the start-up lasts six months, and Victoria's contract ends a month later. The economy hasn't improved much, so we both struggle to find more work. Two weeks after my contract ends, a recruiter calls me with an emergency request to create a performance evaluation form for a client after a vendor failed to deliver on a new system. The project lasts two weeks. Then work dries up again.

Early on a Saturday morning one month later, Emily texts me. "TC's back end went out when he was in the litter box this morning."

It's never good news when a cat loses mobility in his back legs, and I fear the worst. At sixteen, he has outlived my other cats.

I call Emily. "He struggled to get out of the litter box," she says. "He dragged himself to the kitchen and is now lying under the table."

I want to be with him, console him, and make him as comfortable as possible, but the distance between us is too great. All I can do is pray that his suffering ends quickly.

"Please keep me updated. I will check in, too."

Every couple of hours, Emily updates me by text. No changes. Then, at seven-thirty Eastern time, she calls.

"I'm at the animal hospital with TC," she says. "He started struggling with his breathing a half hour ago. The vet wants to talk to you."

She hands the phone to the vet. "TC's system is shutting down," he says. "His lungs have filled up with liquid. We can drain the liquid to keep him comfortable, but I don't expect him to last much longer."

"I don't want him to suffer anymore," I say as my voice cracks and guilt consumes me for not being with him during his final moments. We've been through so much together, and now this. I will never be able to provide a home for him again.

"I understand," the vet says. "We'll set up everything. I'll give you a few minutes with your friend and TC."

He hands the phone back to Emily. "I'll stay with him," she says. "Do you want to talk to him?"

"Yes." It's always hard to say good-bye to a furry friend, but it's even harder when I can't see him. Will he remember my voice after almost eight months?

Emily holds the phone next to TC's ear.

"Hi, TC," I say.

"He's listening," Emily says.

"Hey, TC, you're a sweet kitty. I miss you. I wish I could be with you now, but I'm too far away. I love you very much."

"They're ready," Emily says. "I'll text you later."

I cry the rest of the evening.

The next morning, Emily emails a picture of TC at the animal hospital before the injection. "He died peacefully," she wrote. "I stayed with him until he was gone.

"The vet will call me when he receives TC's ashes, and I'll pick them up. They'll be waiting for you when you return."

I read the message several times before downloading the picture and opening it. The image shows TC lying on his stomach on a towel covering a soft blanket. His chin lays flat on the towel, and his green eyes clearly show his weariness and pain.

My tears flow again.

Marty continues extending his trip overseas, which increases tension between him and Victoria. Whenever they talk via Skype, they argue a lot. I try to avoid listening to their conversations, but it isn't easy, even when I'm in my room. My heart aches for Victoria for her stress and pain.

Victoria finally decides to file for divorce, and with the escalating tension, I'm feeling more uncomfortable. I want to support her, but at the same time, I don't know what to do other than listen if she wants to talk. Often she doesn't, and we stay in our separate rooms. The stress of not working for four months wears on us, too. Although we're drawing unemployment, we're both struggling financially.

I decide it's time to leave, which means returning to my car. Victoria needs space to sort things out, and I feel like I'm in the way. When I'm in the library or logged into Wi-Fi at a coffee shop, I send check-in emails. Sometimes she replies and asks if we can talk by phone, and I never say "no." I remember how grateful I was to have someone to talk to during my toughest moments with Tom after finally opening up to Betty and Lily.

My stay in the car is short this time—less than three weeks. The owner of a local consulting firm calls me about a two-month contract in Minneapolis for writing instructions on how to use a new taxonomy for a catalog one of his teams created for a large retailer. He offers to cover travel and an apartment while I'm there. My only expenses will be food and personal items.

The fully furnished two-bedroom apartment is on the twenty-seventh floor of a high-rise in downtown Minneapolis. Four days a week, a shuttle driver takes the team to an office in Brooklyn Park; the other day, we're working at the corporate headquarters downtown. When I'm not working, I go on long walks in the parks, the skywalks, or along the streets lined with skyscrapers. I discover a jazz club featuring local artists on weeknights for a ten-dollar cover charge two blocks from the apartment building. Across the street, the Minnesota Symphony offers ten-dollar concerts. They're little treats I've missed for a long time.

While I'm in Minneapolis, an agency in Seattle hires me for a remote six-week indexing project for a software company in California. Another agency in Massachusetts sets up an interview for a part-time technical writing contract that will start after my contract in Minneapolis ends. When the hiring manager at the client extends an offer, I accept. After that, I receive more calls for projects, from remote editing work as-needed for a large IT company to developing online help for a construction firm. Many of these opportunities are in Massachusetts and require some onsite work, so I rent a room in an Extended Stay America at a weekly rate for seven months until I find a reasonably priced apartment in Littleton that includes all utilities.

By the time I settle in Littleton, my work among multiple contracts is providing a steady stream of income. Eventually I pay off my bills and slowly start to build my savings. But in the meantime, in Oregon, my mother starts struggling from unpredictable hours as her employer loses orders to competitors, which can produce the same goods at a lower cost. In case I need to be closer to her, I sign a lease on a studio apartment in the same building where I lived twice before in Seattle and start accepting more remote assignments. I keep the apartment in Littleton because I still need to work onsite for some clients.

When I return to Seattle this time, it doesn't feel the same. My old neighborhood is losing its character. Every empty lot is filling with another condominium complex that looks like a bland box, and all the funky beach houses I loved when Tom and I first moved here are gone, except one. It's for sale, so it won't last much longer.

But I've also changed. Now I realize that when I was here the second time, I needed to be here to heal. This time, I've lost the connection, although my desire is to hang on. I struggled for too long to come home, so I don't want to surrender.

You're holding on to the past, Charlotte says. *You need to let go.*

It takes almost two years to understand what she means, but when it happens, the message is clear: I need to move on. Seattle isn't home anymore. It was only a temporary stop in my journey toward healing.

Don's Death

Massachusetts and Pacific Northwest, Spring 2012

I'm in Canton, Massachusetts, today to work one of my two days a week onsite for a client that manufactures appliances for computer networks. They're boxes that remind me of DVD players, except they're thicker. IT people can add code to the boxes, connect them to their network, and run the code to perform a range of tasks. I write and update instructions on how to use these boxes.

It's lunchtime, and I'm sitting in my cubicle, pulling containers of vegetable sticks with dip and fresh blueberries from my bag. Whenever I work here, I bring lunch because the office is too far away from restaurants to grab a bite for a half-hour break.

As soon as I start eating, my cell phone rings. It's Don, calling from his office.

"Hi, Cheryl," he says in a solemn voice. I immediately wonder if something happened to Tom. Usually when Don contacts me, it's after a call from Tom in New York.

"I have some news to share," he continues, "and I wanted you to hear this directly from me." He never starts a conversation like this when he has an update about Tom.

I drop a half-eaten carrot stick into the veggie container. "What is it?" I ask.

"About a month ago, I started having pain in my stomach. It felt like indigestion but steadily grew worse. I went to the doctor, and he ran some tests. When the results came back, he said I have pancreatic cancer."

I'm stunned. Mom's oldest brother died from pancreatic cancer in the 1990s. He lived only two weeks after he was diagnosed. The prognosis for this type of cancer hasn't changed since then; usually by the time it's discovered, it's too late.

Don is semi-retired from his law practice. He plans to travel and play golf. After being a caregiver for so many years, he's looking forward to some relaxation. Now he's battling terminal cancer at sixty-six years old—still young by today's standards. Of all people, why must this happen to him?

"Oh, dear, I'm so sorry," I reply while a lump forms in my throat. I don't know what else to say.

"The doctor said I have up to three months to live," he says. "There's nothing he can do because the cancer has advanced too far."

What appetite I have is gone. I cradle my phone on my shoulder while snapping the lid on the vegetable container.

"I'm so sorry," I say again. "Is there anything I can do? I'm happy to come to Coos Bay if you want." Don is living alone there. The rest of the immediate family either passed away or lives thousands of miles away.

"I talked to my cousin, the doctor who's retired from the Mayo Clinic. He said there's a surgical procedure that shows some promise. He checked with his contacts there, and they believe I'm a good candidate for the procedure."

"What type of procedure?"

"It's a bypass surgery that will help my liver and stomach work properly while they can treat the tumor. They'll connect part of my small intestine to my stomach and the bile duct directly to another part of my small intestine. It's called the *jejunum*, if I recall correctly. The doctor said if this procedure is successful, it will allow me to continue eating solid food during the treatment."

"I've never heard of this surgery," I say. My uncle never sought treatment because he was so distraught from his wife dying suddenly before his diagnosis, he lost the will to live.

But can Don survive the procedure? Since the doctor in Coos Bay said there's nothing anyone could do, would this only prolong Don's suffering if the surgery is successful? One thing's for certain: Don isn't giving up without a fight. He's tackling this with the tenacity he has when he's defending his clients in court.

"I'm flying to Minneapolis next week. I don't know yet when I will be back—it depends on the outcome. Ron will keep everyone updated while I'm there."

The Best I Can Do

After we disconnect, my thoughts can't focus on anything except Don's news. Deep down, Charlotte says that *he'll survive the first battle but won't win the war*. I can't imagine not being able to talk to him anymore. When he's gone, I will also lose my only link to Tom. Whoever becomes Tom's contact will not call me with updates, and it's uncertain whether Tom will contact them. Don is the only person he will talk to.

During the next week, I keep busy writing and editing for my clients, but my thoughts never drift from Don. The day after his surgery, I'm surprised to see his cell number display on my phone screen.

"How did it go?" I ask.

"The bypass wasn't successful," he replies. "The doctor said the cancer is too far advanced. There's nothing they can do."

The second death sentence has been declared. Don sought another opinion from some of the best doctors in the world, who confirmed the doctor's findings in Coos Bay.

"What are your plans now?" I ask.

"I'm going home and will take it from there," he says.

Throughout our conversation, the tone of Don's voice has been calm but upbeat. Why would he be this way at a time like this? My only conclusion is he has accepted his fate and intends to live the time he has left as fully as possible.

I don't want him to suffer long. No one should endure this.

"My offer still stands if you want me to come to Coos Bay," I say.

"I can manage," he replies. "I don't want you to take time off work on my account."

"Most of my clients allow me to work from anywhere. I can make arrangements with the others to work remotely for a while. They won't mind."

Prepare to go, Charlotte says. *He will appreciate it.*

Don and I share one characteristic: We're not the types who can ask for help easily. He didn't when Tess, Al, and Nancy were sick. Before Tom and I moved to the Northeast, before Nancy was diagnosed with cancer, we visited and helped their parents without asking. Don always appreciated us being there whenever we could. He will hire Nancy's former nurse to take care of him, if he decides to live his last days at home, but I can be there to support him.

"I'll think about it," Don says.

I tell my manager about Don's situation. He expresses sympathy, followed by, "Take the time you need." Then I book a flight to Seattle and stay in my apartment there, waiting for more news from Don.

Within two days after flying home from Minneapolis, Don is back in the hospital—this time at Sacred Heart in Eugene for more surgery from complications with the cancer. A friend in Coos Bay took him to the hospital. Now a bag is attached to his body to collect fluids. He's on a diet of clear liquids and will never be able to eat solid food again.

I drive to Eugene to visit him at the hospital and stay with Emily. When I arrive at his room, he smiles and waves me in. Despite his pain and everything else he's going through, he's in good spirits.

"Thank you for coming," he says. "You didn't have to do this on my account."

"I want to be here," I say. "How are you doing?"

"I'm hanging in there, waiting to be released."

"When are they letting you go home?"

"Soon. There's nothing they can do for me."

Tears well in my eyes, and I stare at the foot of the bed to hide them. He won't last much longer.

"My offer still stands if you want me to come to Coos Bay."

"That's okay. Nancy's nurse will be taking care of me, and hospice will check in twice a day."

"Okay. Let me know if you change your mind."

He does, a week later. When I arrive, he's sitting in the family room in his favorite goldenrod recliner, wearing a light blue button-down shirt and pair of khakis. A clear plastic bag, attached to his body with clear plastic cords, hangs over the left arm of the chair. Liquid matching the color of urine trickles into the bag.

It's hard to see him this way.

He smiles at me. "Good to see you! How was the drive?"

"Quiet today. No traffic jams in either Seattle or Portland."

He nods.

"How are you holding up?" I ask, then regret my choice of words. What a ridiculous thing to say when he doesn't have long to live!

"As well as can be expected. I've kept myself busy, making final arrangements." His tone sounds like his "final arrangements" are simply tasks to be marked off an ordinary to-do list. He's at peace with his fate.

The next week passes quickly as Don's closest colleagues and friends stop in to say their good-byes. When they knock on the door, I ask them to wait in the den and check on whether he's feeling well enough to see them. He never turns anyone away.

When Don isn't visiting, he's talking on the phone with people saying their farewells or taking short naps. He never moves from his chair. His nurse and I ask him about it and suggest, "you'll be more comfortable" somewhere else, like his bed.

"I want to stay here," he says. "Nancy passed away in this chair."

During a quiet time when Don and I are alone, he says, "I talked to Tom yesterday. I told him I didn't have much longer."

He must have talked to Tom when I was running some errands while the nurse was here.

"Did he understand?" I ask.

"Not at first. I repeated it a few times, then he seemed to understand."

I wonder if Tom really can comprehend this.

"What did he say after that?"

"Nothing."

Don pauses for a minute, then looks at me and says, "He asked about you."

That's the first time Don mentioned Tom asking about me since our marriage unraveled. Is Tom wondering what happened to me? To us? Can he understand what happened to us?

"What did you tell him?" I ask.

"I said that I don't hear from you anymore," Don replies.

We're silent for a few minutes, Don staring at the fireplace and me watching him.

I still have emotional pain from the destruction mental illness caused in our lives. It's slowly easing over time, but the scars will remain for the rest of my life. Despite my pain, I still love Tom, but even if I could contact him now, nothing would change. Tom's paranoia has advanced so far, he isn't able to get the help he needs. The intruders will haunt and torment him for the rest of his life.

"I told him if he needs anything, he must contact Ron now."

"Did you talk to Ron about this?"

"Yes. It's all set up."

"Did Tom understand that's what he needs to do?"

"I think so. He said he did before we ended the call."

We sit in silence for a long time. Don closes his eyes and naps while I think about our conversation. This was Don's last phone call with Tom and the last time I will receive any reports about Tom. Ron will not update me like Don has—even if Tom contacts him. It's not because Ron and I have a strained relationship; it's simply his nature.

I sleep on the couch in the family room in case Don needs anything in the middle of the night and to check the bag. When the bag fills, I unsnap it from the cord, place a small stainless-steel bowl on the floor under the open end of the cord, and empty and rinse out the bag before snapping it into place again. Throughout this week, less liquid is draining from Don's body.

When Don's private nurse comes for her shifts, I run errands. The hospice nurse stops by for fifteen minutes twice a day to check Don's vitals, get updates, and give instructions. One night, she hands me a small glass bottle of morphine with a dropper.

"Place two drops in the back of his mouth, on the gumline, when he's in pain," she says.

"How often can I give it to him if his pain worsens?" I ask.

"At this point, it doesn't matter," she says. "Give him as much as he needs to be comfortable."

Early afternoon the next day, Don is resting in the recliner. Suddenly he says, "I'm ready."

I don't ask what he means. I know. It's time for him to go.

He closes his eyes and drifts into a deep sleep. During the next four days, his breathing and heartbeat slow gradually until they finally stop. Before he takes his last breath, he raises his arms and stretches them out for a minute, as if he's trying to grab hold of something, then lowers them slowly until they rest on the arms of the recliner. I wonder if he reached out to Nancy and they're reuniting on the other side. Judging by the faint smile on his face, I believe they are.

After almost five years, Don and Nancy are back together while Tom slips farther away from me. I've lost my only remaining connection to Tom with Don's departure.

You still have memories of the happy times you shared with Tom, Charlotte says. *Treasure them.*

Final Journeys

Massachusetts, New York, and Oregon, April-May 2016

It's a beautiful morning in Littleton, Massachusetts—sunny and in the low sixties at nine o'clock. A few daffodils are blooming in Kelly's yard. I'm inside my apartment, across the hallway from the garage on the bottom level of the two-story house, sorting through things to donate to the Salvation Army. This is my second apartment, which I've rented for almost four and a half years as a place to stay when I'm working onsite for clients in New England. But now, I need to spend more time at home with Mom in Vancouver, Washington, so I'm reluctantly letting this apartment go. Kelly has been a wonderful landlord, and I will miss her and her family.

Mom moved in with me three years ago, after the factory where she sewed hats in Wolf Creek, Oregon, closed and she couldn't afford to live in her apartment anymore. She worked at this factory for ten years, after breaking up with her partner. Before we moved in together, she lived in Portland for a year, but the arrangement didn't work out. As the tension grew, I asked her to move into my apartment in Seattle, but she wanted to stay near her grandchildren and great-grandchildren, Julie's offspring, in Portland. I didn't want to move to Portland, so we compromised on living in Vancouver.

I sit on the couch behind the small wooden folding table with my laptop resting on top to check messages. An unread email from Ron, sent this morning, catches my eye. The subject line is "Tom." It's the first time Ron has contacted me since Don's memorial service in Coos Bay almost four years ago.

You need to read this, Charlotte says.

I take a deep breath before opening the message.

Dear Cheryl,
I have some news about Tom. Please call me if you want more information. If you do not respond, I will understand.
Ron

That last sentence puzzles me. Does Ron believe I have hard feelings against Tom? He doesn't know, so he's probably assuming I do. The truth is, I don't, because I understand why Tom changed. He's not the same person I knew and loved before mental illness destroyed our marriage.

Call him, Charlotte says.

Ron picks up on the second ring. His voice sounds exactly like Don's.

"I wish we could talk under more pleasant circumstances," Ron says. "This morning, I received a call from the New York City police. They found Tom passed out on a seat in a subway car. He was dead."

I'm not feeling the usual natural emotional responses to death—no surprise, no shock, not even any sorrow. Ron's words, "He was dead," registers in my mind as only a fact. I'm calm and relieved that Tom's suffering is over. Mental illness has lost its grip. The invisible people who have been following him for the past twenty years are gone. They can't try to harm him anymore.

"Did they say how he died?" I ask. Although I'm at peace with the news, it feels strange asking this question about Tom. He died last night in one of the busiest cities in the world, alone in a subway car. Well, maybe not alone, most likely in the presence of other people who didn't know or care about him. He's just one of hundreds of homeless people in the city who choose to ride the subway for shelter for as long as possible until a police officer catches them and makes them leave.

"They believe he died from an enlarged heart," Ron says. "They will know for sure after the autopsy." He pauses for a second, then asks, "Did Tom have heart problems?"

"The last time he had a checkup in Seattle, the doctor said he had an irregular heartbeat. Did you find out when the coroner will complete the autopsy?"

"Not yet. I will keep you updated, either by email or phone."

Two days later, Ron calls again. "The coroner's office called again today. The autopsy confirmed that Tom died from an enlarged heart. They need copies of his dental records to verify his identity before

The Best I Can Do

the body can be released. Do you have the contact information for his dentist?"

I search online for the name of our last dentist in Seattle, and he's no longer practicing. Tom also saw orthodontists in Seattle and on Staten Island. I look for them, and their offices have closed, too.

I call Ron with the news. "I'll let them know," he says.

The next time I hear from Ron is a week later, when he leaves a voicemail while I'm on a conference call. When I call back, there's frustration in his voice.

"I talked to the coroner's office about Tom's dental records," he says. "They said they can't release Tom's body until they have a positive identification. They need a family member to come to New York to identify his body. If a family member doesn't identify his body within two weeks, they'll bury him in the pauper's grave. I've tried following up several times since then, but the calls go to voicemail. No one is returning my calls."

"That doesn't make sense," I say. "I'd think they'd want to work this out as quickly as possible."

"That's what I thought," Ron says. "They said they need a family member who has seen Tom recently to identify the body. I haven't seen him since the late nineties."

I remember Tom's trip to Nova Scotia. He went there after he drove our Honda Accord cross-country and spent a few days with Ron and his family. I didn't go because I couldn't take time off from my contract at Microsoft.

"I'm the last family member who saw him alive," I say, "although it has been eleven years ago."

"They said he has a full white beard now," Ron says. "I wouldn't recognize him."

Tom never tried to grow a beard when we were together because he said the hair grew unevenly. Now he has one because he didn't have anywhere to shave as a homeless man on the streets of New York City. I wonder what his beard really looks like.

My thoughts return to the coroner's office. Maybe they haven't called Ron because they assume no one in the family can identify Tom's body. Or there's a communication glitch from the cultural differences—the mellow Canadian versus the rushed, stressed-out New Yorkers. If I can talk to them, maybe I can do something. Despite all my struggles with Tom, I still love him and don't want his last resting place to be in a mass grave on Hart Island.

"Would you like me to call them?" I ask.

"It's worth trying," Ron says. He reads his contact's name and phone number at the coroner's office while I write the details on a notepad. "Call me when you find out anything."

I call the coroner's office as soon as we hang up, and a woman answers on the second ring. When I identify myself, she tells me to hold. I hear her place the receiver on a hard surface, probably her desk, and her muffled voice say to someone in the background, "It's the ex-wife!"

They have been waiting for my call! Why didn't they tell Ron they wanted to talk to me?

A minute later, another woman comes on the line and identifies herself. She's Ron's contact. "May I help you?"

"Yes, this is Cheryl Landes, Tom Landes' former wife." I refer to Tom as my "former husband," because I hate the sound of "my ex" and "my ex-husband." Every time I hear those words, I think of the brutal, fatal fight between the husband and wife in the movie, *The War of the Roses*. I filed for divorce to protect myself financially, not because of any hard feelings against Tom.

"My brother-in-law, Ron Landes, gave me your number," I say.

"I'd like to ask you some questions," she says. "Hold on." Papers shuffle in the background.

She asks me to verify Tom's full name and birth date, followed by, "Can you tell me about any unusual birthmarks or any other physical features?"

"He has a dimple in his lower back from a curved spine."

"Is there anything unusual about his teeth?"

"He wore metal braces on his upper teeth to keep two teeth in place. His two upper front teeth were knocked out in high school when someone accidentally hit his mouth with their elbow during a basketball game. His original dentist glued the teeth back in place. They loosened over time. Before we moved to the Northeast, his orthodontist in Seattle applied the braces. The plan was to replace the loose teeth with implants when the rest of the teeth straightened. That never happened."

"Some teeth are missing."

"The orthodontist said that when he takes the braces off, two of Tom's teeth would fall out. Tom was homeless for eleven years, so the braces probably wore out over time. If that's what happened, his two front teeth would be gone."

"Those teeth are missing!" she shouted as if she'd just won a billion-dollar Powerball jackpot.

I'm still not feeling any sadness about Tom's death, but I'm relieved the information I gave to Ron's contact confirms the person they found is really Tom. I know where he is now. He's at peace, and so am I.

"We need a family member to come in and identify the body," the woman says. "We can't release the body until we have a positive ID."

"I'm the last person who saw Tom alive," I say. "I'm in Massachusetts for a few days. The earliest I could come to New York is early next week."

"You need to schedule an appointment. Which borough do you prefer?"

"Staten Island."

She sets an appointment for Tuesday morning. Then I call Ron with an update.

On Monday morning, I leave for Staten Island along a new route—new to me, anyway. I learned about a drive that sounds better than the usual slog through the traffic jams along I-84 across Connecticut. Route 15, also called The Wilbur Cross Parkway, doesn't disappoint. Trees line both sides of the road for as far as I can see. I drive under arch stone bridges instead of bland, boxy concrete overpasses. There isn't much traffic this morning at ten o'clock, either. The scenery calms me despite the task ahead. I don't know what to expect, nor what Tom will look like after eleven years.

The next morning, I call a taxi and ask the driver to take me to the coroner's office and wait to bring me back to the hotel. A few minutes before my appointment time of nine o'clock, we arrive at an ominous granite building in the middle of a forest. At the entrance, I press the silver button on the intercom, and a garbled woman's voice responds.

"My name is Cheryl Landes, and I have an appointment," I say to the speaker.

I hear a buzzer, followed by a click that unlatches the door. I pull it open and walk into a cold lobby with granite walls and floors matching the exterior and four plastic charcoal-colored chairs along one wall. The air smells of chloroform and Pine Sol. I sit in a chair and wait for someone to retrieve me while shivers crawl up my spine and goosebumps cover my arms.

Five minutes later, a tan-skinned woman with short black hair tightly curled against her scalp, dressed in a black shirt, slacks, and loafers, ushers me to a tiny room with walls painted white and a black computer monitor and keyboard on a white tabletop. There are two white plastic chairs, one in front of the monitor and the other behind it.

The woman asks me to sit in the chair behind the monitor. She asks a few questions, such as my name, address, and relationship to Tom, followed by a few personal questions about him, while she types the information into a form on the screen.

After she finishes, she says, "I will show you the first picture on the screen. If you don't recognize him, I have more views."

She turns the monitor, displaying a black screen, toward me. "Are you ready?"

I nod and hold my breath while staring at the empty screen. Out of one corner of my eye, I notice a box of tissues on the table under the monitor and wonder how many people cry in this chair when they're presented pictures of their dead loved ones for the first time.

The first image displays—a headshot of a man. His eyes are closed in his round face. His light brown hair hasn't grayed much and doesn't appear to be receding. The color of his beard isn't white; it matches the shade of the wet sand on the Oregon Coast, where Tom and I took long walks, beachcombed for agates, and sat on driftwood logs to watch the sunsets.

The coroner left the man's mouth open to show the gap where his two front teeth once were. There was even a hint of the smile I fell in love with when he was a regular customer at the 7-Eleven in Eugene—the same place where we met.

"It's Tom," I say. He's safe now.

"Are you sure?" the woman asks.

"Yes."

Tom's tormentors can't harm him anymore. After twenty years of fear, he can rest. Mental illness has stopped controlling his mind and our lives. For that, I'm thankful, but it's sad it took Tom's death to release the grip.

The woman places a printout of the form she completed on the table and points to a line in the bottom left corner.

"Sign here, please," she says. "This confirms you identified the body."

After I finish, she hands a business card to me with Tom's case number neatly written in a fine black marker on a line at the top and the coroner office's contact information at the bottom.

"Call us if you have any questions," she says before escorting me to the cold, empty lobby. Through the windows, I see the taxi parked outside, where the driver waits for me.

That night after I return to Littleton, I write this obituary and email it to Ron to publish in the *Coos Bay World*:

Thomas (Tom) Alan Landes
June 18, 1955–April 16, 2016

On April 16, 2016, Tom Landes passed away in New York City from natural causes. He was 60 years old.

Tom was born in Coos Bay, Oregon, on June 18, 1955, to Theresa Minerva and Alfred Valentine Landes. He was the youngest of four children, all sons.

Tom attended Marshfield High School in Coos Bay and was active as a drummer in the marching band and a tackle for the Pirates football team. After graduation, he attended the University of Oregon and received two bachelor's degrees in General Science and Finance. After he finished his Finance degree, he worked as a sales representative for a *Fortune 500* food company in Seattle, where he received numerous awards for his sales performance and achievements. His territory covered western Washington.

Activities Tom enjoyed were woodworking, hiking, bicycling, and listening to classic rock and jazz music. He also loved chocolate and often joked that chocolate is a major food group.

Tom is survived by his former spouse, Cheryl Landes in Vancouver, Washington; two brothers and their wives, Sam and Nancy Landes in Fountain Valley, California, and Ron and Peggy Landes in Halifax, Nova Scotia; nephew and spouse Don and Kathleen Landes in Montreal, Quebec; and niece Megan Landes and her husband Toby Whitfield in

Toronto, Ontario. His parents and a brother, Don Landes, preceded him in death.

Cremation arrangements are pending, and no services will be held. Tom will be buried at Sunset Memorial Park in Coos Bay.

Then I condense the obituary into one paragraph to publish in the University of Oregon alumni newsletter. Three sentences summarize sixty years of a person's life. I read the words over and over in the body of the email to the editor while thinking about how the years fly by. In terms of our society's greater longevity, Tom's life was short. He probably could have survived longer if he were able to choose a route to recovery. No one will ever know.

You did the best you could do, Charlotte says. *Never forget that.*

I click the Send button and watch the email vanish from my laptop screen.

The sun is shining this early Saturday morning during Memorial Day weekend at Sunset Memorial Park. I'm standing at Tess' grave, looking down at a new black marker encased in concrete in the middle of her grave where Tom's ashes are buried. The marker is decorated in a gold ring of leaves connected by gold vines, which surrounds a knob that's the bottom of a vase stored upside down in an enclosure underground. At the bottom of the ring, there's an inscription with Tom's name, birth date and date of his death, and the words, "Always Loved."

I look around at the other Landes family graves: Al, Don, Nancy, Tess' brother, and Tess' younger sister and husband. A few yards away, two men approach in an olive green vehicle resembling a golf cart with a small truck bed, stopping when they spot certain graves. The driver stops at Don's grave, and the passenger jumps out and pokes the end of a wooden stick attached to a small U.S. flag in the grass in front of his tombstone, followed by Nancy's. They're honoring the veterans who served and their spouses on this holiday weekend.

I look at Tom's marker again and wonder if he can see me, then read the inscription again and stop at "Always Loved." He is still loved. He will always be loved. Did he understand he was loved while he fought the people stalking him in his mind? That his family loves him? That I will always love him?

I turn the knob, pull out the vase, and twist the bottom until it locks in the slots of the holder in the center of the ring. Then I place a bouquet of flowers in the vase and fill it with water.

"I hope you like the flowers," I say. "I'll be back soon."

Cheryl Landes

Appendix

Resources about Mental Health and Finance

Articles

Bonvissuto, Danny. "Coming Out About Mental Illness." WebMD, March 21, 2022, webmd.com/mental-health/features/coming-out-about-mental-illness.

Carey, Benedict. "I Answer the Phone at a Mental Health Hotline. Here's What I've Learned," *The New York Times*, February 12, 2023, nytimes.com/2023/02/12/opinion/health/mental-health-outreach.html.

Carucci, Ron. "How to Tell Your Boss You're Burned Out," *Harvard Business Review*, January 5, 2021, hbr.org/2021/01/how-to-tell-your-boss-youre-burned-out.

Garcia-Navarro, Lulu. "He Was Losing His Mind Slowly, and I Watched It,'" *The New York Times*, February 16, 2023, nytimes.com/2023/02/16/opinion/mental-health-conservatorship.html.

Havermans, B.M., E.P.M. Brouwers, R.J.A. Hoek, et al. "Work stress prevention needs of employees and supervisors," *BMC Public Health*, May 21, 2018, bmcpublichealth.biomedcentral.com/articles/10.1186/s12889-018-5535-1.

HelpGuide.org. "Stress Management: How to Reduce and Relieve Stress," February 5, 2024, helpguide.org/articles/stress/stress-management.htm.

Kaiser Permanente. "Stress Management: Doing Guided Imagery," no date, healthy.kaiserpermanente.org/health-wellness/health-encyclopedia/he.stress-management-doing-guided-imagery-to-relax.uz2270.

Mind Help. "Self-disclosure," *Mind Journal*, no date, mind.help/topic/self-disclosure.

Mokoena, Andile G., Marie Poggenpoel, Chris Myburgh, and Annie Temane. "Lived experiences of couples in a relationship where one partner is diagnosed with a mental illness," *Curationis*, 42(1): 2015. Published online September 19, 2019, at ncbi.nlm.nih.gov/pmc/articles/PMC6779990.

Online Counseling Programs. "Disclosing a Mental Health Condition at Work," February 16, 2021, onlinecounselingprograms.com/resources/disclose-mental-health-condition-at-work.

Raypole, Crystal. "30 Grounding Techniques to Quiet Distressing Thoughts," *Healthline*, January 29, 2024, healthline.com/health/grounding-techniques#mental-techniques.

Shain, Susan and Aiden Gardiner. "What's homelessness really like?" *The New York Times*, February 10, 2023, nytimes.com/interactive/2023/02/10/headway/homelessness-mental-health-us.html.

Slawkowski-Rode, Mikolaj. "It's OK to Never 'Get Over' Your Grief." *The New York Times*, November 25, 2023, nytimes.com/2023/11/25/opinion/grief-mourning-tradition.html.

Tartakovsky, Margarita. "Should You Tell Your Kids about Your Mental Illness?" *PsychCentral*, December 30, 2010, psychcentral.com/blog/should-you-tell-your-kids-about-your-mental-illness#1.

Wright, Becky. "How to Talk to Your Boss About Your Mental Health," *Psycom*, November 18, 2021, psycom.net/how-to-talk-to-your-boss-about-your-mental-health.

Wonders, Lynn. "Avoiding Burnout: 10 Tips for Self-Care," Wonders Counseling & Consulting, no date, wonderscounseling.com/burnout.

Books

Carpenter, Nora Shalaway, and Rocky Callen. *Ab(solutely) Normal: Short Stories that Smash Mental Health Stereotypes*. Somerville, MA: Candlewick Press, 2023. Sixteen authors with a mental health condition share their stories and remind readers that just because someone has a mental illness, they shouldn't be identified by it.

Duckworth, Ken, MD. *you are not alone: The NAMI Guide to Navigating Mental Health.* New York: Zando, 2022. This guide provides information about handling mental health conditions, finding the appropriate care, and which treatments and approaches work based on scientific research. More than one hundred twenty-five people share their mental health journeys.

Hart, Melissa. *Better with Books: 500 Diverse Books to Ignite Empathy and Encourage Self-Acceptance in Tweens and Teens.* Seattle: Sasquatch Books, 2019. This book has a chapter of recommended books about mental health. Another chapter focuses on books about poverty and homelessness. Although these resources are targeted to a younger audience, adults can learn a lot from them, too.

Jacobs, Dr. Sheldon A. *48: An Experiential Memoir on Homelessness.* Bloomington, IN: Archway Publishing, 2020. Dr. Jacobs, a licensed marriage and family therapist and homeless advocate, writes about spending forty-eight hours on the streets of Las Vegas as a homeless man. He chose to do this to better understand the struggles of the homeless and how they survive.

Vikram, Sweta. *The Loss That Binds Us: 108 Tips on Coping with Grief and Loss.* Ann Arbor, MI: Loving Healing Press, 2024. This short book is filled with practical tips and ample resources about coping with grief and loss.

Websites

The Americans with Disabilities Act (ADA) has protections in the workplace for people with a mental illness and their caregivers. By law, accommodations must be made for those with a disability, which includes mental illness, but accommodations are not required for caregivers. But in the "association provision" of the ADA, no one can be discriminated against because of their association or relationship with anyone with a disability. Learn more at eeoc.gov/laws/guidance/questions-answers-association-provision-ada.

The Cleveland Clinic has an excellent page about anosognosia, its symptoms and causes, treatments, and how to live with the condition at my.clevelandclinic.org/health/diseases/22832-anosognosia.

The Fireweed Collective provides online mental health education and support groups through the lenses of healing and disability justice. Learn more about their programs and register at fireweedcollective.org.

The National Alliance on Mental Illness (NAMI), nami.org, has a range of classes and support groups for caregivers of people with mental health issues, as well as their loved ones, along with many other resources. The organization also hosts an annual conference. Most of the services NAMI provides are free, except the conferences.

Madness Radio: Voices and Visions from Outside Mental Health focuses on topics beyond the conventional perspectives on mental illness and mainstream treatments. The show launched in 2005 and has aired more than 200 episodes. Host Will Hall interviews survivors, authors, mental health advocates, professionals, and artists. Stream episodes on the website or through Spotify, Stitcher, iTunes, Pandora, and Google Play. For details about streaming, visit madnessradio.net/about-madness-radio.

Mindspring Mental Health Alliance, a non-profit mental health education, support, and advocacy organization in Des Moines, Iowa, hosts free one-hour webinars three days a week about mental health issues and solutions. A professional social worker and therapist speaks at each webinar. Visit mindspringhealth.org for more information and to register for the webinars you want to watch.

The National Institutes of Mental Health (NIMH) has a web page with information about schizophrenia. Topics include the onset and symptoms of schizophrenia, risk factors, treatments and therapy options, how to help someone you know with schizophrenia, places where help is available, schizophrenia studies recruiting participants, statistics about schizophrenia, and shareable resources. Access this page at nimh.nih.gov/health/topics/schizophrenia.

Rethink Mental Illness has a comprehensive web page about schizophrenia, which includes a definition of the condition, types of schizophrenia, causes, symptoms, treatment options, the future of treatment, and myths. Access this page at rethink.org/advice-and-information/about-mental-illness/learn-more-about-conditions/schizophrenia.

The Schizophrenia & Psychosis Action Alliance, sczaction.org, provides information about what schizophrenia is, the symptoms of schizophrenia, treatment options, a helpline, and support groups.

WebMd has a page describing anosognosia and how this condition affects people's behavior at webmd.com/schizophrenia/what-is-anosognosia. It isn't as detailed as the Cleveland Clinic's page about anosognosia, but it has a good explanation about how anosognosia can interfere with people taking their prescribed medications.

Ramsey Solutions is a financial education organization founded by Dave Ramsey after his experiences recovering from massive debt. His website, ramseysolutions.com, has courses and articles with tips for budgeting and paying off debt. Dave Ramsey also has a popular national radio show focusing on these topics.

Suze Orman is a personal finance expert whose advice is targeted toward women, but men will also find it helpful. Her tips include budgeting, investing, paying off debt, ways to save money, and preparing for retirement. She has a podcast and free weekly newsletter. Sign up for the newsletter and learn more about her podcast at suzeorman.com.

Newsletters

The *Los Angeles Times* had a free weekly newsletter called "Group Therapy," where licensed clinical social worker Laura Newberry answered readers' questions about mental health issues. The newsletter ceased publication in January 2024, but you can read every issue at latimes.com/newsletters/sign-up-for-our-group-therapy-newsletter.

The Washington Post has a free weekly newsletter called "Well+Being," which covers food, fitness, and mental health. Browse articles and register for the newsletter at washingtonpost.com/wellbeing.

Also see the entry for Suze Orman's newsletter in the "Websites" section above.

Videos

A Tale of Mental Illness—From the Inside. Elyn Saks, a legal scholar, talks about her experiences living with schizophrenia in this powerful 14-minute TEDx talk at ted.com/talks/elyn_saks_a_tale_of_mental_illness_from_the_inside.

I See You. This eleven-minute TEDx talk features Joseph ("Joe") A. Smarro, who was one of the original members of the San Antonio Police Department's Mental Health Unit. The unit started in 2009 and became one of the most recognized programs in the country. He talks about how any organization can help contribute to fixing the broken mental health system by focusing on the portion they own and changing it for the better. Joe and his partner, Ernie Stevens, are featured in the award-winning documentary, *Ernie & Joe: Crisis Cops*. Visit ernieandjoethefilm.com for more information, and watch Joe's TEDx talk at ted.com/talks/joseph_a_smarro_i_see_you.

The voices in my head. Eleanor Longden was a college student when her symptoms of schizophrenia started. In this fourteen-minute TEDx talk at ted.com/talks/eleanor_longden_the_voices_in_my_head, she talks about her journey from diagnosis to regaining her mental health.

There's no shame in taking care of your mental health. TED Fellow Sangu Delle talks about learning to cope with his stress by breaking the African male stereotype of not sharing emotions. Watch this nine-minute TEDx talk at ted.com/talks/sangu_delle_there_s_no_shame_in_taking_care_of_your_mental_health.

Acknowledgments

I started writing this book in 2006 but mostly procrastinated on this project for the next fourteen years. Writing life's stories is stepping back in time, reliving everything that happened as much as the memory allows. Following this writing journey was not easy for me—especially recalling the endless moments of Tom's suffering and how it affected us together and separately during the last twenty years of his life.

But Charlotte, that wise inner voice, kept nagging at me. She insisted I write this story because its message can help other caregivers. I listened but struggled until COVID-19 gripped the planet. In March 2020, I realized if I didn't finish this project now, it wouldn't happen. And, of course, Charlotte was more persistent than ever.

I found several virtual writing groups that provided support throughout the process: PDX Writers in Portland; the Power of the Pen meetup in Vancouver, Washington; Wordcrafters in Eugene; and Haven Nest in Montana. I signed up for as many writing sessions as I could fit into my schedule. When the times are blocked out on my calendar and I'm writing with other writers, I'm accountable to someone. We support each other and encourage everyone in our groups to keep going until we reach our finish lines.

I'm also grateful and thankful to so many people who helped along this journey, especially Jennifer Springsteen and Cleo Hehn for their writing prompts and encouragement at the weekly PDX Writers sessions; Melissa Hart for her gentle, but firm prodding to finish and publish essays to promote this book and finish the manuscript; and

William Kenower for his no-excuses motivational messages tailored to writers.

Plus a heartfelt thanks to Claire Johnston and Andrew Zimmerman, who lead the online Friday and Saturday Power of the Pen meetups, respectively, for providing a fun, supportive place to gather and write virtually, and the wonderful friends I've made through this group. Often Andrew schedules additional writing sessions late weekday afternoons to give us "extra credit" or to "catch up." They're all appreciated!

Also thank you to the Braided Creek Crew, my fellow alums from the September 2021 Haven Retreat in Whitefish, Montana, for your continuing support and encouragement. I'm elated we met and formed strong, treasured friendships. We're each other's cheerleaders through our struggles and successes.

Lisa Sasso, my business and life coach, has been with me throughout the process as an accountability partner. Without her, I probably wouldn't have made it this far. Thank you, Lisa, for your belief in me, your support, and your friendship.

And there's my fantastic editor, Laura Munson. I call her my "book coach" because she has been more than an editor. From the beginning, she has helped me find the heart of my story and hone it into a compelling narrative. Laura, you'll never know how much I appreciate your guidance and friendship.

Ryan Forsythe took my concept for a book cover design and transformed it into a beautiful reality. His talents are amazing.

Filmmaker B.J. Bullert and I met during a guided tour of Sedona and the South Rim of the Grand Canyon. When she heard about *The Best I Can Do*, she offered to interview me and give me the recording to promote the book. We quickly finished the interview in a hotel conference room before our guides gave us a ride to the next activity, and she edited the video on her iPhone during the long drive. I'm eternally grateful for her interest in my story and her generosity.

NAMI continues to provide hope and encouragement. I'm grateful I can now give back to this organization by co-facilitating the Creative Writing for Wellness groups and Family to Family classes through NAMI Southwest Washington and train new facilitators for the Family to Family classes at the state level. Thank you to my co-host of Creative Writing for Wellness, Lyssa Orelli, and the many volunteers who are passionate about supporting caregivers and their loved ones facing mental health challenges.

I met Bob Krulish, the author of *When Screams Become Whispers: One Man's Inspiring Victory Over Bipolar Disorder*, at one of his virtual LEAP® (Listen-Empathize-Agree-Partner) workshops co-hosted by the NAMI Eastside and NAMI Thurston/Mason affiliates in September 2021. Thank you, Bob, for recommending mental health resources for this book. I admire your endless dedication to helping others navigate the complexities of mental illness and the mental health system.

Last but not least, I want to thank my family and friends not listed here for your encouragement and support. I love you all.

About the Author

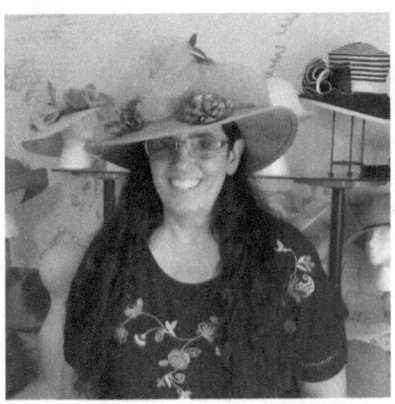

Cheryl Landes is a communications consultant, freelance travel writer, and the author of *The Best I Can Do*, *Rainbows in the Snow*, *Beautiful America's Seattle* (two editions), *Beautiful America's Idaho*, and *Those Wild Northwest Days*. Her articles and essays have appeared in national and regional publications, from *HuffPost* to *Sunset*, and on her Tabby Cat's Pawprints blog. She has also contributed chapters to *The Language of Content Strategy* and *The Language of Technical Communication*.

She volunteers on the marketing and events committees at Animal Aid, a no-kill shelter in Portland, Oregon; co-hosts a Creative Writing for Wellness group; and teaches Family to Family classes for the Southwest Washington affiliate of the National Alliance on Mental Illness (NAMI).

Cheryl lives in Vancouver, Washington, where she enjoys photography, hiking, listening to music, reading, and hanging out with cats (with their permission, of course).

Visit Cheryl's website at tabbycatco.com and her travel blog at tabbycatspawprints.com.

www.ingramcontent.com/pod-product-compliance
Lightning Source LLC
Chambersburg PA
CBHW030816190426
43197CB00036B/503